The Kinetics of Psychiatric Drugs

Edited by
JOSEPH C. SCHOOLAR, PH.D., M.D.
Director, Texas Research
Institute of Mental Sciences
Houston, Texas

and

JAMES L. CLAGHORN, M.D.
Assistant Director, Texas Research
Institute of Mental Sciences
Houston, Texas

PROCEEDINGS OF THE ELEVENTH ANNUAL SYMPOSIUM,
NOVEMBER 28-30, 1977
TEXAS RESEARCH INSTITUTE OF MENTAL SCIENCES

BRUNNER/MAZEL, Publishers • New York

Library of Congress Cataloging in Publication Data
Main entry under title:

The Kinetics of Psychiatric drugs.

Includes bibliographies and index.
1. Psychotropic drugs—Complications and sequelae—Congresses. 2. Movement disorders—Congresses. I. Schoolar, Joseph Clayton. II. Claghorn, James, 1935- III. Texas Research Institute of Mental Sciences. [DNLM: 1. Psychotropic drugs—Pharmacodynamics—Congresses. 2. Kinetics—Congresses. QV77 K51 1977]
RC483.K52 615'.788 78-27200
ISBN 0-87630-189-8

Published by
BRUNNER/MAZEL, INC.
19 Union Square West
New York, New York 10003

MANUFACTURED IN THE UNITED STATES OF AMERICA

CONTENTS

INTRODUCTION

One often hears that patients are being treated for emotional dysfunction by more and more physicians, nonpsychiatrists as well as psychiatrists, with more and more drugs. The accuracy of such a statement is surprisingly difficult to document. It is evident, however, that the kinetics of psychiatric drugs are a matter of increasing importance, not only in research institutes and psychiatric hospitals where patient selection dictates a neurobiological emphasis, but in public and private outpatient clinics as well.

What are the usual metabolic and kinetic patterns of the commonly used psychotropic drugs, and what are the implications of these patterns for treatment, both with respect to clinical response and the future physical well-being of the patient? Does the blood level of a drug correlate in any useful way with therapeutic response? Is the patient's response predictable, especially early in treatment? What biological factors underlie the so-called "nonresponse" of a patient? To what degree and under what conditions may these agents be used safely in conjunction with other medications?

Questions like these have long been asked by therapists and researchers. Fortunately, laboratory technology has advanced to the stage at which answers can begin to be expected. One needs to be able to design the best therapeutic regimen for patients, integrating drug treatment with environmental, psychodynamic, and behavioral methods. Further, one must think of long-term therapy and its potential effect on the patient, both beneficial and detrimental. Think, for example, of the possible prevention of tardive dyskinesia if equally effective treatments can be designed using significantly lower dosages of drugs, or of changes in vision or cardiac function that can be avoided.

Knowledge of drug-drug interaction is of vital importance at each pharmacological stage. At present not enough is known about the effects of prescribed and over-the-counter medications on psychotropic agents, and vice versa. We need information on altered absorption gradients, enzyme induction, and excretion rates.

In selecting *The Kinetics of Psychiatric Drugs* as the topic of our eleventh annual symposium, we at the Texas Research Institute of Mental Sciences had questions such as these foremost in mind. The conference was designed to proceed from a presentation of basic-foundation studies to topics of clinical usefulness—first those of general application, then a consideration of the unique needs of special patient populations. Conclusions drawn from the entire series of papers will be beneficial in formulating new research directions and treatment practices.

In his overview, Leo E. Hollister reviews current methods used in treatment for the major psychiatric diagnostic entities from the standpoint of new drugs and their action, as well as possible complications. Although he concludes that progress is slower than we would like it to be, the advances already made are significant. His introduction lays the groundwork for the preclinical and clinical papers that follow.

In the preclinical section, Claude F. Baxter presents an incisive review of principles known to influence strategies for pharmacological control of neurotransmitter function, discussing 12 critical areas. This is followed by elaborations of techniques and states of knowledge useful in kinetic studies: radioimmuno-assay by Sydney Spector, a review of catecholamine transmitter systems and receptor specificity by Floyd E. Bloom and his associates, pharmacologic differentiation of GABA-receptive sites by Ernest J. Peck, and finally an extensive review of neuroendocrinology and psychiatric drug interaction and association by J. Mark Ordy.

The papers on clinical studies cover the entire spectrum of neuroleptic, antidepressant, and anxiolytic agents. Carl Kinard, John M. Davis, and their associates discuss blood levels of neuroleptic drugs and clinical response in acutely psychotic patients, while Robert C. Smith et al. focus on blood levels in chronic nonresponding schizophrenic patients. Completing the discussion of neuroleptics is the paper by Edward F. Domino on the usefulness of blood-level monitoring in treatment of schizophrenic patients.

The findings of the Boston Collaborative Drug Surveillance Program on drug-drug interactions, including their association with renal function, allergic skin reactions, and potassium-sparing or -depletion, are reported by Hershel Jick. Stanley A. Kaplan and Margaret L. Jack explain pharmacokinetic parameters applicable to minor tranquilizers, especially the benzodiazepines and propanediols.

The value of plasma drug concentrations in assessing the effects of tricyclic antidepressants is discussed by Samuel G. Siris, Alexander H. Glassman, and Fay Stetner. They report on not only therapeutic response but on potential cardiovascular complications when tricyclic antidepressants are given to patients with preexisting heart disease.

The last part, on special populations, emphasizes groups of patients who not only have unique needs but for whom treatment programs are less well developed, especially in public caregiving systems. W. Edwin Dodson outlines the kinetics of antiepileptic drugs in children, stressing the wide variability of therapeutic range and the consequent need for monitoring treatment. William E. Fann and Jannine C. Wheless are concerned with special aspects of psychopharmacology in the elderly; K. D. Charalampous and D. S. McCaul present data on the pharmacokinetics of ethyl alcohol in conjunction with sedatives and anxiolytic agents.

Thus the entire volume treats topics and imparts information of immediate interest and relevance to basic scientists and clinicians alike.

Acknowledgments

We owe thanks for the success of the conference and the comprehensiveness of this book not only to the authors, but to our institute's staff, particularly Frank Womack, administrator, our secretaries Dixie Hahn and Myrna Harlan who helped to organize the meeting, and to the volunteers who joined us as hosts. Thanks to Lore Feldman for editing the manuscript with Marsha Recknagel's assistance.

For their financial support of the symposium we are grateful to Abbott Laboratories, Endo Laboratories, the George and Mary Josephine Hamman Foundation, Houston National Bank, Ives Laboratories, Lederle Laboratories, Merrell-National Laboratories, Roche Laboratories, Sandoz Pharmaceuticals, Searle Laboratories, and Wyeth Laboratories.

Joseph C. Schoolar
James L. Claghorn

CONTRIBUTORS

CLAUDE F. BAXTER, Ph.D.
Chief, Neurochemistry Laboratories, Veterans Administration Hospital, Sepulveda, California; Research Professor, Department of Psychiatry, University of California School of Medicine, Los Angeles

FLOYD E. BLOOM, M.D.
Director, The Arthur Vining Davis Center for Behavioral Neurobiology, The Salk Institute, La Jolla, California

SIDNEY CHANG, M.D.
Chief, Psychopharmacology Research Ward, Illinois State Psychiatric Institute, Chicago

K.D. CHARALAMPOUS, M.D.
Professor of Psychiatry, Baylor College of Medicine, Houston; now Chairman, Department of Psychiatry, Texas Tech University Medical School, Lubbock

JAMES L. CLAGHORN, M.D.
Assistant Director, Texas Research Institute of Mental Sciences; Assistant Professor of Psychiatry, Baylor College of Medicine; Associate Professor of Mental Sciences, The University of Texas Graduate School of Biomedical Sciences, Houston

JOHN W. CRAYTON, M.D.
Assistant Professor of Psychiatry, University of Chicago; Chief, Clinical Investigation Unit, Manteno State Hospital, Manteno, Illinois

JOHN M. DAVIS, M.D.
Director of Research, Illinois State Psychiatric Institute, Chicago; Professor of Psychiatry, University of Chicago

HAROUTUNE DEKIRMENJIAN, Ph.D.
Chief, Biological Psychiatry Laboratories, Research Division, Illinois State Psychiatric Institute, Chicago; Research Associate, University of Chicago

W. EDWIN DODSON, M.D.
Assistant Professor of Pediatrics and Neurology, Washington University School of Medicine and St. Louis Children's Hospital, St. Louis, Missouri

EDWARD F. DOMINO, M.D.
Professor of Pharmacology, The University of Michigan Medical School, Ann Arbor; Head, Pharmacology Laboratories, Lafayette Clinic, Detroit

WILLIAM E. FANN, M.D.
Professor of Psychiatry and Associate Professor of Pharmacology, Baylor College of Medicine; Chief, Psychiatry Service, Veterans Administration Hospital, Houston, Texas

DAVID GARVER, M.D.
Associate Director of Research, Illinois State Psychiatric Institute, Chicago; Associate Professor of Psychiatry, University of Cincinnati College of Medicine, Cincinnati, Ohio

ALEXANDER H. GLASSMAN, M.D.
Chief, Unit for Psychopharmacology, and Associate Professor of Psychiatry, New York State Psychiatric Institute, New York

S. J. HENRIKSEN, Ph.D.
Staff Scientist, The Arthur Vining Davis Center for Behavioral Neurobiology, The Salk Institute, La Jolla, California

LEO E. HOLLISTER, M.D.
Chief, Psychopharmacology, Veterans Administration Hospital; Professor of Medicine and Psychiatry, Stanford University School of Medicine, Palo Alto, California

MARGARET L. JACK, M.S.
Senior Scientist, Department of Biochemistry and Drug Metabolism, Hoffmann La Roche Inc., Nutley, New Jersey

HERSHEL JICK, M.D.
Associate Professor of Medicine, Boston University School of Medicine; Director, Boston Collaborative Drug Surveillance Program, Boston University Medical Center, Boston, Massachusetts.

STANLEY A. KAPLAN, Ph.D.
Associate Director, Department of Biochemistry and Drug Metabolism, Hoffmann-LaRoche Inc., Nutley, New Jersey

CARL KINARD, M.D.
Research Psychiatrist, Illinois State Psychiatric Institute, Chicago

ROY J. MATHEW, M.D.
Psychiatrist and Chief of the Psychosomatic Laboratory, Texas Research Institute of Mental Sciences, Houston

D. S. MCCAUL, B.S.
Medical Student, Baylor College of Medicine, Houston, Texas

J. MARK ORDY, Ph.D.
Head, Neurobiology, Delta Regional Primate Research Center, Tulane University, Covington, Louisiana

ERNEST J. PECK, JR., Ph.D.
Associate Professor, Department of Cell Biology, Baylor College of Medicine, Houston, Texas

LINDA D. ROBERTS, M.A.
Research Assistant, Therapeutic Research, Texas Research Institute of Mental Sciences, Houston

JOSEPH C. SCHOOLAR, Ph.D., M.D.
Director, Texas Research Institute of Mental Sciences; Professor of Pharmacology, Chief, Division of Psychopharmacology, and Professor of Psychiatry, Baylor College of Medicine; Associate Professor of Mental Sciences, The University of Texas Graduate School of Biomedical Sciences, Houston

J. E. SCHULTZ, Ph.D.
Professor, The Pharmaceutical Institute, University of Tübingen, Tübingen, German Federal Republic

G. R. Siggins, Ph.D.
Associate Director, The Arthur Vining Davis Center for Behavioral Neurobiology, The Salk Institute, La Jolla, California

Samuel G. Siris, M.D.
Associate Director, Department of Clinical Psychopharmacology, New York State Psychiatric Institute, New York

Robert C. Smith, M.D., Ph.D.
Chief, Behavioral Neurochemistry Section, Texas Research Institute of Mental Sciences, Houston

Sydney Spector, Ph.D.
Head, Department of Physiological Chemistry and Pharmacology, Roche Institute of Molecular Biology, Nutley, New Jersey

Fay Stetner, M.S.
Research Coordinator, Department of Clinical Psychopharmacology, New York State Psychiatric Institute, New York

Carol Tamminga, M.D.
Assistant Professor of Psychiatry, University of Chicago; Consultant, Manteno State Hospital, Manteno, Illinois; now Visiting Scientist, National Institute of Neurological Diseases and Stroke, Bethesda, Maryland

Jeanine C. Wheless, B.A.
Evaluation Coordinator, Alcohol and Drug Dependency Treatment Unit, Veterans Administration Hospital/ Atlanta, Decatur, Georgia

I.
OVERVIEW

1

THE IMPORTANCE OF NEW PHARMACOLOGICAL DEVELOPMENTS TO CLINICAL TREATMENT

LEO E. HOLLISTER, M.D.

One of the curious aspects of psychopharmacology is that the drugs we use for treating patients are also tools with which we may better understand what we treat. Effective drug therapy for many major psychiatric disorders has provided psychiatric research the ability to propose and to test hypotheses. Psychiatry has become a scientific discipline for the first time.

I shall now review briefly some pharmacological developments that bear on new approaches to treatment and new tools for understanding illnesses as provided by each of the four major categories of psychotherapeutic drugs.

Treatment for Schizophrenia

New Drugs

With more than 200 antipsychotic drugs on the market throughout the world, the search continues for compounds with different chemical structures or spectra of pharmacological activity. Many of the new structures resemble the typical 6-6-6 or 6-7-6 tricyclic ring structures of the most prevalent current drugs, but others differ markedly from it. Extensive variations in side chains are also being tried.

Although none of the drugs seems to be more effective overall than present drugs, some are of great interest. Clozapine, for instance, possesses little propensity for inducing extrapyramidal motor reactions or tardive dyskinesias, despite having excellent credentials as an antipsychotic drug.

Quite possibly this drug does not work primarily through dopaminergic mechanisms (Bürki et al., 1975). Unfortunately, the drug produces agranulocytosis, which may limit its use. An older drug, oxypertine, also an effective antipsychotic, chiefly reduces noradrenergic rather than dopaminergic transmission. Although possibly not as effective overall as chlorpromazine, it was especially useful in combating inertia in schizophrenics (van Praag, Dols, and Schut, 1975).

These observations with drugs with unusual pharmacologic properties suggest that the emphasis on dopaminergic mechanisms in schizophrenia, so fashionable in recent years, may be wrongly placed. Although the circumstantial evidence for involvement of dopamine is great, it should have been abundantly clear that dopamine could only have been part of the story. Our patients, even when treated with drugs which strongly block dopamine receptors, are far from well. Some other systems must also be involved. Reports of the efficacy of high doses of propranolol as a treatment for schizophrenia also raise interesting questions (Atsmon et al., 1972; Yorkston et al., 1974). If propranolol helps schizophrenia, it would probably act through noradrenergic beta-receptor blockade, again adding evidence that we must look toward other neurotransmitters as being involved in schizophrenia.

Alterations of Neurotransmitters

Attempts to reduce further dopamine transmission in schizophrenic patients have met with questionable success. The enzyme inhibitor, alphamethylparatyrosine (AMPT), which blocks dopamine synthesis, was said to reduce the requirement for thioridazine in chronic patients (Carlsson et al., 1973). Our own experience with AMPT alone as a treatment for newly admitted schizophrenic patients was entirely negative (Gershon et al., 1967). Methyldopa, which might form a false transmitter for either dopamine or norepinephrine, was said to potentiate haloperidol, but the results were difficult to interpret (Chouinard et al., 1973). In short, it is not proved that further reduction of dopamine transmission over what can be accomplished with adequate doses of antipsychotic drugs advances clinical treatment.

In the experience of most of us, substantial doses of levodopa, such as 2 to 8 g daily, aggravate schizophrenia. Thus, it was puzzling when a Japanese group averred that low doses (under 1200 mg daily without a concomitant aromatic amino acid decarboxylase inhibitor) were of benefit when added to treatment with antipsychotics (Inanaga et al., 1972). We have tried this procedure and find that even such small doses may aggravate schizophrenia. It is still possible that other dopamine agonists may act preferentially at presynaptic receptors. A favorable report of the effects of apomorphine needs to be tested further.

Other Neurotransmitters

Every few years a new neurotransmitter catches the fancy of the scientific community and comes into fashion. Currently the neurotransmitter of the year is gamma-aminobutyric acid (GABA). It was not long before a clinical report indicated that a GABA-like compound, baclofen, was effective in treating schizophrenic patients (Frederiksen, 1975). The claim was short-lived. Our own studies indicated that it makes most patients worse, quite possibly because it acts more like beta-phenethylamine than like GABA (Davis et al., 1976). The rush to get on the GABA bandwagon was so great, however, that some investigators, with no data whatever, even speculated that diazepam might be an antipsychotic drug, something for which there was absolutely no evidence.

Hormonal Treatment

Even though hormones have been used for decades as treatments for various mental disorders, the possibility that thyrotropin-releasing hormone (TRH) would help schizophrenia opened up new approaches to treatment (Wilson, Lara, and Prange, 1973). Our experience with TRH in these patients indicates that it has no benefit, and in a substantial number aggravates the psychosis (Davis, Hollister, and Berger, 1975). As might be expected, the discovery of a new set of brain hormones, the endorphins, has set off a flurry of quick and dirty experiments to determine their effects on various mental disorders, including schizophrenia. Results are highly controversial and many of the studies are poorly done. The endorphins may be "hysterogenic," at least among investigators in this field.

Metabolism and Kinetics

I shall not discuss these matters in great detail as they will be covered extensively in other chapters. A few summary points are worth some mention.

Although chlorpromazine and thioridazine form at least one active metabolite, only in the case of the side chain metabolite of the latter drug, mesoridazine, does the activity approach (and in this case exceed) that of the parent drug. While metabolites may ultimately prove to be important in regard to certain side effects, active metabolites are not essential to the therapeutic action, provided adequate amounts of the parent drug are present. Active metabolites of other antipsychotics, if they occur at all, seem to be of little importance clinically.

Absorption of some antipsychotics is highly variable. Chlorpromazine is the worst offender; anything that delays its transit in the gut, whether it be a pharmaceutical preparation of the drug or another drug with anticholinergic activity, sharply reduces its bioavailability (Hollister et al., 1970). The recent tendency to use parenteral doses of drug initially makes sense, but it is only feasible with potent drugs such as fluphenazine, haloperidol, or thiothixene. We used loading doses of chlorpromazine and reserpine in our first studies in 1954. The results were quite satisfactory except for local pain induced by chlorpromazine; the newer drugs are much better tolerated intramuscularly.

Marked interpatient variability is seen in the peak plasma concentrations attained and in the plasma half-lives of these drugs. The plasma concentrations may vary considerably even in the same patient during steady-state conditions, following the dosing pattern. Such observations cast some doubt on the meaning of plasma concentrations of drug except as they may indicate acute drug effects. The plasma half-life often has little relation to the actual biological half-life of these drugs, which may be quite long, especially after chronic administration.

Although a therapeutic range of plasma concentrations has been proposed for chlorpromazine, its validity has not been established, either for that drug or for others (Rivera-Calimlim et al., 1976). The great hope of clinical pharmacologists is that plasma concentrations of drugs will mirror clinical results, but that is sometimes difficult to realize with certain drugs. Measurements of plasma concentrations may be more valuable for determining poor compliance of patients or for detecting undertreatment, as well as helping to elucidate possible side effects of the drug.

Complications of Treatment

For the past several years, tardive dyskinesia has been the most important complication of antipsychotic drug treatment. Current belief is that it evolves from a compensatory mechanism by which the drug-induced block of postsynaptic dopamine receptors is overcome by development of supersensitivity of receptors because of pharmacologic denervation. Of the treatments proposed for decreasing dopaminergic transmission, none has been entirely reliable or safe in clinical practice (Kobayashi, 1977). Evaluation of treatment is difficult because of spontaneous remission in many patients. Recent attempts to increase cholinergic activity, using such precursors of acetylcholine as dimethylaminoethanol (deanol) or choline, must still be considered experimental. Clinical experience with choline suggests that it is more reliably effective than deanol (Davis et al., 1976).

Does this pharmacologically induced change occur only in a single dopaminergic system? Although one may clinically see the disappearance of extrapyramidal motor reactions during continuous treatment with these drugs, tolerance to the antipsychotic effects is not so evident. Thus, it may be postulated that this homeostatic mechanism is more developed in the nigrostriatal than in the mesolimbic dopamine systems of the brain. This comforting belief may not be true; evidence indicates that receptor supersensitivity also develops in the nucleus accumbens, a portion of the mesolimbic system (Ungerstedt and Ljungberg, 1977). The clinical implications are fearsome: patients may truly develop tolerance to the antipsychotic effects of these drugs; they may require increasing dosages to attain the same degree of remission; they may become dependent upon these drugs to avoid relapse into a mental state worse than that with which they started. So far, these are simply possibilities, but they are a source of considerable concern. What seems to be increasingly evident is that we should use these powerful drugs sparingly, knowing as little as we do about their long-term effects.

Treatment of Depressed Patients

New Drugs

Clomipramine is one of several new drugs that may be specific in blocking the amine pump reuptake of serotonin. It is simply the chloro homolog of imipramine, but others with such properties have rather different structures, sometimes assuming a bicyclic configuration. Such drugs may be important for testing theories about the types of neurotransmitter disorder that may underlie various types of endogenous depressions.

A number of new tricyclic compounds has been studied. Iprindole has a 6-5-8 ring structure, in contrast to the 6-7-6 configuration of most tricyclics. It is important to determine whether this drug, which does not block the amine pump, is effective in seriously ill patients with endogenous depression. So far, its main efficacy has been in outpatients with depression (Rickels et al., 1973). Doxepin is a tricyclic with a relatively weak action on the amine pump, yet it is said to be effective clinically. If this drug and iprindole really work, then we would have to reexamine our ideas about the importance of the amine pump for the antidepressant action of these drugs.

Maprotiline has a tetracyclic structure with the fourth ring lying perpendicular to the others, but with a side chain similar to that of the tricyclics. The drug is said to be as good as amitriptyline, as judged by several studies (Pinder et al., 1977). Trazadone is the most different of all the current new drugs, being a phenylpiperazine derivative. It also seems to be effective, although its efficacy in relation to other drugs has not been defined (Amin, Ban, and Klingner, 1973).

The discovery that tricyclic antidepressant drugs differ in their effects on the amine pump has spurred attempts to resolve the question of whether serotonin or norepinephrine is involved in endogenous depression. Tertiary amines, such as amitriptyline, block uptake of serotonin preferentially, while secondary amines, such as desipramine, show a preference for blocking norepinephrine uptake (Carlsson et al., 1969a and b). The next advance was the identification of 3-methoxy-4-hydroxyphenylglycol (MHPG) as a urinary metabolite which most clearly reflected the activity of norepinephrine in the brain (Maas, Dekirmenjian, and Fawcett, 1974). Using MHPG excretion as an index, several laboratories have shown that depression may be associated with either a low excretion of MHPG (presumably due to deficiency of norepinephrine) or with normal or high excretion of MHPG (presumably associated with a deficiency of serotonin). Depressed patients with presumed norepinephrine deficiency tended to respond better to imipramine (which tends to be metabolized predominantly to its secondary amine metabolite, desipramine) while those presumed to be deficient in serotonin responded better to amitriptyline (Maas, 1975; Beckmann and Goodwin, 1975).

Whether or not this biochemical classification of endogenous depression as well as the selective responses to drug therapy will be confirmed awaits further work. If these observations are confirmed, the implication would be that a biochemical test could distinguish between clinically similar depressed states and predict the proper drug for treatment.

During the past several years, two forms of monoamine oxidase (MAO) have been found in brain and other tissues, now termed MAO type A and type B. Type A monoamine oxidase inhibitors use serotonin and norepinephrine as preferred substrates. These drugs might be more specific for treating depressed patients than the current group of MAO inhibitors, which largely affect both types of MAO (Neff and Yang, 1974). Whether or not this will prove to be the case is a problem for future study.

Alterations of Neurotransmitters

Serotonin precursors, either l-tryptophan or 5-hydroxytryptophan, have been tried as treatment for depression, with the idea that increasing brain serotonin is desirable. Neither has proved to be especially effective, although more trials need to be done (Herrington et al., 1976; Puhringer et al., 1976). Possibly results might be better if patients were screened to identify those presumed to have serotonin-deficient depressions. Another possibility would be to couple the use of the serotonin precursor with a drug like clomipramine, which selectively blocks serotonin uptake, as was reported in a blind, controlled clinical trial (Walinder et al., 1976). Such clinical findings would be of theoretical interest in supporting the concept of a heterogeneous group of "endogenous" depressions with different biochemical bases.

Other Neurotransmitters

The central anticholinergic action of tricyclic antidepressants has generally been discounted as simply producing unwanted side effects. Some workers have suggested that increasing acetylcholine content in the brain by administering the cholinesterase inhibitor, physostigmine, aggravates depression (Janowsky, El-Yousef, and Davis, 1974). Such a phenomenon would be consonant with a balance between norepinephrine or serotonin and acetylcholine in the brain, in which a deficiency of one of the former neurotransmitters would lead to a relative preponderance of the latter. A similar balance has been proposed in the striatum between dopamine and acetylcholine, as is evident in Parkinson's disease. Thus, not only might one treat depression by increasing one type of neurotransmitter but possibly also by decreasing activity of another. Few attempts have been made to treat depression with anticholinergic drugs alone. The idea that anticholinergic effects may play a role in the action of antidepressants has been reviewed, but evidence is fragmentary at best (Berger, 1975).

Hormonal Treatment

As depression is so common in postmenopausal women, the deficiency of estrogens that accompanies this state seemed to be a logical cause. From time to time, treatment with estrogens is revived. The most recent study claimed that estrogens have weak action in inhibiting MAO. Why one would prefer to use a weak MAO inhibitor, when so many potent ones are available, is difficult to understand.

Thyrotropin-releasing hormone (TRH) was said to produce rapid and lasting relief of depression when given to women in intravenous doses, but we have been unable to confirm this effect (Hollister et al., 1974). Triiodothyronine (T_3) has also been used in an attempt to potentiate the antidepressant effects of tricyclics, but few clinicians seem to use this procedure in practice.

One can be certain that the endorphins will be given a full play in treating depression, especially as some believe that they may serve reward systems in the brain. It is still too early to be sure what uses they may have.

Metabolism and Kinetics

As this subject is discussed in detail elsewhere in this volume, I shall make only a few summary statements.

First, unlike in the case of the antipsychotic drugs, active metabolites of tricyclic antidepressants play a major role in their action. Their production is highly variable, so that among different patients a manifold variation may occur in the ratio of secondary amine metabolites to the parent tertiary amine drugs. If the two types act somewhat differently, it is easy to see how this uncontrollable variable might confound attempts to assess the efficacy of these compounds in various types of depression. Amitriptyline is less amenable to such conversion than imipramine and is thus more specific as a serotonin-uptake blocker. On the other hand, the availability of the secondary amines as separate drugs makes them useful as selective blockers of norepinephrine uptake, desipramine being the preferred agent.

Second, the enormous interpatient variation in steady-state plasma concentrations reported early on has persisted throughout many studies. The important clinical conclusion to be drawn is that dosages of drugs for patients must be highly individualized, as doses often correlate poorly with the plasma concentrations attained. Third, the bioavailability of oral forms of these agents is modified by an extensive first-pass effect from passage through the liver (Gram and Christiansen, 1975). Fourth, plasma concentrations seem to relate to clinical effects in an inverted U-shaped fashion in the case of nortriptyline, but in a linear fashion in the case of amitriptyline. Thus, a range of effective plasma concentrations for nortriptyline of 50 to 150 ng/ml has been suggested (Kragh-Sorensen, Asberg, and Eggert-Hansen, 1973). With amitriptyline, on the other hand, patients with a combined concentration of amitriptyline and nortriptyline of 95 ng/ml showed progressive improvement as the concentrations increased to 250 ng/ml (Ziegler, Fuller, and Biggs, 1976). Fifth, the biological half-lives of antidepressants also show little correlation with the measured plasma half-lives.

To date, the most important use of measurements of plasma concentrations of tricyclics has been to determine when a patient is being undertreated or to confirm a suspected side effect. They have also been useful in monitoring treatment of overdoses.

Treatment for Manic-Depressive Disorder

New Drugs

The success of lithium in treating manic-depressive disorder has been so great that virtually no attempts have been made to find new treatments that might supplant it. Nor has the pharmacology of lithium, as it is known to date, provided any solid leads upon which new drug treatments might be designed.

Alterations of Neurotransmitters

According to current theory, mania may represent a state in which the balance of neurotransmission in the brain favors catecholaminergic transmission. Clinically, mania may be precipitated by a variety of drugs, such as sympathomimetic stimulants, MAO inhibitors, tricyclic antidepressants and levodopa. All these drugs increase catecholaminergic transmission. On the other hand, both lithium and antipsychotic drugs are therapeutic, while experimental studies suggest that alphamethylparatyrosine, a tyrosine hydroxylase inhibitor that blocks catecholamine synthesis, may also alleviate mania. Thus, a decrease in catecholaminergic transmission, by whatever means it is achieved, seems to be central to the treatment of mania.

The neurotransmitter explanation has as much appeal for explaining manic-depressive disorder as it has for explaining schizophrenia or endogenous depression. The abrupt change from mania to depression, or vice versa, is presumed to be caused by a switch process in which the prevailing balance of these transmitters is altered in the opposite direction. Just what would trigger such sudden switches (for the phases may even oscillate on a daily cycle) remains unexplained.

Other Neurotransmitters

Many years ago, diisopropylfluorophosphate was used both acutely and chronically in the treatment of mania, with apparent success (Rountree, Nevin, and Wilson, 1950). More recently another cholinesterase, physostigmine, has been used to reverse manic symptoms (Janowsky et al., 1973). We have been able to confirm this observation. Whether cholinergic mechanisms are directly involved in mania or only involved by a secondary effect on catecholamines remains undetermined.

The precursor of serotonin, l-tryptophan, has also been reported to be useful in treating mania. The hypothesis was that serotonin acted in a "permissive" fashion in affective disorders, allowing them to occur; their exact manifestation, either mania or depression, depended on the level of concurrent catecholaminergic activity (Prange et al., 1974).

What seems clear from all studies of neurotransmitters in mental disorders is that one must consider various aspects of the synthesis, storage, release, accessibility to receptors, and uptake simultaneously. This must be done in the context of several transmitters rather than a single one. We use a lot of shorthand to depict enormously complicated events.

Pharmacokinetics

The kinetics of lithium are simple in relation to those of other psychotherapeutic drugs. Lithium is well absorbed, is distributed mainly in body water, is not metabolized and is excreted unchanged almost totally by the kidney. This simple kinetic pattern is in marked contrast to that of the antipsychotics and antidepressants. Reliance on measurement of plasma lithium concentrations often seems to be overly done. Surely, having these determinations to guide treatment is a boon. Sometimes one sees clinicians who rely more on laboratory reports than on their observations of patients. Lithium toxicity may occur even at so-called "therapeutic" levels of the drug. Whenever it is suspected on clinical grounds, the laboratory report should not be considered a license to continue treatment unless one can find another explanation for the toxic manifestations. Conversely, some clinicians worry when the lithium concentrations are reported to be at subtherapeutic plasma levels, even though the patient may be doing well. Laboratory tests are never a substitute for good clinical observations and good clinical judgment.

Measurement of lithium concentrations in erythrocytes has not been widely adopted. Initially, it was thought that these concentrations might be more readily correlated with clinical response than those in plasma. Later studies found no difference in the ratios of erythrocyte to serum lithium among patients with manic-depressive disorder and endogenous depression, with considerable variability being found over time (Rybakowski et al., 1974). This variability may be due to the fact that the ratio can either decrease or increase with changing plasma lithium levels (Lee et al., 1975). For the moment, determination of plasma concentration should be adequate.

Treatment of Anxious Patients

New Drugs

A host of new drugs is vying for a place on the market, but most of these are various modifications of the benzodiazepine group. As we currently have benzodiazepine drugs promoted specifically for almost all known indications, it is difficult to justify more.

The use of propranolol as an antianxiety drug is of great theoretical interest. A peripheral point of pharmacologic attack on anxiety would represent a departure in treatment and one that could be used easily in combination with existing centrally active drugs. Clinical results have ranged from negative to questionable to effective. Part of the problem may be that anxiety has both a "psychic" and "somatic" component and that only the latter is affected by beta-adrenergic blocking drugs (Tyrer and Lader, 1974). One is almost forced back to the original observation that patients who have tachycardia as well as anxiety may feel less anxious as the beta blocker slows their heart rate.

Other beta blockers which have been tried include oxoprenolol and practolol. Any benefit from the latter drug must be considered the result of a peripheral mode of action, but so far clinical results from this drug have not been spectacular (Bonn, Turner, and Hicks, 1972).

Metabolism and Kinetics

Do differences in the kinetics of benzodiazepines make one or another the drug of choice for a particular indication? The rapid absorption of diazepam when given orally, as well as its long duration of action through its major metabolite, N-desmethyldiazepam, seems to provide the best of both worlds. Slower absorption of other benzodiazepines may be the clue to the overwhelming preference for diazepam. The high lipid solubility of the drug probably accounts for its rapid entry into the brain with a fairly fast termination of its acute action by redistribution to the lipid compartments of the body. The fact that diazepam can be given intravenously, unlike some of the others, makes it especially valuable for the acute treatment of epilepsy or alcohol withdrawal reactions. Chlordiazepoxide, which most resembles diazepam, is less favored by patients for reasons which are not clear. Its long span of action is also mediated by formation of long-lived metabolites; lesser lipid solubility may, however, make termination of its acute action less prompt.

Oxazepam has been believed to be of special value in treating alcohol-withdrawal reactions; theoretically, it is eliminated more rapidly than diazepam since it is already a metabolite of diazepam and needs only to be conjugated. Such ready elimination might protect patients with advanced liver disease against possible precipitation of hepatic coma. The lack of a suitable intravenous dosage form severely limits this application, even if the basic assumptions were correct. Lorazepam might conceivably remedy the matter, as it is available for intravenous administration, but if its amnesic effect is as strong as purported, that might be a disadvantage.

Assuming that dosage schedules are geared to kinetic differences and to the response of patients, one might assume that most patients would gain therapeutic benefit from any of these drugs. The choice might be left to the patient.

SUMMARY

Progress in developing effective drugs is always slower than clinicians would like it to be. Quantum leaps are unusual, and they are followed by a period of consolidation in which the properties of the drugs are explored for their best clinical use. For much of the past several years we have been in the exploratory stage with psychotherapeutic drugs. Only by looking back to see how far we have come can we appreciate the progress being made. Psychotherapeutic drugs have provided abundant new leads about the disorders that they are used to treat. Soon we may be able to take advantage of this knowledge to tailor new drugs to fit our patients' needs.

REFERENCES

AMIN, M., BAN, T. A., and KLINGNER, A. 1973. Trazodone in the treatment of affective disorders. *Curr. Ther. Res.* 15:781-788.

ATSMON, A., BLUM, I., STEINER, M., LATZ, A., and WIJSENBEEK, H. 1972. Further studies with propranolol in psychotic patients. *Psychopharmacologia* 27:249-254.

BECKMANN, H., and GOODWIN, F. K. 1975. Antidepressant response to tricyclics and urinary MHPG in unipolar patients. *Arch. Gen. Psychiatry* 32:17-21.

BERGER, F. M. 1975. Commentary: Depression and antidepressant drugs. *Clin. Pharmacol. Ther.* 18:241-248.

BONN, J. A., TURNER, P., and HICKS, D. C. 1972. Beta-adrenergic-receptor blockade with practolol in treatment of anxiety. *Lancet* 1,814-815.

BÜRKI, H. F. EICHENBERGER, E. SAYERS, A. C., and WHITE, T. G. 1975. Clozapine and the dopamine hypothesis of schizophrenia, a critical appraisal. *Pharmakopsychiatrie* 8:115-121.

CARLSSON, A. CORRODI, H., FUXE, K., and HOKFELT, T. 1969b. Effects of some antidepressant drugs on the depletion of intraneuronal brain catecholamine stores caused by 4-methyl-alpha-ethyl-meta-tyramine. *Eur. J. Pharmacol.* 5:357-366.

CARLSSON, A., CORRODI, H., FUXE, K., and HOKFELT, T. 1969b. Effects of some antidepressant drugs on the depletion of intraneuronal brain catecholamine stores caused by 4-alpha-dimethyl-meta-tyramine. *Eur. J. Pharmacol.* 5:367-373.

CARLSSON, A., ROOS, B.-E., WALINDER, J., and SKOTT, A. 1973. Further studies on the mechanism of antipsychotic action: Potentiation by a-methyltyrosine of thioridazine effects in chronic schizophrenics. *J. Neural Transm.* 34:125-132.

CHOUINARD, G., PINARD, G., SERRANO, M., and TETREAULT, L. 1973. Potentiation of haloperidol by a-methyldopa in the treatment of schizophrenic patients. *Curr. Ther. Res.* 15:473-483.

DAVIS, K. L., HOLLISTER, L. E., and BERGER, P. A. 1975. Thyrotropin-releasing hormone in schizophrenia. *Am. J. Psychiatry* 132:951-953.

DAVIS, K. L., HOLLISTER, L. E., and BERGER, P. A. 1976. Baclofen in schizophrenia. Letter. *Lancet* 1:1245.

DAVIS, K. L., HOLLISTER, L. E., BARCHAS, J. D., and BERGER, P. A. 1976. Choline in tardive dyskinesia and Huntington's disease. *Life Sci.* 19:1507-1516.

FREDERIKSEN, P. K. 1975. Baclofen in the treatment of schizophrenia. Letter. *Lancet* 1:702.

GERSHON, S., HEKIMIAN, L. J., FLOYD, A., JR., and HOLLISTER, L. E. 1967. a-Methyl-p-tyrosine (AMT) in schizophrenia. *Psychopharmacologia* 11:189-194.

GRAM, L. F., and CHRISTIANSEN, J. 1975. First-pass metabolism of imipramine in man. *Clin. Pharmacol. Ther.* 17:555-563.

HERRINGTON, R. N., BRUCE, A., JOHNSTONE, E. C., and LADER, M. H. 1976. Comparative trial of l-tryptophan and amitriptyline in depressive illness. *Psychol. Med.* 6:673-678.

HOLLISTER, L. E., BERGER, P. A., OGLE, F. L., ARNOLD, R. C., and JOHNSON, A. 1974. Protirelin (TRH) in depression. *Arch. Gen. Psychiatry* 31:468-470.

HOLLISTER, L. E., CURRY, S. H., DERR, J. E., and KANTER, S. L. 1970. Studies of delayed-action medication V. Plasma levels and urinary excretion of four different dosage forms of chlorpromazine. *Clin. Pharmacol. Ther.* 11:49-59.

INANAGA, K., INOUE, K., TACHIBANA, H., OSHIMA, M., and KOTORII, T. 1972. Effect of L-dopa in schizophrenia. *Folia Psychiatrica et Neurologica Japonica* 26:145-157.

JANOWSKY, D. S., EL-YOUSEF, M. K., DAVIS, J. M., and SEKERKE, H. J. 1973. Parasympathetic suppression of manic symptoms by physostigmine. *Arch. Gen. Psychiatry* 28:542-547.

JANOWSKY, D. S., EL-YOUSEF, M. K., and DAVIS, J. M. 1974. Acetylcholine and depression. *Psychosom. Med.* 36:248-257.

KOBAYASHI, R. M. 1977. Drug therapy of tardive dyskinesia. *Drug Therapy* 296:257-260.

KRAGH-SORENSEN, P., ASBERG, M., and EGGERT-HANSEN, C. 1973. Plasma-nortriptyline levels in endogenous depression. *Lancet* 1:113-115.

LEE, C. R., HILL, S. E., DIMITRAKOUDI, M., JENNER, F. A., and POLLITT, R. J. 1975. The relationship of plasma to erythrocyte lithium levels in patients taking lithium carbonate. *Brit. J. Psychiatry* 127:596-598.

MAAS, J. W. 1975. Biogenic amines and depression. Biochemical and pharmacological separation of two types of depression. *Arch. Gen. Psychiatry* 32:1357-1361.

MAAS, J. W., DEKIRMENJIAN, H., and FAWCETT, J. A. 1974. MHPG excretion by patients with affective disorders. *Int. Pharmacopsychiatry* 9:14-26.

NEFF, N. H., and YANG, H.-Y.T. 1974. Another look at the monoamine oxidases and the monoamine oxidase inhibitor drugs. *Life Sci.* 14:2061-2074.

PINDER, R. M., BROGDEN, R. N., SPEIGHT, T. M., and AVERY, G. S. 1977. Maprotiline: A review of its pharmacological properties and therapeutic efficacy in mental depressive states. *Drugs* 13:321-352.

PRANGE, A. J., WILSON, I. C., LYNN, C. W., ALLTOP, L. B., and STIKELEATHER, R. A. 1974. L-tryptophan in mania: Contribution to a permissive hypothesis of affective disorders. *Arch. Gen. Psychiatry* 30:56-62.

PUHRINGER, W., WIRZ-JUSTICE, A., GRAW, P., LACOSTE, V., and GASTPAR, M. 1976. Intravenous 1-5-hydroxytryptophan in normal subjects: An interdisciplinary precursor loading study. *Pharmakopsychiatr. Neuropsychopharmakol.* 9:260-268.

RICKELS, K., CHUNG, H. R., CSANALÓSI, I., SABLOSKY, L., and SIMON, J. H. 1973. Iprindole and imipramine in non-psychotic depressed out-patients. *Brit. J. Psychiatry* 123:329-339.

RIVERA-CALIMLIM, L. 1976. Effect of lithium on gastric emptying and absorption of oral chlorpromazine. *Psychopharmacol. Commun.* 2:263-272.

ROUNTREE, D. W., NEVIN, S., and WILSON, A. 1950. The effects of diisopropylfluorophosphate in schizophrenia and manic-depressive psychosis. *J. Neurol. Neurosurg. Psychiatry* 13:47-59.

RYBAKOWSKI, J., CHLOPOCKA, M., KAPELSKI, Z., HERNACKA, B., SZAJNERMAN, Z., and KASPRZAK, K. 1974. Red blood cell lithium index in patients with affective disorders in the course of lithium prophylaxis. *Int. Pharmacopsychiatry* 9:166-171.

TYRER, P. J., and LADER, M. H. 1974. Response to propranolol and diazepam in somatic and psychic anxiety. *Brit. Med. J.* 2:14-16.

UNGERSTEDT, U., and LJUNGBERG, T. 1977. Behavioral patterns related to dopamine neurotransmission: Effect of acute and chronic antipsychotic drugs. In E. Costa and G. L. Gessa (eds.), *Non-Striatal Dopaminergic Neurons. Advances in Biochemical Psychopharmacology vol. 16*, pp. 193-199. New York: Raven Press.

VAN PRAAG, H. M., DOLS, L. C. W., and SCHUT, T. 1975. Biochemical versus psychopathological action profile of neuroleptics: A comparative study of chlorpromazine and oxypertine in acute psychotic disorders. *Compr. Psychiatry* 16:255-263.

WALINDER, J., SKOTT, A., CARLSSON, A., NAGY, A., and ROOS, B.-E. 1976. Potentiation of the antidepressant action of clomipramine by tryptophan. *Arch. Gen. Psychiatry* 33:1384-1389.

WILSON, I. C., LARA, P. P., and PRANGE, A. J. JR. 1973. Thyrotropin-releasing hormone in schizophrenia. *Lancet* 2:43-44.

YORKSTON, N. J., ZAKI, S. A., MALIK, M. K. U., MORRISON, R. C., and HAVARD, C. W. 1974. Propranolol in the control of schizophrenic symptoms. *Brit. Med. J.* 4:633-635.

ZIEGLER, V. E., FULLER, T. A., and BIGGS, J. T. 1976. Nortriptyline and 10-hydroxynortriptyline plasma concentrations. *J. Pharm. Pharmacol.* 28:849-850.

II.
PRECLINICAL STUDIES

2

AN EVALUATION OF SOME CRITICAL POINTS FOR DRUG ACTION

CLAUDE F. BAXTER, PH.D.

Drugs used for the treatment of neurological and psychiatric illness should be specific in their action without producing unwanted side effects. To design such drugs and use them correctly requires considerable insight into their mode of action and a detailed knowledge of the biochemical processes which they may modify. This chapter focuses upon actual or potential control points at which the function of putative (suspected) neurotransmitter agents in the central nervous system could be modified by pharmacological agents, by age, or by disease.

Acetylcholine was the first chemical neurotransmitter to be discovered almost 60 years ago. In the years that followed, a vast array of physiological, pharmacological, biochemical, and morphological research has established the existence of other neurotransmitters as functional entities at select synaptic nerve endings. Today, the neuroscientific literature is glutted with reports of compounds with properties that suggest their function as a neurotransmitter (or modulator) at specific nerve endings in select neurological systems. In the mammalian nervous system, the list includes not only amino acids such as γ-aminobutyric acid (GABA), glutamic acid, glycine, aspartic acid, histidine, proline, taurine, and the biogenic amines related metabolically to phenylalanine and tyrosine, but also small peptides such as carnosine and substance P. In addition, purine-related compounds such as ATP and cyclic nucleotides have been implicated.

This chapter is designed to elucidate the broader, more universal, principles that influence the strategies for the pharmacological regulation of

It is a pleasure to acknowledge the meticulous help of Louise V. Eaton in the production of the manuscript. Some of the research described and the preparation of this review have been supported by the Medical Research Service of the Veterans Administration.

neurotransmitter function. The few putative neurotransmitters discussed thus represent a very small fraction of the total and have been selected to serve only as illustrative examples.

An Overview of Pharmacological Control Points

Many early attempts to alter brain function were influenced by models of enzyme kinetics in which the rate of a chemical reaction sequence was controlled by a rate-limiting reaction. This concept is illustrated by analogy in Figure 1. The maximal rate of flow through a pipe is regulated by its narrowest point, which in the analogy would correspond to the rate-limiting reaction of a sequence of enzymatically catalyzed reactions occurring in an amorphous soup such as a tissue homogenate. Since the nervous system is not an amorphous soup but a highly specialized *structured*

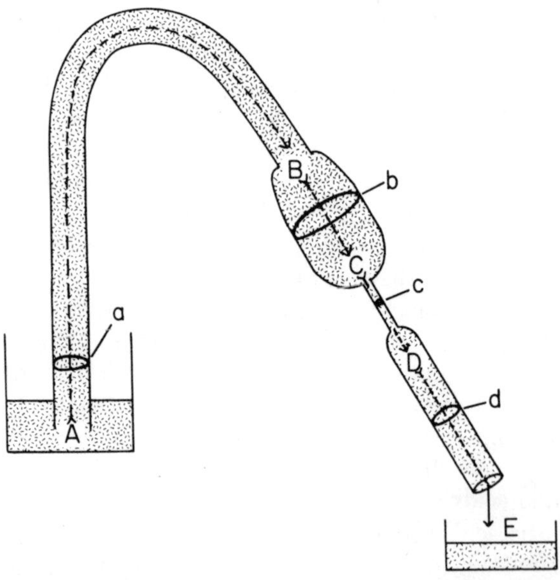

Figure 1. *Hydraulic design as an analog for an enzyme reaction sequence*: The maximum rate of flow of a liquid through pipes of different sizes (a, b, c, d) is a function of the size of their internal circumference (a, b, c, d). For a system in which these pipes are connected to each other, the maximal flow rate is determined by the pipe with the smallest circumference (c). The analogy is to an enzymatic reaction sequence from compound A to E. Reaction A to B is endothermic and requires energy for initial priming (like a siphon). The overall reaction rate is limited by the rate at which compound C is converted to compound D; that is, (c) is the rate-limiting reaction of the sequence and, therefore, potentially the most important for pharmacological regulation of the metabolic pathway from A to E.

tissue, compartmentalized at many cellular and subcellular levels, the above analogy of a classical enzyme kinetic model has at best only limited applicability for the conceptualization of control points that regulate neurotransmitter activity.

A conceptual model of neurochemical events must take into account concurrently morphological and biochemical factors. With this in mind, the potential points for the regulation of neurotransmitter function have been organized to fit into 12 categories, each representing an *area* of control (Figures 2 and 3). These categories are arbitrary but are presented in a logical sequence, starting with the availability of the building blocks for

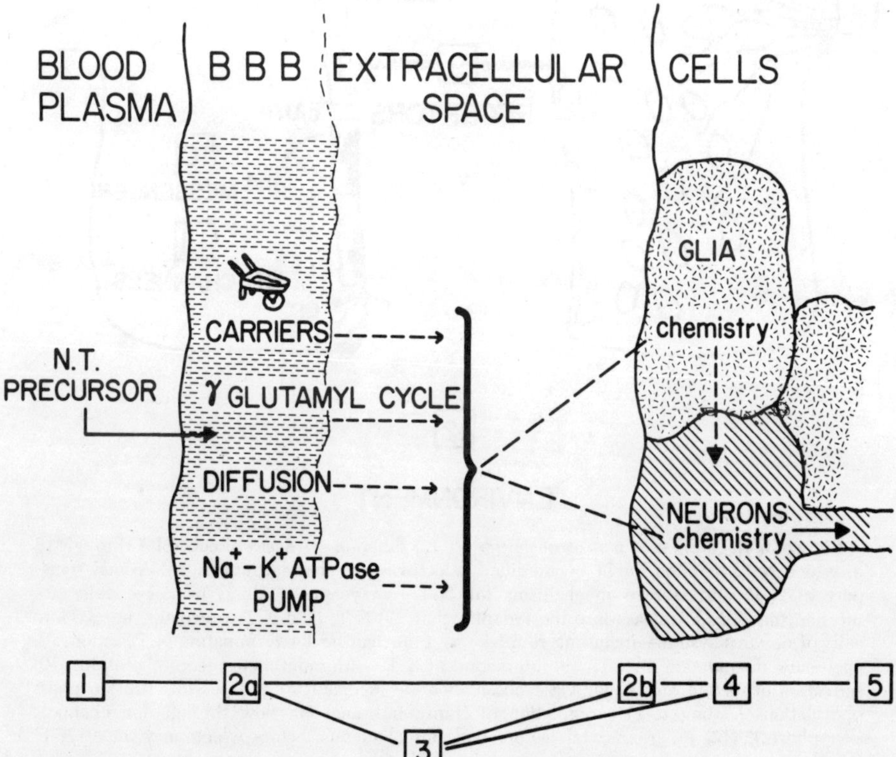

Figure 2. *Regulation of neurotransmitter (N.T.) function I*: The first five control areas in which N.T. function might be modified selectively by pharmaceuticals: (1) Precursor availability; (2) transport across the blood-brain barrier (BBB), (3) energy and oxygen requirements, (4) N.T. biosynthetic mechanism, (5) axonal transport of N.T. and storage mechanisms for N.T. in synaptic endings of nerve cells.

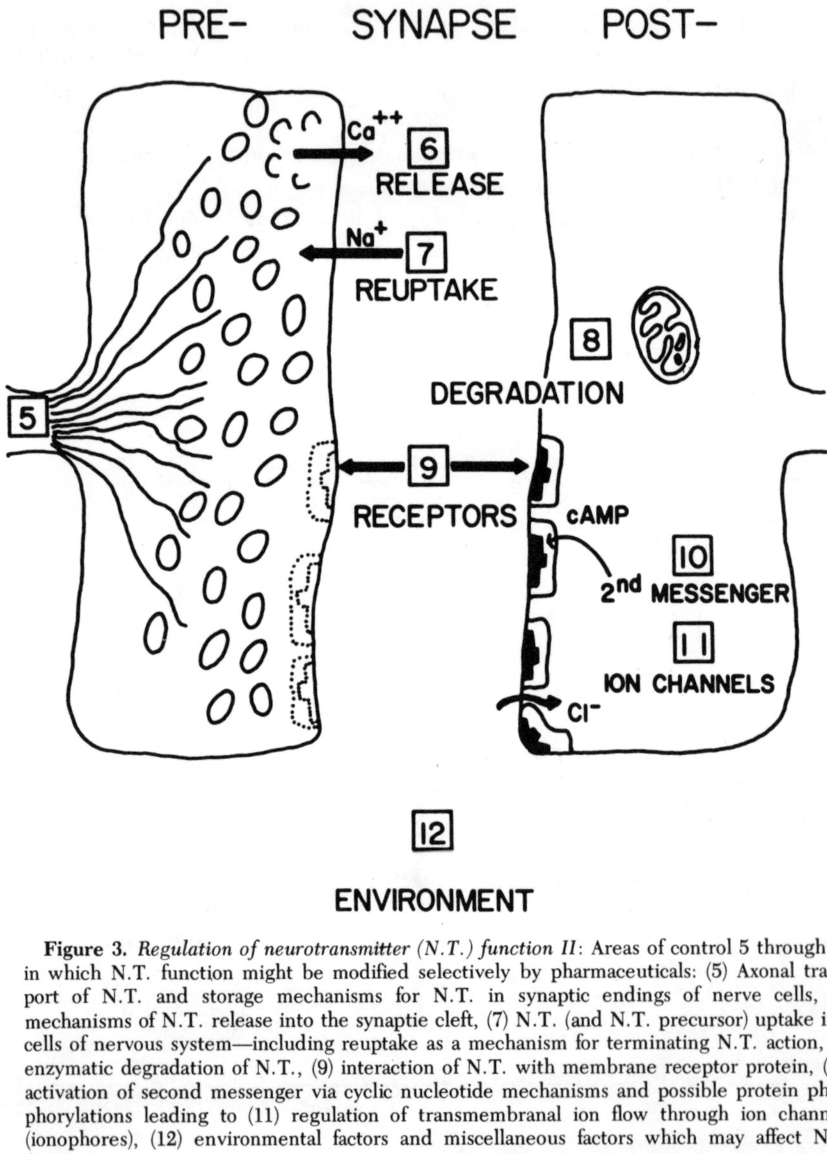

Figure 3. *Regulation of neurotransmitter (N.T.) function II*: Areas of control 5 through 12 in which N.T. function might be modified selectively by pharmaceuticals: (5) Axonal transport of N.T. and storage mechanisms for N.T. in synaptic endings of nerve cells, (6) mechanisms of N.T. release into the synaptie cleft, (7) N.T. (and N.T. precursor) uptake into cells of nervous system—including reuptake as a mechanism for terminating N.T. action, (8) enzymatic degradation of N.T., (9) interaction of N.T. with membrane receptor protein, (10) activation of second messenger via cyclic nucleotide mechanisms and possible protein phosphorylations leading to (11) regulation of transmembranal ion flow through ion channels (ionophores), (12) environmental factors and miscellaneous factors which may affect N.T. function.

neurotransmitters (categories 4-5), and release into the synaptic cleft (category 6). The next five areas of control (7-11) (Figure 3) relate to the means by which neurotransmitters exert their action postsynaptically (categories 9 to 11) and the means by which their action is terminated (categories 7 and 8). Finally, the influences of the tissue environment upon the action of neurotransmitters are grouped together as a twelfth category.

Many papers and reviews have been written concerning each one of these areas of control. The following are selected illustrations of the way in which neurotransmitter function can be regulated within each one of these 12 broad areas.

Precursor Availability

First Area of Control: Dietary

The levels of amino acids in any specific area of the mature central nervous system (CNS) are quite constant under most physiological conditions. Lajtha and co-workers showed 20 years ago that whereas radioactively labeled amino acids are taken up from the blood into brain tissue at a rapid rate, artificially elevated levels of amino acids (particularly glutamate) in the blood do not increase the level in brain tissues (see Lajtha, Berl, and Waelsch, 1959, and Roberts, 1964, for pertinent references). These observations created the impression that, except for extraordinary conditions, dietary levels of amino acids had little effect upon the rather constant amino acid levels in brain tissues (Guroff, 1972).

More recently, however, such a generalized concept has been challenged. Studies in Wurtman's laboratory have shown that levels of choline in the diet of rats can affect levels of choline and acetylcholine in the brain tissues of these animals (Hirsch, Growdon, and Wurtman, 1977). Similarly, dietary levels of protein can affect in brain tissues the levels of tryptophan, serotonin, and 5-hydroxyindoleacetic acid (Fernstrom and Wurtman, 1972).

Second Area of Control: Uptake into Brain Tissues

The availability of precursors for neurotransmitter biosynthesis depends upon the ability of such precursors to move from the blood into the brain tissues. At least two barriers with different properties impede free movement for most substances: the blood-brain barrier and the membrane barriers surrounding individual cells.

The blood-brain barrier. The blood-brain barrier is manifest in at least three sites of the adult animal brain: the choroid plexus, the arachnoid villi, and the capillary walls of cerebral blood vessels (for details, see Rapoport, 1976). The capillaries in brain tissue comprise a huge surface area which has been estimated at 240 cm^2/g tissue (Crone, 1963). Movement through the capillary walls into the extracellular space of the brain is usually by "passive facilitated diffusion," "passive" because it is from an area of high concentration to an area of lower concentration and "facilitated" because a saturable carrier is involved. For amino acids, six different stereospecific carriers have been identified (Christensen and Riggs, 1952). Also, a carrier for nucleic acid precursors (Cornford and Oldendorf, 1975) and three carriers for other groups of compounds have been reported.

Since there is only one specific carrier for neutral amino acids, these amino acids compete with each other for transport into the brain, especially at times when the carrier capacity becomes rate-limiting. When levels of neutral amino acids (phenylalanine, leucine, isoleucine, tyrosine, methionine, valine, and threonine) in the blood are high, they compete with tryptophan for transport across the blood-brain barrier; as a consequence, a high level of dietary (and blood) tryptophan per se does not assure a high availability of this amino acid for the synthesis of neurotransmitter within brain tissues. This consideration is important for an understanding of the etiology of some diseases. For example, patients with phenylketonuria (PKU) have a greatly elevated level of phenylalanine in their blood which competes with other neutral amino acids for uptake into brain tissues (Wiltse and Menkes, 1972). The result is a drop in levels of neutral amino acids (other than phenylalanine) within the brains of untreated PKU patients (McKean, Boggs, and Petersen, 1968; Hughes and Johnson, 1977). At the same time, it is likely that the excessively high level of phenylalanine in the brain inhibits protein synthesis (Siegel, Aoki, and Colwell, 1971; MacInnes and Schlesinger, 1971; Taub and Johnson, 1975) by shifting the balance from polyribosomes (essential entities for the protein-synthetic process) to monosomes. When phenylalanine is eliminated from the diet, blood levels of this amino acid are reduced and usually neurological symptoms of PKU (including seizures) and mental retardation can be avoided. But not in all cases. A patient with PKU was described recently in whom accumulation of phenylalanine was the result of a deficiency in the reduced cofactor for the enzyme that hydroxylates phenylalanine (Friedman, Cappelman, and Kaufman, 1974). The absence of the reduced cofactor, tetrahydrobiopterin, was in turn the result of a deficiency in brain and liver of the enzyme dihydropterdine reductase (Koslow and Buttler, 1977).

The blood-brain barrier is of direct concern not only for an understanding of the etiology of diseases related to neurotransmitters but also for the use of drugs that can exert their effect upon neurotransmitter-related cellular mechanisms within the brain. The ability of a specific drug to enter the brain depends upon its affinity for plasma protein, its affinity for a carrier (protein), and its lipid-water partition coefficient (Oldendorf, 1976). In addition, consideration must be given to what happens to a drug before it traverses the blood-brain barrier. Two examples in which drug action upon neurotransmitter function is modified by blood-brain barrier permeability may be illustrative: In patients afflicted with Parkinson's disease, dopamine (a putative neurotransmitter) is deficient in the CNS, due to the destruction of dopaminergic neurons in the nigrostriatal pathway. Since dopamine does not cross the blood-brain barrier to an appreciable extent, its precursor dihydroxyphenylalanine (DOPA), which enters the brain, normally would be an obvious choice as a drug for the treatment of Parkinsonian patients. However, DOPA is decarboxylated very rapidly to dopamine *outside* of the brain, thereby preventing this precursor of dopamine from entering the CNS. To overcome this difficulty, treatment prior to 1968 required the injection into Parkinsonian patients of heroic doses of DOPA to assure that just a little would end up in their brain tissues. In 1967, it was discovered that α-methyldopahydrazine would inhibit the peripheral DOPA decarboxylase, without itself crossing the blood-brain barrier to inhibit the *intracerebral* DOPA decarboxylase (Bartholini, Burkard, and Pletscher, 1967). This discovery paved the way for today's treatment of Parkinsonian patients with Sinemet, a drug marketed by Merck since 1973 which contains both DOPA and the peripheral DOPA decarboxylase inhibitor.

Another DOPA analog is the drug Aldomet (α-methyl DOPA) which is used in the treatment of hypertension. The drug traverses the blood-brain barrier on the neutral amino acid carrier. Its rate of absorption into brain tissues and subsequent pharmacological effect is, therefore, very much affected by the nutritional state of a patient taking the drug (Markovitz and Fernstrom, 1977). Aldomet absorption into the brain is rapid in the postabsorptive state and slow after a high-protein meal.

Efforts have been made to alter the blood-brain barrier and thereby affect the rate of transfer of drugs and compounds related to putative neurotransmitters. Hypertonic solutions of 2.5 M lactamide, 1.8 M arabinose, and various concentrations of urea have been used to open up the blood-brain barrier without apparent damage to brain function (see Rapoport, 1976, pp. 112-113, for references).

Stereospecific transport mechanisms are part of the blood-brain barrier also in the choroid plexus. In contrast to the blood capillaries, however, the transport across the membranes of the choroid plexus appears to be active and requires energy. Active transport with energy requirements also characterizes transport across cellular membranes of the cells in brain tissues. A number of models for active transport have been proposed. Of these, the NA^{+}-K^{+}ATPase sodium pump mechanism is the best documented (see Swanson and Stahl, 1972, for review) and is distributed widely in nature. In 1970, Orlowski and Meister proposed the presence of an ingenious cycle involving four enzymes (γ-glutamyl transpeptidase, γ-glutamyl cyclotransferase, 5-oxoprolinase, and a peptidase) that with the help of ATP could move amino acids across a membrane barrier. Some information has accumulated to support the existence of this so-called γ-glutamyl cycle. All of the above-mentioned enzymes have been detected in the choroid plexus and in brain capillaries (Orlowski, Sessa, and Green, 1974; Okonkwo, Orlowski, and Green, 1974) and, in patients with polyglutamic acidurias, the absence of one of these enzymes (5-oxoprolinase) is accompanied by mental retardation (Eldjarn, Jellum, and Stokke, 1972). On the negative side, it has been pointed out that the cycle is an "energy guzzler" and unable to account per se for either the transport of amino acids or group-specific transport mechanisms. For these reasons, the γ-glutamyl cycle is discounted by some investigators as a potential transport mechanism (Rapoport, 1976).

Uptake across cellular membrane barriers. The synthesis of a putative neurotransmitter within a cell is dependent upon precursor compounds entering such a cell. In addition to the blood-brain barrier, the membrane barriers surrounding each cell constitute another barrier for such compounds as well as for the neurotransmitter itself during the reuptake phase (see Seventh Area of Control). Since the mechanisms that appear to regulate reuptake are the same as or similar to mechanisms that regulate uptake of neurotransmitter or neurotransmitter precursors, these topics will be discussed jointly under the heading of "reuptake" (see Seventh Area of Control).

Energetics

Third Area of Control: Glucose Metabolism

Energy in the form of ATP is required not only for the active transport, uptake, and reuptake of neurotransmitters or their precursors, but also in processes related to their synthesis, degradation, and transmitter action at the postsynaptic receptor site. Glucose carbon atoms may become precursors of the carbon skeleton of several putative neurotransmitter amino acids. Thus, many drugs and physiological conditions that affect glucose metabolism of the brain may indirectly affect neurotransmitter function.

Whereas a full discussion of this topic is beyond the scope of this chapter, a thumbnail sketch of an important recent technological breakthrough is described briefly; it concerns the localization of changes in energy metabolism as a function of neuronal activity.

[^{14}C]Deoxyglucose is an analog of glucose and is carried into brain tissue by the normal glucose carrier mechanisms. Within brain tissues, [^{14}C]deoxyglucose is phosphorylated just like glucose, but the [^{14}C]deoxyglucose-6-phosphate *cannot* be metabolized any further; that is, it cannot be converted to [^{14}C]deoxyfructose-6-phosphate. Consequently, the [^{14}C]deoxyglucose-6-phosphate formed is trapped within the tissue and serves as a marker for the site of glucose metabolism as determined by autoradiography. Furthermore, the amount of [^{14}C]deoxyglucose-6-phosphate trapped in the tissue can be correlated with the rate of regional glucose metabolism (Sokoloff et al., 1977) if one assumes that the hexokinase step is rate-determining. Using the [^{14}C]deoxyglucose technique, it has been shown unequivocally that *functional* activity in specific components of the mammalian CNS is related to the rate of energy metabolism. The evidence has been summarized in a Neurosciences Research Program Bulletin (Plum, Gjedde, and Samson, 1976). Selective stimulation of a specific cerebral functional activity increases the rate of glucose utilization in specific brain areas related to that function, whereas reduced functional activity decreases glucose utilization.

Two examples from the work of Sokoloff's group epitomize these findings. An autoradiographic visualization of the effect of an altered auditory input on the glucose utilization in central auditory structures of the rat is shown in Figure 4. The normal rat is compared with the rat in which one or both auditory canals are obstructed (Sokoloff et al., 1976, p. 489), and it is clear that the loss of hearing is correlated with a loss of glucose utilization in a specific cerebral area. Similar changes in regional glucose utilization have been observed also in rats with otitis media (Sokoloff, personal communication). Glucose utilization in the visual cortex of the rhesus monkey with normal binocular vision, with monocular vision, or with no vision (Sokoloff, 1977) is depicted in Figure 5. The coronal sections of the monkey in which vision in one eye was occluded are shown in Figure 5C. These sections show dark and light striations which correspond to the ocular dominance columns discovered by Hubel and Wiesel (1968) using much more laborious electrophysiological techniques. More recently, these authors have conducted experiments using [^{14}C]deoxyglucose and confirm the visualization of ocular dominance columns by this method (Hubel, Wiesel, and Stryker, 1977). The dominance columns delineate the interdigitation of representations from the two retinae upon the visual

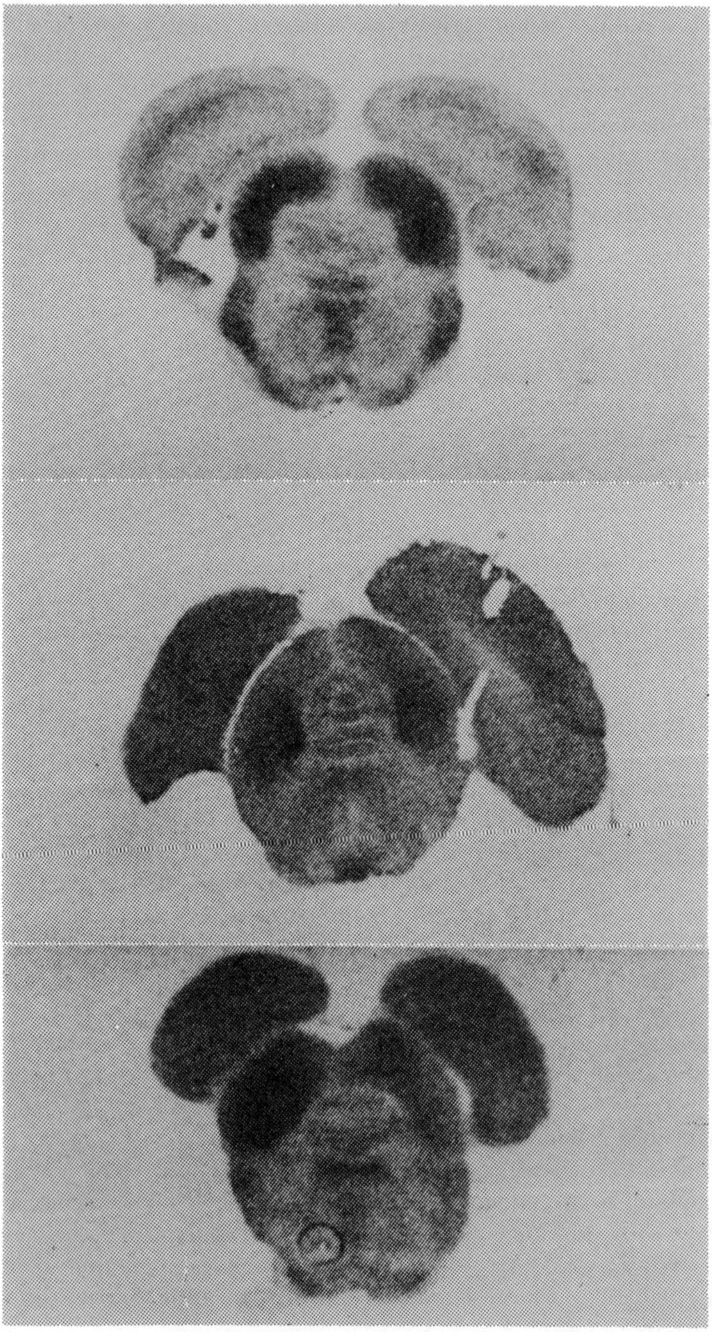

cortex. The dark columns are generated by the normal eye and the light columns by the occluded eye. The latter generates little or no stimulated functional activity in the visual cortex, and the corresponding ocular dominance columns are light in color, indicating little or no deposition of [^{14}C]deoxyglucose-6-phosphate.

The [^{14}C]deoxyglucose technique has been applied also to localize the effect of drugs on energy metabolism (Sokoloff, 1977). Glucose utilization is preferentially reduced in the gray matter of brain by γ-buterolactone. Agents that stimulate dopamine release (such as amphetamines) and dopamine agonists (such as apomorphine) increase glucose consumption in areas of brain that are known to contain cells with dopamine receptors. Some psychomimetic drugs cause dose-dependent reductions of glucose utilization in specific structures of the brain, and others such as lysergic acid diethylamide counteract the generalized morphine-induced reduction in glucose utilization in just one area of rat brain, the habenula.

Preliminary experiments by Reivich and colleagues (Reivich, 1976) and in the laboratories of D. Phelps and D. E. Kuhl at the University of California-Los Angeles (UCLA) suggest that the ^{18}fluoro derivative of deoxyglucose may be used in conjunction with topographic techniques as a diagnostic tool for determining differential regional cerebral metabolism in man.

Does an altered cerebral blood flow affect cerebral energy metabolism? If it does, then the [^{14}C]deoxyglucose method might be measuring changes in circulation. There is no doubt that the innervation of cerebral blood vessels is profuse, involving adrenergic, cholinergic, and possibly catecholaminergic mechanisms (Edvinsson and MacKenzie, 1977). Many of these mechanisms are affected by drugs that alter blood flow. However, there is no clear-cut evidence that an altered cerebral blood flow is *necessarily* related to the rate of cerebral glucose metabolism. Evidence to the contrary is available. The *normal* needs of cerebral tissues for glucose appear well below the glucose which is available from the circulation. When

Figure 4. *Effects of auditory deprivation on cerebral glucose utilization of some components of the auditory system of the albino rat: Upper,* autoradiograph of section of brain from normal conscious rat with intact bilateral hearing in ambient noise of laboratory. The autoradiograph shows the inferior colliculi, the lateral lemnisci, and the superior olives, all of which exibit bilateral symmetry of optical densities. *Middle,* autoradiograph of comparable section of brain from rat with bilateral occlusion of external auditory canals with wax and kept in sound-proof room. Note the virtual disappearance of the inferior colliculi, lateral lemnisci, and superior olives. *Lower,* autoradiograph of comparable section of brain from rat with almost symmetrical intermediate reductions of densities in the lateral lemnisci and superior olives. The ear that was blocked was contralateral to the inferior colliculus that was markedly depressed. From M. H. Des Rosiers, C. Kennedy, and L. Sokoloff (unpublished obserbations), as reported by Sokoloff (1977).

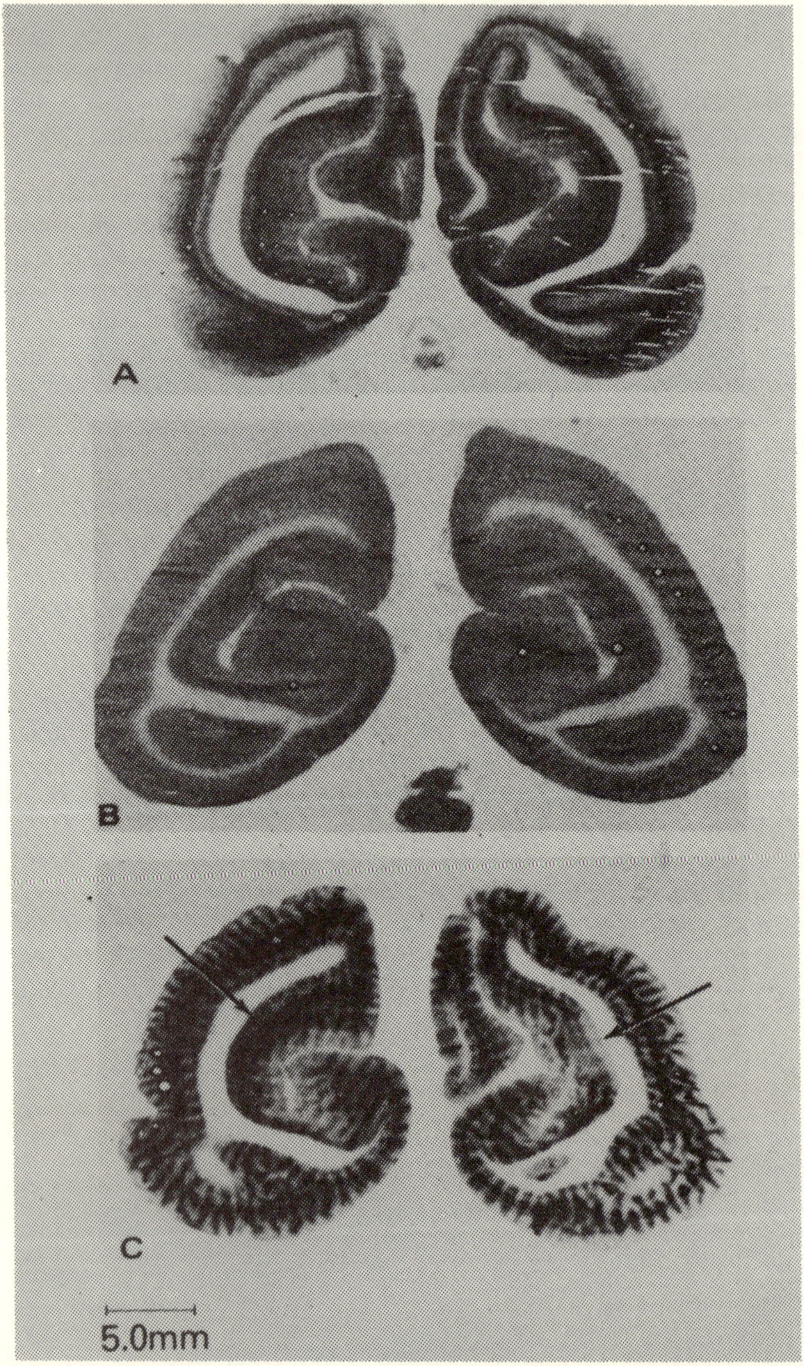
A
B
C
5.0mm

glucose levels in the circulation drop (as under conditions of hypoglycemia), the levels of high-energy phosphate compounds in brain tissues are not reduced appreciably (Gorell, Dolkart, and Ferrendelli, 1976). Other experimental data also suggest that, under most conditions, the rate of glucose metabolism in the nervous system is not regulated by the availability of glucose from the circulation. Thus, it seems reasonable to assume that changes in the metabolism of [^{14}C]deoxyglucose usually reflect changes in glucose metabolism. A more detailed understanding of the regional relationship between brain metabolism and blood flow will be required to eliminate all ambiguities.

Metabolism

Fourth Area of Control: Neurotransmitter Biosynthesis and Turnover

Since this is a vast area, one neurotransmitter, GABA, will be considered in this section as a prototype. Iversen and Bloom (1972) have calculated that 40 percent of the synapses in the brain are GABAergic, making GABA the most universal neurotransmitter in the CNS.

Regulation of GAD. One enzyme, glutamic acid decarboxylase (GAD), is responsible for the bulk of the GABA synthesized in the nervous system. This enzyme is, therefore, a prime point of control for GABA metabolism and physiological action (see Baxter, 1976, for review). GAD is dependent in its activity upon pyridoxal phosphate (PLP) as a cofactor. Recent studies suggest that in rat brain *in vivo*, the GAD apoenzyme is only 35 percent saturated with the vitamin B_6 cofactor (Miller, Walters, and Martin, 1977). Thus, the availability of the PLP cofactor may regulate *in vivo* the level of GAD activity.

Many investigators have shown that GAD activity and the resultant GABA levels are altered by a variety of pharmacological agents that can

Figure 5. *Autoradiographs of coronal brain sections from rhesus monkeys at the level of the striate cortex:* (A) Animal with normal binocular vision. Note the laminar distribution of the density; the dark band corresponds to Layer IV. (B) Animal with bilateral visual deprivation. Note the almost uniform and reduced relative density, especially the virtual disappearance of the dark bank corresponding to Layer IV. (C) Animal with right eye occluded. The half-brain on the left side of the photograph represents the left hemisphere contralateral to the occluded eye. Note the alternate dark and light striations, each about 0.3 to 0.4 mm in width, representing the ocular dominance columns. These columns are most apparent in the dark lamina corresponding to Layer IV but extend through the entire thickness of the cortex. The arrows point to regions of bilateral asymmetry where the ocular dominance columns are absent. These are presumably areas with normally only monocular input. The one on left, contralateral to occluded eye, has a continuous dark lamina corresponding to Layer IV which is completely absent on the side ipsilateral to the occluded eye. These regions are believed to be the loci of the cortical representations of the blind spots. From Kennedy et al. (1976) and Sokoloff (1977).

interact with PLP (carbonyl-trapping agents) or that appear to interact with the receptor site for PLP on the apoenzyme (for review, see Tapia, 1975; Wu and Roberts, 1974; Bayón et al., 1977; Bayón, Possani, and Tapia, 1977). The kinetics of inhibitor interaction with GAD is complicated by the apparent presence of two types of GAD apoenzymes with different requirements for PLP (Bayón et al., 1977). The reader should be cautioned also concerning the validity of *some* of the earlier studies. Within seconds after death, there is a rapid conversion of some glutamate in brain tissue to GABA (Minard and Mushawar, 1966), and some of the drugs shown as having an effect on GAD *in vivo* may have exerted their effect, instead, by preventing the flux of glutamate to GABA immediately after death! Very recent observations suggest also that GAD not only continues to operate after death, but is actually activated by decapitation and homogenization (Miller, Walters, and Martin, 1977). Such an effect was postulated some time ago on the basis of experiments related to PLP availability (Baxter, 1969).

The many different ways in which the activity of GAD may be changed both by physiological or pharmacological means have been discussed in detail elsewhere (Tapia, 1975; Baxter, 1976). Recently, the work of Miller and Walters (1977) has refocused attention upon the earlier observations of Tursky (1970) that ATP competes for, or interferes with, the interaction of GAD apoenzyme with the PLP coenzyme; the possibility cannot be excluded that, under certain conditions, ATP may regulate GAD activity *in vivo*. Attention is being focused also upon the possibility that under certain physiological or pathological conditions some naturally occurring substances, intrinsic to the nervous system, exert a regulating effect upon GAD. One of the more recent regulators of this kind to be discovered is uric acid (Baxter et al., 1978) which was identified as an intrinsic inhibitor of GAD in the insect nervous system.

An understanding of the GAD control point requires a detailed knowledge of the localization of this enzyme. Drugs and other biologically active compounds enter different brain tissues or areas at different rates. Thus, exact localization of GAD is of importance not only for the interpretation of the action of existing drugs, but also for the design of drugs that can act specifically upon GAD. In the last three years, methods have been developed that permit fairly exact localization of GAD. For this purpose, labeled antibody to pure GAD has been prepared and, in conjunction with regular microscopic and electron microscopic techniques, the localization of GAD at specific nerve endings has been demonstrated (Ribak et al., 1976).

Enzyme and substrate compartmentation. Control of GAD by pharmacological agents is influenced by yet another consideration: the compartmentalization of the enzyme substrate. When a tracer dose of ^{14}C-labeled glutamate is injected into the brain of an animal, the specific activity of cerebral glutamine is invariably higher than that of the glutamate precursor. This effect is observable within the short time that is required for the tracer dose to mix with the glutamate pool into which the tracer has been injected. The results have been interpreted as indicating the existence of two distinct glutamate pools within the brain tissues. A small pool of glutamate, primarily in glial cells, is labeled preferentially by the injected tracer dose of [^{14}C]glutamate. In sampling and extracting amino acids from brain tissue, the glutamate from the large and small pools is mixed, giving rise to glutamate in the extract that has a lower specific activity than glutamine. Based on these and similar observations, Van den Berg et al. (1975) constructed a scheme (Figure 6) in which glutamate is converted to glutamine in glial cells. That such a reaction does occur in glial cells has been confirmed (Martinez-Hernandez, Bell, and Norenberg, 1977). According to the scheme, the glutamine is transported from the glial cells into the neuronal cells where it is reconverted to glutamate. This glutamate serves as the substrate for the formation of GABA in the

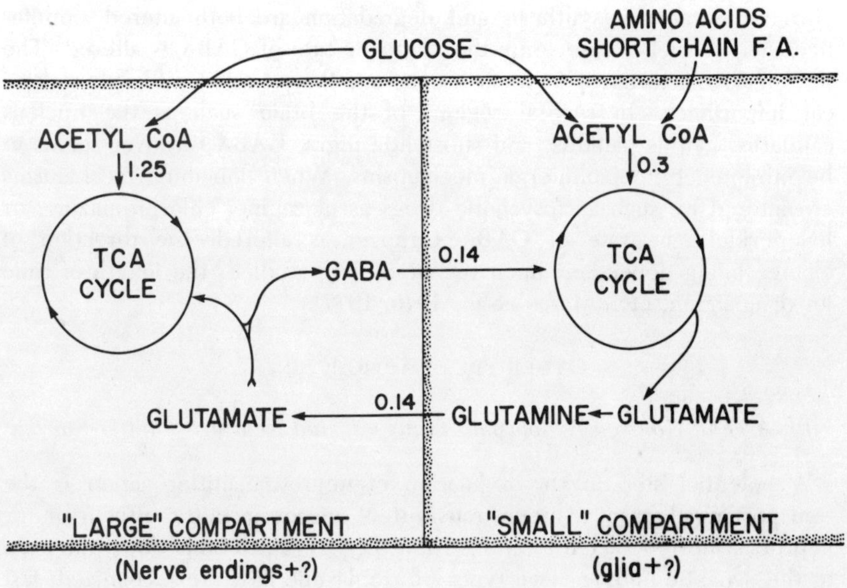

Figure 6. *Compartmentation and metabolism of GABA, glutamate and glutamine.* From Van den Berg et al. (1975), as modified by Baxter (1976).

neuron (Ribak et al., 1977). In Van den Berg's scheme (Figure 6), the glutamine pool is cast as a more immediate precursor of GABA than is the *large* glutamate pool. The scheme suggests that glutamine metabolism and transport might, under certain circumstances, become a rate-limiting step in the regulation of glutamate and GABA biosynthesis (Shank and Aprison, 1977). It has been suggested, for example, that the nervous system depressant 1-hydroxy-3-amino-pyrrolidone-2 not only depresses glucose metabolism but also disrupts the communication, via glutamine, between the glial and neuronal compartments (Möhler et al., 1975). The scheme in Figure 6 places into focus the possibility that that portion of the large glutamate pool, which may act as a neurotransmitter at certain nerve endings (for references, see Johnston, 1976), could be under the control of such enzymes as glutaminase (Bradford and Ward, 1976). Such a possibility has not been considered seriously before, because glutamine has been looked upon as the product rather than the precursor of neuronal glutamate (see, for example, Benjamin and Quastel, 1974; for review, see Baxter, 1976.)

GABA turnover. Under steady-state conditions, the level of GABA in brain tissues remains constant presumably because the rate of its synthesis and degradation are the same. However, the level may remain constant also if the rates of synthesis and degradation are both altered simultaneously. In such a case, only the turnover rate of GABA is altered. The rate of GABA turnover in brain tissues may have considerable physiological importance. In several regions of the brain such as the nucleus caudatus, globus pallidus, and substantia nigra, GABA turnover seems to be inhibited by dopaminergic mechanisms. When dopamine mechanisms are altered by such antipsychotic drugs as clozapine, chlorpromazine, or haloperidol, the rate of GABA turnover is altered—the direction of change being dependent upon the brain area studied, the length of time for drug action, etc. (Marco et al., 1976, 1977).

Other Presynaptic Events

Fifth Area of Control: Axoplasmic Transport and Neurotransmitter Storage

A potential step in the regulation of neurotransmitter action is the transport mechanism of neurotransmitter, neurotransmitter precursor, or neurotransmitter-related enzymes from the nerve cell body down the axon to the synaptic ending. Two types of axoplasmic flow are recognized: fast and slow. Axoplasmic flow is Ca^{2+}-dependent and is inhibited by a number of vinca alkaloids, which cause microtubular disassembly. It is premature to make any definitive statements about this potential control point. Its importance is uncertain because of the lack of evidence that *selective* neurotransmitter transport can be regulated at this point. Further complications are inherent in the observations that some neurotransmitters can be synthesized along the whole nerve and in the axon terminal. In invertebrates, there appears to be a glial-neuronal interrelationship along the axon that may include the transfer of neurotransmitter, its precursor, or related enzymes from glial cells to a portion of the nerve. For GABA and other amino acids, there is the additional uncertainty of exactly how these putative neurotransmitters are stored at the axon terminal. (For reviews of these topics, refer to Ochs, 1975, and Holtzman, 1977.)

Sixth Area of Control: Release of Neurotransmitter (into the synaptic cleft)

A voluminous literature describes the release of neurotransmitters from nerve endings. Several mechanisms may be involved including heteroexchange, homoexchange, and carrier-mediated transport (Raiteri et al., 1975). In a Na^+-containing medium, release can be both Ca^{2+}-independent and carrier-mediated Ca^{2+}-dependent (Levi, Redburn and Cotman, 1973; Levi, Haycock, and Cotman, 1974; Redburn, Shelton, and Cotman, 1976; Nadler et al., 1977). Carrier-mediated release of GABA is blocked by 2,4-diaminobutyric acid, a GABA analog (Levi, Rusca, and Raiteri, 1976). This is not the same release mechanism that operates when GABA is released by depolarizing concentrations of K^+ or ouabain, both of which affect the sodium pump mechanism.

GABA efflux is accelerated by such metabolic inhibitors as cyanide, dinitrophenol, and by such pharmacological agents as chlorpromazine and proveratin (Cherayil, Kandera, and Lajtha, 1967). There is evidence now that benzodiazepines like the anticonvulsants diazepam and flurazepam act by facilitating the release of GABA through their action upon the *presynaptic* membrane (Curtis et al., 1976; Choi, Farb, and Fischbach, 1977; Tremblay and Grenon, 1977). These drugs at concentrations of about 3×10^{-5} M increase the Ca^{2}-independent and decrease the Ca^{2+}-dependent efflux of GABA from mouse brain synaptosomes (Olsen, Lamar, and Bayless, 1977). Whether barbiturates alter efflux (Cutler, Markowitz, and Dudzinski, 1974) by a similar mechanism remains in doubt (Nicoll et al., 1975; Steiner and Felix, 1976; Curtis et al., 1976; Kozhechkin and Ostrovskaya, 1977). In the case of dopamine, which may regulate the release of GABA (Reubi, Iversen, and Jessell, 1977), an impressive correlation has been shown to exist between the ability of certain antipsychotic drugs to block the efflux of dopamine from dopaminergic terminals and the clinical efficacy of these drugs (Seeman and Lee, 1975). This relationship depends upon a number of debatable variables including "average clinical dose" and the definition of "efficacy." Other bits of evidence suggest alternative, equally feasible, mechanisms by which antipsychotic drugs might exert their action. Data in a recently published paper suggested that these drugs might interact with receptor sites on glial membranes (Henn, Anderson, and Sellström, 1977).

Release mechanisms seem to regulate select populations of neurotransmitter molecules. Physiologically important release mechanisms appear to act preferentially upon those compartments in the neurotransmitter pool that contain the most recently synthesized or acquired neurotransmitter (Ryan and Roskoski, 1975). Thus, the reuptake of neurotransmitter (see Seventh Area of Control) may be a rather important source for the stimulus-releasable neurotransmitter. In such a case, the mechanisms regulating release and reuptake of neurotransmitter at presynaptic nerve terminals might be quite closely interrelated. In any case, the incomplete evidence illustrates the unquestioned importance of neurotransmitter release mechanisms as a control point of neurotransmitter action.

Inactivation of Neurotransmitter

Seventh Area of Control: Pre- and Postsynaptic Uptake and Reuptake as a Mechanism for Terminating Neurotransmitter Effect

When acetylcholine is released into the cleft (neuromuscular junction) between nerve and muscle, the degradative enzyme acetylcholine esterase, in the cleft, *helps* to terminate the neurotransmitter action and assures that the neurotransmitter will have its effect for only a short, finite time period. No degradative enzymes have been shown to exist in the synaptic cleft for such other putative neurotransmitters as catecholamines and amino acids. Therefore, enzymatic degradation does not play a major role in the rapid termination of the effect of these putative neurotransmitters secreted into the cleft. The work of Axelrod and coworkers (Hertting and Axelrod, 1961) was the first to provide evidence that rapid reuptake of putative neurotransmitter from the synaptic cleft could be a most effective mechanism for terminating neurotransmitter action. Subsequent pharmacological studies emphasized that this inactivating mechanism for catecholamines was subject to regulation by a number of drugs (Iversen, 1967). Recently, a very large number of studies attest to the fact that active uptake and reuptake mechanisms for putative amino acid neurotransmitters (such as GABA, glutamate, glycine, and aspartate) are operative in brain tissues.

Uptake of any one amino acid into the cellular compartments of the tissue seems to be facilitated by two transport mechanisms distinguishable by their different affinity (high and low) for the amino acid (Snyder et al., 1973). Unlike transport across the blood-brain barrier, the uptake of amino acids into the cells of central nervous system tissues is against a very steep concentration gradient and requires Na^+ and energy (Martin, 1973; Teller et al., 1977). An example of this is shown in Figure 7. Glutamate, GABA, and aspartate are taken up by toad brain tissues against a steep concentration gradient which may be as high as 1:3800 for glutamate (Shank, Whiten, and Baxter, 1973; Baxter and Baldwin, 1978). Similar experiments have been performed with mammalian brain tissues and show somewhat lower concentration gradients. The apparently steeper gradients for toad brain as compared to gradients in mammalian brain tissues *in vitro* may be an indication of less postmortem deterioration of the amphibian brain. For the experiment in Figure 7, the live toads were cooled to a temperature of 2° to 4°C before the brains were excised (Shank and Baxter, 1975) and used for uptake studies at higher temperatures. Such a procedure is not feasible with mammals.

High-affinity uptake of putative neurotransmitter amino acids is the property not only of neuronal cells but also of glial cells (Henn and Hamberger, 1971; Schousboe, Hertz, and Svenneby, 1977). In the GABA system, the development of high-affinity uptake does not parallel the time course for the development of glutamate decarboxylase and GABA levels (Coyle and Enna, 1976; Redburn, Broome, and Enna, 1977). Furthermore, some compounds not presently known to be putative neurotransmitters can be transported into cells via the high-affinity carrier. Consequently, the premise that high-affinity uptake may be used as a screening tool for putative neurotransmitters (Bennett, Logan, and Snyder, 1973) seems to be untenable.

The uptake of amino acids into brain tissues and brain structures such as synaptosomes has been studied extensively. Energy, Na^+, and to some extent K^+ are required for this process. The rate of uptake is not uniform in different regions of the brain nor for different amino acids (Kandera, Levi, and Lajtha, 1968; Iversen and Kelly, 1975). Such uptake mechanisms may be blocked pharmacologically, thereby prolonging the effect of a neurotransmitter secreted into the synaptic cleft. Tricyclic antidepressants, phenothiazines (such as chlorpromazine), butyrophenones (such as haloperidol) and various other compounds, including ethanol, block amino acid uptake to a greater or lesser extent. However, the effects of these pharmacological agents appear to lack specificity for the uptake of any one amino acid or for other putative neurotransmitters (Harris, Hopkin, and Neal, 1973; Roach et al., 1973; Beart and Johnston, 1973).

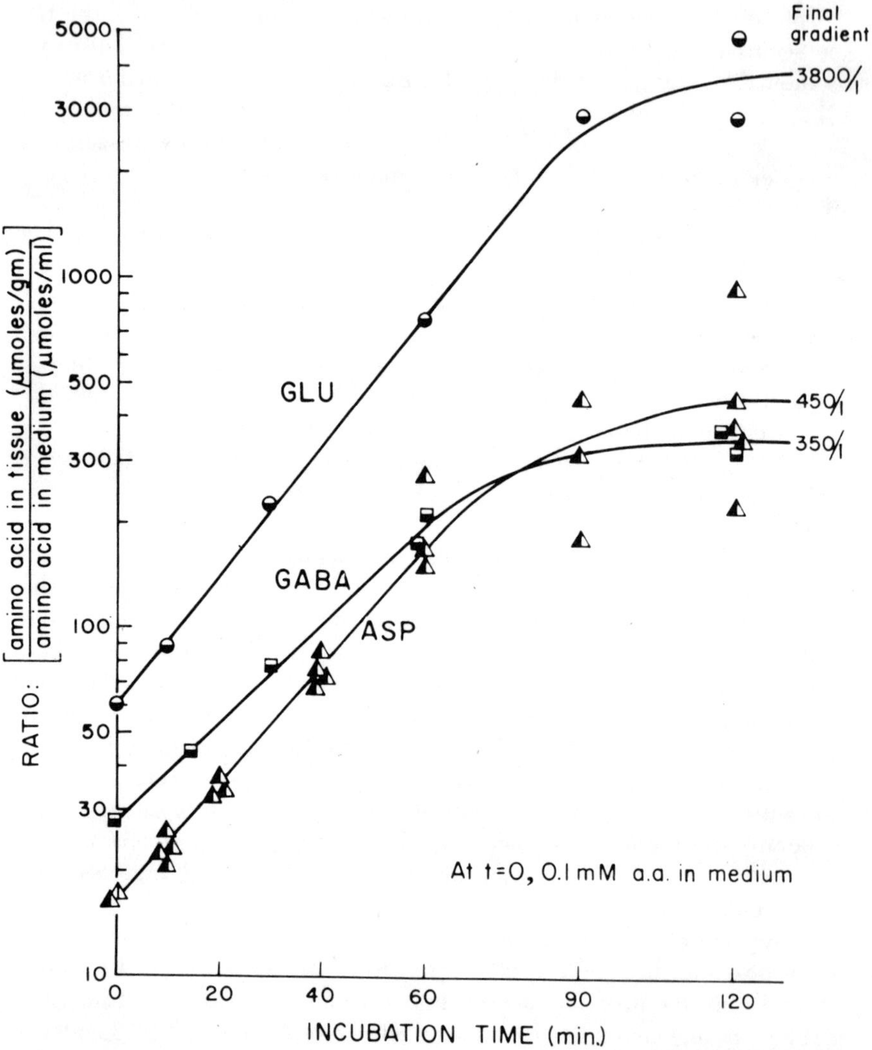

Figure 7. *Uptake in vitro of glutamate (GLU), γ-aminobutyrate (GABA), and aspartate (ASP) by hemisections of toad brain*: Concentration gradients established during incubation in oxygenated buffer medium for two hours at 25°C. For details of methodology, see Shank and Baxter (1975).

In the GABA system, 2,4-diaminobutyric acid and ß-alanine seem to inhibit the uptake of GABA into neuronal and glial cells, respectively (Schon and Kelly, 1975). More recent results, however, cast some doubt upon this specificity for neuronal and glial cells in *all* areas of the brain.

It is claimed that GABA analogs, in which charged zwitterionic centers are separated by no less than about 0.54 nm, inhibit selectively GABA transport into neuronal cells (Neal and Bowery, 1977). The inhibitor cis 1,3,-aminocyclohexane carboxylic acid (Beart, Johnston, and Uhr, 1972; Bowery, Jones, and Neal, 1976) meets this requirement. One of the most potent, if not entirely specific, inhibitors of the high-affinity GABA uptake system (that has been described to date) is nipecotic acid (piperidine-3-carboxylic acid). This constituent of betel nut is an isoxazole, related structurally to muscimol (see binding-site antagonists). Johnston and coworkers have studied nipecotic acid and other related compounds in some detail (Krogsgaard-Larsen and Johnston, 1975; Johnston et al., 1976).

Eighth Area of Control: Enzymatic Degradation of Putative Neurotransmitter

Since this is a vast area of research, only GABA degradation and its regulation will be discussed here as an example of neurotransmitter degradation and its regulation. The enzyme GABA-α-ketoglutarate transaminase (GABA-T; technical name: 4-aminobutyrate:2-oxoglutarate aminotransferase) is the major enzyme catalyzing the degradation of GABA and is, to a large extent, located in mitochondria. It is coupled to the enzyme succinic semialdehyde dehydrogenase, so that GABA is converted via a two-step reaction to succinic acid. The reaction sequence as well as the characteristics of the two enzymes and their inhibitors have been described in reviews by me (Baxter, 1970, 1976), by others, and in recent papers (Wu, 1976; De Boer and Bruinvels, 1977).

The inhibition of GABA-T or succinic semialdehyde dehydrogenase (without a concomitant and equal inhibition of glutamate decarboxylase) will tend to elevate the intrinsic levels of GABA in brain tissues. Since succinic semialdehyde requires NAD^+, the degradation of GABA is oxygen-dependent. Immediately after the death of an animal, the enzyme that synthesizes GABA continues to function anaerobically at a time when the degradation via GABA-T has stopped. This then accounts for the elevation of GABA levels in nervous tissues within seconds after death (Alderman and Shellenberger, 1974; Tappaz, Brownstein, and Kopin, 1977). Similarly, any other form of anoxia, whether caused by reduced circulation, obstructed respiration, drugs, or anesthetics, has the capacity to inhibit the degradation of GABA and elevate GABA levels in brain tissues (Thorn, Grieshaber, and Junge, 1973).

Many, but not all, of the drugs that elevate the level of GABA in the brain tend to have anticonvulsant effects (Wood and Peesker, 1975). For this reason, there is an extensive literature on GABA-T inhibitors (Tapia, 1975). Many of these inhibitors are highly reactive carbonyl-trapping agents with potential effects upon membrane permeability and upon a variety of enzymatic reactions. They act upon the GABA system by virtue of their high affinity for the pyridoxal phosphate cofactor of the GAD and GABA-T enzymes.

Of those inhibitors that cross the blood-brain barrier, aminooxyacetic acid, a selective inhibitor of GABA-T (Wallach, 1961; Baxter and Roberts, 1961), is most effective in elevating the levels of GABA in the central nervous system. In addition, this drug has the capacity to inhibit GABA uptake (Johnston and Balcar, 1974) so that its anticonvulsant action might be related to a prolonged physiological effectiveness of GABA secreted into the synaptic cleft. Other compounds that have been shown to inhibit GABA-T *in vivo* include: L-glutamic acid-γ-hydrazide, a convulsant (Tapia et al., 1967); phenelzine, a monoamine oxidase inhibitor (Popov and Matthies, 1969; Perry and Hansen, 1973); hydrazinoproprionic acid (Van Gelder, 1969); isonicotinic acid hydrazide (INH) (Wood and Peesker, 1972; Perry and Hansen, 1973); possibly sodium n-dipropylacetate (Simler et al., 1973; but see also Emson, 1976); and branched-chain fatty acids such as 2-methyl-2-ethyl caproic acid and 2,2-dimethyl valeric acid (Ciesielski, Cash, and Mandel, 1977). Most of these compounds are either carbonyl reagents or substrate competitors.

To facilitate penetration of the blood-brain barrier, nonpolar drugs were designed which would be hydrolyzed to form an active GABA-T inhibitor *within* the tissues of the CNS. For example, 5-ethyl-5-phenyl-2-pyrrolidinone (Carvajal et al., 1964) is hydrolyzed to form 5-ethyl-5-phenyl-2-GABA, an active but not very potent inhibitor of GABA-T. Such compounds as phenelzine and phenylhydrazine inhibit GABA-T but are much better inhibitors of monoamine oxidase (Popov and Matthies, 1969). Another GABA analog, as well as a phenylethylamine, is lioresal (ß-p-chloro-phenyl-GABA, marketed as Baclofen). Although this compound is only a weak inhibitor of GABA-T, it is claimed to be a strong inhibitor of the action of substance P (a putative peptide neurotransmitter) (Saito, Konishi, and Otsuka, 1975). However, this claim is disputed (Fotherby, Morrish, and Ryall, 1976).

A real breakthrough in designing enzyme inhibitors was made on the basis of an idea formulated by Konrad Bloch and his colleagues some 11 years ago (Kass and Bloch, 1967). They suggested that the most specific inhibitors of any enzyme would be those compounds that could be activated by the target enzyme to become inhibitors of the enzyme (i.e., the enzyme essentially commits suicide). The kinetic requirements for such irreversible suicide substrate/inhibitors and the conditions for unmasking the latent receptive groupings on the substrate by the target enzyme were described in detail some three years ago (Rando, 1975). Several such compounds have now been reported. They include ethanolamine-O-sulfate (Fowler and John, 1972) which is impractical for use *in vivo* because of its poor penetration of the blood-brain barrier; more recently, GABAculine (Kobayashi, Miyazawa, and Terahara, 1976; Rando and Bangerter, 1976) and, most recently, γ-acetylenic GABA and γ-vinyl GABA (4-amino-hex-5-ynoic acid and 4-amino-hex-5-enoic acid, respectively) have been shown to be inhibitors of GABA-T both *in vitro* and *in vivo* (Jung et al., 1977a, b). The γ-vinyl GABA is most specific for GABA-T acting on the lysine residue of the apoenzyme, but a high dosage level (1500 mg/kg body weight intraparenterally) is required to elevate cerebral levels of GABA to 700 μg/g tissue, wet weight. γ-Vinyl GABA is strongly anticonvulsant, and its weak inhibitory effect on GAD might be indirect via a biofeedback mechanism triggered by the high level of GABA in the tissues (Sze and Lovell, 1970). It is important to note that *in vivo* these rather specific GABA-T inhibitors can be shown to have other effects as well. This may be the result of the modulatory role of GABA on dopaminergic pathways in the nigrostriatal and limbic systems and on serotonergic pathways in the cerebral hemisphere and midbrain. Thus, γ-acetylenic GABA has been shown to affect dopamine, norepinephrine, and serotonin turnover (Palfreyman, Sylvie, and Schechter, 1977).

GABA degradation might be inhibited also by blocking the succinic semialdehyde dehydrogenase step. Specific inhibition has been achieved with 4-hydroxy benzaldehyde (Maitre, Ossola, and Mandel, 1976) but, in general, inhibitors tested have lacked specificity. Jeng and Guillory (1975) have synthesized arylazido analogs of adenine and pyridine nucleotides, compounds which, upon photolysis, generate highly reactive arylnitrene. This compound bonds covalently to amino acid side chains and, thus, can become an irreversible inhibitor of enzymes (such as succinic semialdehyde dehydrogenase), which require pyridine nucleotides for their operation (Russell, Jeng, and Guillory, 1976). Recently, arylazido-β-alanine was coupled to tetrodotoxin in a similar way. The complex that was formed bound irreversibly to receptor sites on excitable membranes. The receptor sites were associated with the Na^+ channels (Guillory, Rayner, and D'Arrigo, 1977), making the complex an excellent marker for Na^{2+} channels (see also the Eleventh Area of Control).

Effects on and in Synaptic Membranes

Ninth Area of Control: Neurotransmitter Membrane Receptors

Neurotransmitters secreted into the synaptic cleft exert their effect by interacting with receptor sites on postsynaptic (and, in some cases, presynaptic) membranes. This mechanism of neurotransmitter action parallels a similar action of hormones upon membrane receptor sites. Similar also to hormonal action, the effectiveness of a neurotransmitter may be altered by the number and the sensitivity of receptor sites that are available for interaction over a specific area of the target organ. At times, the actions of hormones and neurotransmitters seem to overlap as, for example, in hyperthyroid patients whose hearts appear to be more susceptible to *normal* levels of catecholamines because of an increase in the number of catecholamine receptor sites in their heart cells (Lefkowitz and Williams, 1976). The binding of neurotransmitter to transport proteins is distinguished from binding to receptor sites by the assumption that the binding of neurotransmitter to a receptor site does not require the presence of Na^+ (Young et al., 1976). Obviously, the receptor site is an ideal specific control point for the regulation of neurotransmitter function. It is affected by many drugs and by a number of diseases.

Specificity is well illustrated by the following example: Kainic acid (a ketocyclic analog of glutamate) will cause degeneration of cells in the cerebellum which contain glutamate receptors (e.g., Purkinje, basket, stellate, and Golgi-2-type cells) without affecting the integrity of the cells in the cerebellum which contain glutamate (Young et al., 1974; McBride et al., 1976; Herndon and Coyle, 1977). Similarly, an increase in the number of dopamine receptor sites in the nervous system of patients with tardive dyskinesia may be the reason for long-term receptor supersensitivity (Burt, Creese, and Snyder, 1977; Creese, Burt, and Snyder, 1977).

The subject of GABA receptor sites and their interaction with drugs such as bicuculline, imidazole acetic acid, and the new alkaloid muscimol is discussed by Ernest Peck in this volume (Chapter 5) and will not be covered here. Changes have been observed in the number and sensitivity of GABA receptor sites during some disease conditions. In Parkinson's disease, there appear to be fewer receptor sites for GABA in the substantia nigra (Lloyd, Shemen, and Hornykiewicz, 1977) and binding capacity is decreased. On the other hand, in patients with Huntington's chorea, the binding capacity for GABA per unit of brain tissue seems to increase (Enna et al., 1976a, b), perhaps as a compensatory mechanism for the loss of GAD and GABA.

Tenth Area of Control: The Second Messenger

A number of putative neurotransmitters is known to activate adenylate cyclases. The elevated activity of these enzymes leads to an increased production of cyclic nucleotides. There is a large body of literature concerning the role of cyclic AMP and cyclic GMP in the functions of the nervous system (see Phillis, 1977, for a recent review). In particular, it has been suggested that they may function as facilitators (second messengers) of neurotransmitter actions (Greengard, 1976). Both the activation and degradation of cyclic nucleotides are mediated by enzymes which in one way or another are themselves controlled by Ca^{2+} or calcium-dependent regulators (see Egrie et al., 1977, for earlier references). Thus, in addition to the cyclic adenine nucleotides, some investigators consider CA^{2+} to be a potential second messenger (Rasmussen and Goodman, 1977).

Compounds that are capable of activating brain adenylate cyclase have been reviewed recently (Nathanson, 1977). They include norepinephrine and dopamine (reviewed by Iversen, 1977), some preparations sensitive to serotonin (von Hungen, Roberts, and Hill, 1975), and histamine (Hegstrand, Kanof, and Greengard, 1976), as well as some excitatory amino acids (Ferrendelli, Chang, and Kinscherf, 1974).

Despite all of the correlations of putative neurotransmitters with the activation of adenine cyclases—which in turn reflect upon protein phosphorylation mechanisms in synaptic membranes (see Greengard, 1975, and Mahler, 1977, for reviews)—there is no clear-cut experimental consensus that these "second messenger mechanisms" are *closely* linked to the opening and closing of the ionic channels within, and ion fluxes through, the synaptic membranes.

Eleventh Area of Control: Ion Channels and Ion Flux

Membrane potentials are the manifestation of electrical activity in the nervous system, and membrane hyperpolarization, depolarization, or the maintenance of the membrane potential is the end product of neurotransmitter function. Membrane potentials are the product of differential distribution of ions on opposite sides of a membrane, and changes in potential require a redistribution of these ions. According to present beliefs, ions traverse through the membrane via pores or channels (ionophores) which are ion-specific. It has been possible to show the existence of such pores in the membrane and the importance of Ca^{2+} for the regulation of ionic movement through the pores. (For reviews, see Abood, 1972;

Llinás, 1977; Blaustein et al., 1977.) It was not feasible, until quite recently, to distinguish between the action of any drug upon neurotransmitter receptor sites versus its action upon the closely associated ion channels (ionophores). This topic is covered to some extent by Floyd Bloom in this volume (Chapter 4), and only one or two highlights will be mentioned here.

Of particular interest have been the findings that tetrodotoxin specifically blocks Na^+ channels (Henderson, Richie, and Strichartz, 1974). The ability to label such channels with a tetrodotoxin analog has already been mentioned (see Eighth Area of Control). An opposite effect is obtained with kainic acid (the structurally restricted analog of glutamate) and with veratridine which, like glutamate, are depolarizing agents and increase Na^+ permeability, presumably by opening the Na^+ ionophores. Other evidence strongly suggests that picrotoxin, penicillin, bicuculline, and pentylene tetrazol exert their effects by modulating chloride conductance rather than acting directly upon receptors in the membrane (Hochner, Spira, and Werman, 1975; Pellmar and Wilson, 1977 [quoting Yarowsky and Carpenter]). Similarly, the blockage of glycine receptor action by strychnine now appears to be mediated via the effect of this drug upon the related Cl^- channels (Young and Snyder, 1974).

Pellmar and Wilson (1977) suggest on the basis of the findings in invertebrate nervous systems that many convulsant agents may act by blocking chloride ionophores and, thereby, exert their effect via a selective reduction of transmitter-induced chloride conductance. Such a suggestion, while provocative, should be viewed with caution. Some pharmacological agents that interact with ionophores—for example, kainic acid—display markedly different properties in vertebrate and invertebrate nervous systems (Constanti and Nistri, 1975; Walker, 1976).

Other Regulatory Mechanisms

Twelfth Area of Control: Miscellaneous and Environmental Modulators

A final area of control has been added to this chapter in order to provide a catchall for direct and indirect factors that help to regulate and modulate neurotransmitter function but are unmentioned in other parts of this chapter.

A list of such factors would include internal environmental regulators such as pH, osmolality, and hormones. It would include the little understood actions of trophism and neuronal-glial metabolic interrelationships, the reciprocal relationships of neurotransmitters with the lipid constituents of membranes, and the interactions of neurotransmitters with each other, both as agonists and antagonists. Some data suggesting all of these effects may be found in the literature. Recently, some experimental results have suggested that a single neuron may release more than one neurotransmitter. Should this challenge to Dale's principle be confirmed, it will further complicate the definition of selective control points for the regulation of individual neurotransmitter function. This as well as some other topics are still too preliminary to deserve any comment here.

The information provided on the preceding pages constitutes a fragmentary survey. Some parts are somewhat simplistic (even perhaps naive) and all are incomplete. But it is my hope that this chapter is a Venus de Milo to which other contributors to this volume will be adding some of the missing parts.

SUMMARY

The potentials of pharmacological regulation of neurotransmitter func-

TABLE 1. AREAS OF NEUROTRANSMITTER REGULATION

Areas of Control	Examples
(1) PRECURSOR AVAILABILITY	nutrition
(2) BRAIN BARRIERS	transport mechanisms and carriers; precursor uptake
(3) ENERGY AND OXYGEN REQUIREMENTS	circulation, carbohydrate metabolism, anoxia, hypoxia, etc.
(4) N.T. SYNTHESIS	enzyme cofactors, biofeedback, neural-glial interrelations, compartmentation, intrinsic inhibitors, etc.
(5) N.T. TRANSPORT, STORAGE	axoplasmic flow, vesicles
(6) N.T. RELEASE	efflux mechanisms, Ca^{2+} regulation
(7) N.T. UPTAKE	presynaptic reuptake, Na^{+} regulation
(8) N.T. DEGRADATION	enzyme cofactors, turnover, etc. [see (4), above]
(9) N.T. RECEPTORS	receptor-sites: sensitivity, density, specificity
(10) SECOND MESSENGER AND MEMBRANE MODIFICATION	cyclic AMP, cyclic GMP, protein phosphorylation
(11) ION CHANNELS AND ION FLUX	Na^{+}, K^{+}, Ca^{2+}, Cl^{-}
(12) GENERAL ENVIRONMENTAL FACTORS	pH, osmolality, CO_2, hormones, etc.

N.T. = neurotransmitter.

tion have been presented within a framework of 12 general areas of control. These areas range from the availability of metabolic precursors for neurotransmitter biosynthesis to the interaction of neurotransmitter or second messenger with the opening and closing of specific ion channels in excitable membranes. The 12 areas of control as well as the more specific points of regulation are summarized in Table 1. Some points, where modification is the cause of disease or where specific drugs may modify neurotransmitter function, have been documented and discussed. Emphasis has been placed upon providing recent references in the more readily available research literature of neuroscience.

REFERENCES

ABOOD, L. G. 1972. Excitation and conduction in the neuron. In R. W. Albers, G. J. Siegel, R. Katzman, and B. W. Agranoff (eds.), *Basic Neurochemistry*, pp. 41-65. Boston: Little, Brown.

ALDERMAN, J. L., and SHELLENBERGER, M. K. 1974. γ-Aminobutyric acid (GABA) in the rat brain: Reevaluation of sampling procedures and the post-mortem increase. *J. Neurochem.*, 22:937-940.

BARTHOLINI, G., BURKARD, W. P., and PLETSCHER, A. 1967. Increase of cerebral catecholamines caused by 3,4-dihydroxyphenylalanine after inhibition of peripheral decarboxylase. *Nature*, 215:852-853.

BAXTER, C. F. 1969. Changes in gamma-aminobutyric-acid-shunt enzymes and substrates after administration of carbonyl reagents and vitamin B_6 *in vivo*: An apparent discrepancy in assay techniques. *Ann. N.Y. Acad. Sci.*, 166:267-280.

BAXTER, C. F. 1970. The nature of γ-aminobutyric acid. In A. Lajtha (ed.), *Handbook of Neurochemistry*, vol. 3, pp. 289-353. New York: Plenum Press.

BAXTER, C. F. 1976. Some recent advances in studies of GABA metabolism and compartmentation. In E. Roberts, T. N. Chase, and D. B. Tower (eds.), *GABA in Nervous System Function*, pp. 61-87. New York: Raven Press.

BAXTER, C. F., and BALDWIN, R. A. 1978. A functional role for amino acids in the adaptation of tissues from the nervous system to alterations in environmental osmolality. In F. Fonnum (ed.), *Amino Acids as Chemical Transmitters*. pp. 599-627. New York: Plenum Press.

BAXTER, C. F., and ROBERTS, E. 1961. Elevation of γ-aminobutyric acid in brain: Selective inhibition of γ-aminobutyric-α-ketoglutaric acid transaminase. *J. Biol. Chem.*, 236:3287-3294.

BAXTER, C. F., MORIN, A. M., KOVARIK, R. A., and OZAKI, L. K. 1978. Identification of intrinsic glutamate decarboxylase inhibitor in roach. *Trans. Am. Soc. Neurochem.*, 9:54.

BAYÓN, A., POSSANI, L. D., and TAPIA, R. 1977. Kinetics of brain glutamate decarboxylase inhibition studies with N-(5′-phosphopyridoxyl) amino acids. *J. Neurochem.*, 29:513-517.

BAYÓN, A., POSSANI, L. D., TAPIA, M., and TAPIA, R. 1977. Kinetics of brain glutamate decarboxylase interactions with glutamate, pyridoxal 5′-phosphate and glutamate-pyridoxal 5′-phosphate schiff base. *J. Neurochem.*, 29:519-525.

BEART, P. M., and JOHNSTON, G. A. R. 1973. GABA uptake in rat brain slices: inhibition by GABA analogues and by various drugs. *J. Neurochem.*, 20:319-324.

BEART, P. M., JOHNSTON, G. A. R., and UHR, M. L. 1972. Competitive inhibition of GABA uptake in rat brain slices by some GABA analogues of restricted conformation. *J. Neurochem.*, 19:1855-1861.

BENJAMIN, A. M., and QUASTEL, J. H. 1974. Fate of L-glutamate in the brain. *J. Neurochem.*, 23:457-464.

BENNETT, J. P. JR., LOGAN, W. J., and SNYDER, S. H. 1973. Amino acids as central nervous transmitters: The influence of ions, amino acid analogues and ontogeny on transport systems for L-glutamic acid and L-aspartic acids and glycine into central nervous synaptosomes of the rat. *J. Neurochem.*, 21:1533-1550.

BLAUSTEIN, M. P., KENDRICK, N. C., FRIED, R. C., and RATZLAFF, R. W. 1977. Calcium metabolism at the mammalian presynaptic nerve terminal: lessons from the synaptosome. *Neurosciences Symposium*, 2:172-194.

BOWERY, N. G., JONES, G. P., and NEAL, M. J. 1976. Selective inhibition of neuronal GABA uptake by cis 1,3,-amino-cyclohexane carboxylic acid. *Nature*, 264:281-284.

BRADFORD, H. F., and WARD, H. K. 1976. On glutaminase activity in mammalian synaptosomes. *Brain Res.*, 110:115-125.

BURT, D. R., CREESE, I., and SNYDER, S. H. 1977. Antischizophrenic drugs: Chronic treatment elevates dopamine receptor binding in brain. *Science*, 196:326-328.

CARVAJAL, G., RUSSEK, M., TAPIA, R., and MASSIEU, G. 1964. Anticonvulsive action of substances designed as inhibitors of γ-aminobutyric acid α-ketoglutaric acid transaminase. *Biochem. Pharmacol.*, 13:1059-1069.

CHERAYIL, A., KANDERA, J., and LAJTHA, A. 1967. Cerebral amino acid transport *in vitro*. IV. The effect of inhibitors on exit from brain slices. *J. Neurochem.*, 14:105-115.

CHOI, D. W., FARB, D. H., and FISCHBACH, G. D. 1977. A mechanism of action of benzodiazepines: Effect of chlordiazepoxide upon GABA chemosensitivity and synaptic activity in spinal tissue culture. *Society for Neuroscience Annual Meeting Abstracts*, 3:405.

CHRISTENSEN, H. N., and RIGGS, T. R. 1952. Concentrative uptake of amino acids by the Ehrlich mouse ascites carcinoma cell. *J. Biol. Chem.*, 194:57-68.

CIESIELSKI, L., CASH, C., and MANDEL, P. 1977. Branched chain fatty acids effects on human, rat, mouse purified GABA transaminase and succinic semialdehyde dehydrogenase. *Proc. Int. Soc. Neurochem.*, 6:521.

CONSTANTI, A., and NISTRI, A. 1975. A comparative study of the effects of glutamate and kainate on the lobster muscle fibre and the frog spinal cord. *Br. J. Pharmacol.*, 57:359-368.

CORNFORD, E. M., and OLDENDORF, W. H. 1975. Independent blood-brain barrier transport systems for nucleic acid precursors. *Biochim. Biophys. Acta*, 394:211-219.

COYLE, J. T., and ENNA, S. J. 1976. Neurochemical aspects of the ontogenesis of GABAnergic neurons in the rat brain. *Brain Res.*, 111:119-133.

CREESE, I., BURT, D. R., and SNYDER, S. H. 1977. Dopamine receptor binding enhancement accompanies lesion-induced behavioral supersensitivity. *Science*, 197:596-598.

CRONE, C. 1963. The permeability of capillaries in various organs as determined by the use of the "indicator diffusion" method. *Acta Physiol. Scand.*, 58:292-305.

CURTIS, D. R., LODGE, D., JOHNSTON, G. A. R., and BRAND, S. J. 1976. Central actions of benzodiazepines. *Brain Res.*, 118:344-347.

CUTLER, R. W. P., MARKOWITZ, D., and DUDZINSKI, D. S. 1974. The effect of barbiturates on [^{3}H]GABA transport in rat cerebral cortex slices. *Brain Res.*, 81:189-197.

DE BOER, T., and BRUINVELS, J. 1977. Assay and properties of 4-aminobutyric-2-oxoglutaric acid transaminase and succinic semialdehyde dehydrogenase in rat brain tissue. *J. Neurochem.*, 28:471-478.

EDVINSSON, L., and MACKENZIE, E. T. 1977. Amine mechanisms in the cerebral circulation. *Pharmacol. Rev.*, 28:275-348.

EGRIE, J. C., CAMPBELL, J. A., FLANGAS, A. L., and SIEGEL, F. L. 1977. Regional, cellular and subcellular distribution of calcium-activated cyclic nucleotide phosphodiesterase and calcium-dependent regulator in porcine brain. *J. Neurochem.*, 28: 1207-1213.

ELDJARN, L., JELLUM, E., and STOKKE, O. 1972. Pyroglutamic aciduria: Studies on the enzymic block and on the metabolic origin of pyroglutamic acid. *Clin. Chim. Acta*,

40:461-476.

EMSON, P. C. 1976. Effects of chronic treatment with amino-oxyacetic acid or sodium n-dipropylacetate on brain GABA levels and the development and regression of cobalt epileptoform foci in rats. *J. Neurochem.*, 27:1489-1494.

ENNA, S. J., BENNETT, J. P. JR., BYLUND, D. B., SNYDER, S. H., BIRD, E. D., and IVERSEN, L. L. 1976a. Alterations of brain neurotransmitter receptor binding in Huntington's chorea. *Brain Res.*, 116:531-537.

ENNA, S. J., BIRD, E. D., BENNETT, J., BYLUND, D. B., YAMAMURA, H. I., IVERSEN, L. L., and SNYDER, S. H. 1976b. Huntington's chorea: Changes in neurotransmitter receptors in the brain. *New Engl. J. Med.*, 294:1305-1309.

FERNSTROM, J. D., and WURTMAN, R. J. 1972. Brain serotonin content: physiological regulation by plasma neutral amino acids. *Science*, 178:414-416.

FERRENDELLI, J. A., CHANG, M. M., and KINSCHERF, D. A. 1974. Elevation of cyclic GMP levels in central nervous system by excitatory and inhibitory amino acids. *J. Neurochem.*, 22:535-540.

FOTHERBY, K. J., MORRISH, N. J., and RYALL, R. W. 1976. Is Lioresal (Baclofen) an antagonist of substance P? *Brain Res.*, 113:210-213.

FOWLER, L. J., and JOHN, R. A. 1972. Active-site-directed irreversible inhibition of rat brain 4-aminobutyrate aminotransferase by ethanolamine O-sulfate *in vitro* and *in vivo*. *Biochem. J.*, 130:569-573.

FRIEDMAN, P. A., CAPPELMAN, A. H., and KAUFMAN, S. 1974. Partial purification and characterization of tryptophan hydroxylase from rabbit hindbrain. *J. Biol. Chem.*, 247:4165-4173.

GORELL, J. M., DOLKART, P. H., and FERRENDELLI, J. A. 1976. Regional levels of glucose, amino acids, high energy phosphates and cyclic nucleotides in the central nervous system during hypoglycemic stupor and behavioral recovery. *J. Neurochem.*, 27:1043-1049.

GREENGARD, P. 1975. Cyclic nucleotides, protein phosphorylation and neuronal function. In G. I. Drummond, P. Greengard, and G. A. Robison (eds.), *Advances in Cyclic Nucleotide Research*, vol. 5, pp. 585-602. New York: Raven Press.

GREENGARD, P. 1976. Possible role for cyclic nucleotides and phosphorylated membrane proteins in postsynaptic actions of neurotransmitters. *Nature*, 260:101-108.

GUILLORY, R. J., RAYNER, M. D., and D'ARRIGO, J. S. 1977. Covalent labeling of the tetrodotoxin receptor in excitable membranes. *Science*, 196:883-885.

GUROFF, G. 1972. Transport and metabolism of amino acids. In R. W. Albers, G. J. Siegel, R. Katzman, and B. W. Agranoff (eds.), *Basic Neurochemistry*, pp. 191-206. Boston: Little, Brown.

HARRIS, M., HOPKIN, J. M., and NEAL, M. J. 1973. Effect of centrally acting drugs on the uptake of γ-aminobutyric acid (GABA) by slices of rat cerebral cortex. *Br. J. Pharmacol.*, 47:229-239.

HEGSTRAND, L. R., KANOF, P.D., and GREENGARD, P. 1976. Histamine-sensitive adenylate cyclase in mammalian brain. *Nature*, 260:163-165.

HENDERSON, R., RITCHIE, J. M., and STRICHARTZ, G. R. 1974. Evidence that tetrodotoxin and saxitoxin act as a metal cation binding site in the sodium channels of nerve membrane. *Proc. Nat. Acad. Sci. USA*, 71:3936-3940.

HENN, F. A., and HAMBERGER, A. 1971. Glial cell function: Uptake of transmitter substances. *Proc. Nat. Acad. Sci. USA*, 68:2686-2690.

HENN, F., ANDERSON, D. J., and SELLSTRÖM, A. 1977. Possible relationship between glial cells, dopamine and the effect of antipsychotic drugs. *Nature*, 266:637-638.

HERNDON, R. M., and COYLE, J. T. 1977. Selective destruction of neurons by a transmitter agonist. *Science*, 198:71-72.

HERTTING, G., and AXELROD, J. 1961. Fate of tritiated noradrenaline at sympathetic nerve endings. *Nature*, 192:172-173.

HIRSCH, M. J., GROWDON, J. H., and WURTMAN, R. J. 1977. Increase in hippocampal acetylcholine after choline administration. *Brain Res.*, 125:383-385.

HOCHNER, B., SPIRA, M. E., and WERMAN, R. 1975. Penicillin decreases chloride conductance in crustacean muscle: a model for the epileptic neuron. *Brain Res.*, 107:85-103.

HOLTZMAN, E. 1977. The origin and fate of secretory packages, especially synaptic vesicles. *Neuroscience*, 2:327-355.

HUBEL, D. H., and WIESEL, T. N. 1968. Receptive fields and functional architecture of monkey striate cortex. *J. Physiol.*, 195:215-243.

HUBEL, D. H., WIESEL, T. N., and STRYKER, M. P. 1977. Orientation columns in macaque monkey visual cortex demonstrated by the 2-deoxyglucose autoradiographic technique. *Nature*, 269:328-330.

HUGHES, J. V., and JOHNSON, T. C. 1977. Hyperphenylalanemia: Effect on brain polyribosomes can be partially reversed by other amino acids. *Science*, 195:402-404.

IVERSEN, L. L. 1967. *The Uptake and Storage of Noradrenaline in Sympathetic Nerves.* London: Cambridge University Press.

IVERSEN, L. L. 1977. Catecholamine-sensitive adenylate cyclases in nervous tissues. *J. Neurochem.*, 29:5-12.

IVERSEN, L. L., and BLOOM, F. E. 1972. Studies of the uptake of ^{3}H-GABA and [^{3}H]glycine in slices and homogenates of rat brain and spinal cord by electron microscopic autoradiography. *Brain Res.*, 41:131-143.

IVERSEN, L. L., and KELLY, J. S. 1975. Uptake and metabolism of γ-aminobutyric acid by neurons and glial cells. *Biochem. Pharmacol.*, 24:933-938.

JENG, S. J., and GUILLORY, R. J. 1975. The use of aryl azido ATP analogs as photoaffinity labels for myosin ATPase. *J. Supramol. Struct.*, 3:448-468.

JOHNSTON, G. A. R. 1976. Glutamate and aspartate as transmitters in the spinal cord. *Adv. Biochem. Psychopharmacol.*, 15:175-184.

JOHNSTON, G. A. R., and BALCAR, V. J. 1974. Amino-oxyacetic acid: a relatively nonspecific inhibitor of uptake of amino acids and amines by brain and spinal cord. *J. Neurochem.*, 22:609-610.

JOHNSTON, G. A. R., KROGSGAARD-LARSEN, P., STEPHANSON, A. L., and TWITCHIN, B. 1976. Inhibition of the uptake of GABA and related amino acids in rat brain slices by the optical isomers of nipecotic acid. *J. Neurochem.*, 26:1029-1032.

JUNG, M. J., LIPPERT, B., METCALF, B. W., BÖHLEN, P., and SCHECHTER, P. J. 1977a. γ-Vinyl GABA (4-amino-hex-5-enoic acid), a new selective irreversible inhibitor of GABA-T: effects on brain GABA metabolism in mice. *J. Neurochem.*, 29:797-802.

JUNG, M. J., LIPPERT, B., METCALF, B. W., SCHECHTER, P. J., BÖHLEN, P., and SJOERDSMA, A. 1977b. The effect of 4-amino-hex-5-ynoic acid (γ-acetylenic GABA, γ-ethynyl GABA), a catalytic inhibitor of GABAtransaminase, on brain GABA metabolism *in vivo*. *J. Neurochem.*, 28:717-723.

KANDERA, J., LEVI, G., and LAJTHA, A. 1968. Control of cerebral metabolite levels. II. Amino acid uptake and levels in various areas of the rat brain. *Arch. Biochem. Biophys.*, 126:249-260.

KASS, L. R., and BLOCH, K. 1967. On the enzymatic synthesis of unsaturated fatty acids in Escherichia coli. *Proc. Nat. Acad. Sci. USA*, 58:1168-1173.

KENNEDY, C., DES ROSIERS, M. H., SAKURADA, O., SHINOHARA, M., REIVICH, M., JEHLE, J. W., and SOKOLOFF, L. 1976. Metabolic mapping of the primary visual system of the monkey by means of the autoradiographic [^{14}C]deoxyglucose technique. *Proc. Nat. Acad. Sci. USA*, 73:4230-4242.

KOBAYASHI, K., MIYAZAWA, S., and TERAHARA, A. 1976. Gabaculine: γ-aminobutyrate aminotransferase inhibitor of microbial origin. *Tetrahedron Lett.*, 7:537-540.

KOSLOW, S. H., and BUTTLER, I. J. 1977. Biogenic amine synthesis defect in dihydropterdine reductase deficiency. *Science*, 198:522-523.

KOZHECHKIN, S. N., and OSTROVSKAYA, R. U. 1977. Are benzodiazepines GABA antagonists? *Nature*, 269:72-73.

KROGSGAARD-LARSEN, P., and JOHNSTON, G. A. R. 1975. Inhibition of GABA uptake in rat brain slices by nipecotic acid, various isoxazoles and related compounds. *J. Neurochem.*, 25:797-802.

LAJTHA, A., BERL, S., and WAELSCH, H. 1959. Amino acid and protein metabolism of the brain. IV. The metabolism of glutamic acid. *J. Neurochem.*, 3:322-332.

LEFKOWITZ, R. J., and WILLIAMS, L. T. 1976. [as quoted by Kolata, G. B.] Hormone receptors: How are they regulated? *Science*, 196:747-800.

LEVI, W. B., HAYCOCK, J. W., and COTMAN, C. W. 1974. Effects of polyvalent cations on stimulus-coupled secretion of (^{14}C) gamma-aminobutyric acid from isolated brain synaptosomes. *Molec. Pharmacol.*, 10:438-449.

LEVI, W. B., REDBURN, D. A., and COTMAN, C. W. 1973. Stimulus-coupled secretion of γ-aminobutyric acid from rat brain synaptosomes. *Science*, 181:676-678.

LEVI, G., RUSCA, G., and RAITERI, M. 1976. Diaminobutyric acid: A tool for discriminating between carrier mediated and non-carrier mediated release of GABA from synaptosomes? *Neurochem. Res.*, 1:581-590.

LLINÁS, R. R. 1977. Calcium and transmitter release in squid synapse. *Neuroscience Symposium*, 2:139-160.

LLOYD, K. G., SHEMEN, L., and HORNYKIEWICZ, O. 1977. Distribution of high affinity sodium-independent [^{3}H]gamma-aminobutyric acid ([^{3}H]GABA) binding in the human brain: alterations in Parkinson's disease. *Brain Res.*, 127:269-278.

MACINNES, J. W., and SCHLESINGER, K. 1971. Effects of excess phenylalanine on in vitro and in vivo RNA and protein synthesis and polyribosome levels in brains of mice. *Brain Res.*, 29:101-110.

MAHLER, H. R. 1977. Proteins of the synaptic membrane. *Neurochem. Res.*, 2:119-147.

MAITRE, M., OSSOLA, L., and MANDEL, P. 1976. In vitro studies into the effect of inhibition of rat brain succinic semialdehyde dehydrogenase on GABA synthesis and degradation. *FEBS Lett.*, 72:53-57.

MARCO, C. C., CHENEY, D. L., MARCO, E., REVUELTA, A., and COSTA, E. 1977. Turnover times of gamma-aminobutyric acid and acetylcholine in nucleus caudatus, nucleus accumbens, globus pallidus and substantia nigra: effects of repeated administration of haloperidol. *Brain Res.*, 132:375-379.

MARCO, E., MAO, C. C., CHENEY, D. L., REVUELTA, A., and COSTA, E. 1976. The effects of antipsychotics on the turnover rate of GABA and acetylcholine in rat brain nuclei. *Nature*, 264:363-365.

MARKOVITZ, D. C., and FERNSTROM, J. D. 1977. Diet and uptake of Aldomet by brain: Competition with natural large neutral amino acids. *Science*, 197:1014-1015.

MARTIN, D. L. 1973. Kinetics of the sodium-dependent transport of gamma-aminobutyric acid by synaptosomes. *J. Neurochem.*, 21:345-356.

MARTINEZ-HERNANDEZ, A., BELL, K. P., and NORENBERG, M. D. 1977. Glutamine synthetase: Glial localization in brain. *Science*, 195:1356-1358.

MCBRIDE, W. J., NADI, N. S., ALTMAN, J., and APRISON, M. H. 1976. Effects of selective doses of X-irradiation on the levels of several amino acids in the cerebellum of the rat. *Neurochem. Res.*, 1:141-152.

MCKEAN, C. M., BOGGS, D. E., and PETERSEN, N. A. 1968. The influence of high phenylalanine and tyrosine on the concentrations of essential amino acids in brain. *J. Neurochem.*, 15:235-241.

MILLER, L. P., and WALTERS, J. R. 1977. Effect of depolarizing agents on the percent saturation of glutamate decarboxylase (GAD) with pyridoxal-5′-phosphate (PLP) in rat substantia nigra synaptosomes. *Society for Neuroscience Annual Meeting Abstracts*, 3:410.

MILLER, L. P., WALTERS, J. R., and MARTIN, D. L. 1977. Post-mortem changes implicate adenine nucleotides and pyridoxal-5′-phosphate in regulation of brain glutamate decarboxylase. *Nature*, 266:847-848.

MINARD, F. N., and MUSHAWAR, I. K. 1966. Synthesis of γ-aminobutyric acid from a pool of glutamic acid in brain after decapitation. *Life Sci.*, 5:1409-1413.

MÖHLER, H., PATEL, A. J., JOHNSON, A. L., REYNOLDS, A. P., and BÁLAZS, R. 1975. Metabolic compartmentatation in the brain: Effects of a central nervous system depressant, l-hydroxy-3-amino-pyrrolidone-2. *J. Neurochem.*, 24:865-873.

NADLER, J. V., WHITE, W. F., VACA, K. W., REDBURN, D. A., and COTMAN, C. W. 1977. Characterization of putative amino acid transmitter release from slices of rat dentate gyrus. *J. Neurochem*, 29:279-290.

NATHANSON, J. A. 1977. Cyclic nucleotides and nervous system function. *Physiol. Rev.*, 57:157-256.

NEAL, M. J., and BOWERY, N. G. 1977. Cis-3-aminocyclohexane carboxylic acid: a substrate for the neuronal GABA transport system. *Brain Res.*, 138:169-174.

NICOLL, R. A., ECCLES, J. C., OSHIMA, T., and RUBIA, F. 1975. Prolongation of hippocampal inhibitory postsynaptic potentials by barbiturates. *Nature*, 258:625-627.

OCHS, S. 1975. Axoplasmic transport. In D. B. Tower (ed.), *The Nervous System*, vol. 1, pp. 137-146. New York: Raven Press.

OLDENDORF, W. H. 1976. Certain aspects of drug distribution to brain. In G. Levi, L. Battistin, and A. Lajtha (eds.), *Transport Phenomena in the Nervous System*, pp. 103-109. New York: Plenum.

OKONKWO, P. O., ORLOWSKI, M., and GREEN, J. P. 1974. Enzymes of the γ-glutamyl cycle in the choroid plexus and brain. *J. Newrochem.*, 22:1053-1058.

OLSEN, R. W., LAMAR, E. E., and BAYLESS, J. D. 1977. Calcium induced release of γ-aminobutyric acid from synaptosomes: effects of tranquilizer drugs. *J. Neurochem.*, 28:299-305.

ORLOWSKI, M., and MEISTER, A. 1970. The γ-glutamyl cycle: A possible transport system for amino acids. *Proc. Nat. Acad. Sci. USA*, 67:1248-1255.

ORLOWSKI, M., SESSA, G., and GREEN, J. P. 1974. γ-Glutamyl transpeptidase in brain capillaries: Possible site of a blood-brain barrier for amino acids. *Science*, 184:66-68.

PALFREYMAN, M. G., SYLVIE, H., and SCHECHTER, P. J. 1977. The effect of γ-acetylenic GABA, a new inhibitor of GABA-transaminase, on catechol and indoleamine systems in rat brain. *Proceedings of the International Society of Neurochemistry*, 6:642.

PELLMAR, T. C., and WILSON, W. A. 1977. Synaptic mechanism of pentylenetetrazole: Selectivity for chloride conductance. *Science*, 197:912-914.

PERRY, T. L., and HANSEN, S. 1973. Sustained drug-induced elevation of brain GABA in the rat. *J. Neurochem.*, 21:1167-1175.

PHILLIS, J. W. 1977. The role of cyclic nucleotides in the C.N.S. *J. Can. Sci. Neurol.*, 4:153-195.

PLUM, E., GJEDDE, A., and SAMSON, F. E. (eds.) 1976. *Neurosciences Research Program Monograph: Neuroanatomical Functional Mapping by the Radioactive 2-Deoxy-D-Glucose Method*. Cambridge, Mass.: MIT Press.

POPOV, N., and MATTHIES, H. 1969. Some effects of monoamine oxidase inhibitors on the metabolism of γ-aminobutyric acid in rat brain. *J. Neurochem.*, 16:899-907.

RAITERI, M., FEDERICO, R., COLETTI, A., and LEVI, G. 1975. Release and exchange studies relating to the synaptosomal uptake of GABA. *J. Neurochem.*, 24:1243-1250.

RANDO, R. R. 1975. Chemistry and enzymology of K_{cat} inhibitors. *Science*, 185:320-324.

RANDO, R. R., and BANGERTER, F. W. 1976. The irreversible inhibition of mouse brain γ-aminobutyric acid (GABA-α-ketoglutaric acid transaminase by Gabaculine. *J. Am. Chem. Soc.*, 98:6762-6764.

RAPOPORT, S. I. 1976. *Blood-Brain Barrier in Physiology and Medicine.* New York: Raven Press.

RASMUSSEN, H., and GOODMAN, D. B. 1977. Relationships between calcium and cyclic nucleotides in cell activation. *Physiol. Rev.*, 57:421-509.

REDBURN, D. A., BROOME, D. S., and ENNA, S. J. 1977. Ontogenesis of calcium-dependent GABA release in rat brain. *Society for Neuroscience Annual Meeting Abstracts*, 3:412.

REDBURN, D. A., SHELTON, D., and COTMAN, C. W. 1976. Calcium dependent release of exogenously loaded γ-amino-[U-^{14}C]butyrate from synaptosomes: time course of stimulation by potassium, veratridine and the calcium ionophore A23187. *J. Neurochem.*, 26:297-303.

REIVICH, M. 1976. Application of the deoxyglucose method to human cerebral dysfunction.

In F. Plum, A. Gjedde, and F. E. Samson (eds.), *Neurosciences Research Program Monograph: Neuroanatomical Functional Mapping by the Radioactive 2-Deoxy-D-Glucose Method*, vol. 14, pp. 502-504. Cambridge, Mass.: MIT Press.

REUBI, J.-C., IVERSEN, L. L., and JESSELL, T. M. 1977. Dopamine selectively increases ^{3}H-GABA release from slices of rat substantia nigra *in vitro*. *Nature*, 268:652-654.

RIBAK, C. E., VAUGHN, J. E., SAITO, K., BARBER, R., and ROBERTS, E. 1976. Immunocytochemical localization of glutamate decarboxylase in rat substantia nigra. *Brain Res.*, 116:287-298.

RIBAK, C. E., VAUGHN, J. E., SAITO, K., BARBER, R., and ROBERTS, E. 1977. Glutamate decarboxylase localization in neurons of the olfactory bulb. *Brain Res.*, 126:1-18.

ROACH, M. K., DAVIS, D. L., PENNINGTON, W., and NORDYKE, E. 1973. Effect of ethanol on the uptake by rat brain synaptosomes of [^{3}H]DL-norepinephrine, [^{3}H]5-hydroxytryptamine, [^{3}H]GABA and [^{3}H]glutamate. *Life Sci.*, 12:433-441.

ROBERTS, E. 1964. Comparative aspects of the distribution of ninhydrin-positive constituents in nervous tissue. In D. Richter (ed.), *Comparative Neurochemistry*, pp. 167-183. New York: Macmillan.

RUSSELL, J., JENG, S. J., and GUILLORY, R. J. 1976. Arylazido aminopropionyl ATP, an active site directed photoaffinity reagent for mitochondrial adenosine triphosphatase. *Biochem. Biophys. Res. Commun.*, 70:1225-1234.

RYAN, L. D., and ROSKOSKI, R. JR. 1975. Selective release of newly synthesized and newly captured GABA from synaptosomes by potassium depolarization. *Nature*, 258:254-255.

SAITO, K., KONISHI, S., and OTSUKA, M. 1975. Antagonism between Lioresal and substance P in rat spinal cord. *Brain Res.*, 96:177-180.

SCHON, F., and KELLY, J. S. 1975. Selective uptake of [^{3}H]ß-alanine by glia: Association with the glial uptake system for GABA. *Brain Res.*, 86:243-257.

SCHOUSBOE, A., HERTZ, L., and SVENNEBY, G. 1977. Uptake and metabolism of GABA in astrocytes cultured from dissociated mouse brain hemispheres. *Neurochem. Res.*, 2:217-229.

SEEMAN, P., and LEE, T. 1975. Antipsychotic drugs: Direct correlation between clinical potency and presynaptic action on dopamine neurons. *Science*, 188:1217-1219.

SHANK, R. P., and APRISON, M. H. 1977. Glutamine uptake and metabolism by the isolated toad brain: Evidence pertaining to its proposed role as a transmitter precursor. *J. Neurochem.*, 28:1189-1196.

SHANK, R. P., and BAXTER, C. F. 1975. Uptake and metabolism of glutamate by isolated toad brains containing different levels of endogenous amino acids. *J. Neurochem.*, 24:641-646.

SHANK, R. P., WHITEN, J. T., and BAXTER, C. F. 1973. Glutamate uptake by the isolated toad brain. *Science*, 181:860-862.

SIEGEL, F. L., AOKI, K., and COLWELL, R. E. 1971. Polyribosome disaggregation and cell-free protein synthesis in preparations from cerebral cortex of hyperphenylalaninemic rats. *J. Neurochem.*, 18:537-547.

SIMLER, S., CIESIELSKI, L., MAITRE, M., RANDRIANARISOA, H., and MANDEL, P. 1973. Effect of sodium n-dipropylacetate on audiogenic seizures and brain γ-aminobutyric acid level. *Biochem. Pharmacol.*, 22:1701-1708.

SNYDER, S. H., YAMAMURA, H. I., PERT, C. B., LOGAN, W. J., and BENNETT, J. P. 1973. Neuronal uptake of neurotransmitters and their precursors: Studies with "transmitter" amino acids and choline. In A. J. Mandell (ed.), *New Concepts in Neurotransmitter Regulation*, pp. 195-222. New York: Plenum Press.

SOKOLOFF, L. 1977. Relation between physiological function and energy metabolism in the central nervous system. *J. Neurochem.*, 29:13-26.

SOKOLOFF, L., REIVICH, M., KENNEDY, C., DES ROSIERS, M. H., PATLAK, C. S., PETTIGREW, K. D., SAKURADA, O., and SHINOHARA, M. 1977. The [^{14}C]deoxyglucose method for the measurement of local cerebral glucose utilization: Theory, procedure, and normal values in the conscious and anesthetized albino rat. *J. Neurochem.*, 28:897-916.

SOKOLOFF, L., SHARP, F. R., SHEPHERD, G. M., REIVICH, M., and COLLINS, R. C. 1976. In F. Plum, A. Gjedde, and F. E. Samson (eds.), *Neurosciences Research Program Monograph: Neuroanatomical Functional Mapping by the Radioactive 2-Deoxy-D-Glucose Method*, vol. 14, pp. 466-518. Cambridge, Mass.: MIT Press.

STEINER, F. A., and FELIX, D. 1976. Antagonistic effects of GABA and benzodiazepines on vestibular and cerebellar neurones. *Nature*, 260:346-347.

SWANSON, P. D., and STAHL, W. L. 1972. Ion transport. In R. W. Albers, G. J. Siegel, R. Katzman, and B. W. Agranoff (eds.), *Basic Neurochemistry*, pp. 21-40. Boston: Little, Brown.

SZE, P. Y., and LOVELL, R. A. 1970. Reduction of level of L-glutamic acid decarboxylase by γ-aminobutyric acid in mouse brain. *J. Neurochem.*, 17:1657-1664.

TAPIA, R. 1975. Biochemical pharmacology of GABA in CNS. In L. L. Iversen, S. D. Iversen, and S. H. Snyder (eds.), *Handbook of Psychopharmacology*, vol. 4, pp. 1-58. New York: Plenum.

TAPIA, R., PASANTES, H., PEREZ DE LA MORA, M., ORTEGA, B. G., and MASSIEU, G. H. 1967. Free amino acids and glutamate decarboxylase activity in brain of mice during drug-induced convulsions. *Biochem. Pharmacol.*, 16:483-496.

TAPPAZ, M. L., BROWNSTEIN, M. J., and KOPIN, I. J. 1977. Glutamate decarboxylase (GAD) and γ-aminobutyric acid (GABA) in discrete nuclei of hypothalamus and substantia nigra. *Brain Res.*, 125:109-121.

TAUB, F., and JOHNSON, T. C. 1975. The mechanism of polyribosome disaggregation in brain tissue by phenylalanine. *Biochem. J.*, 151:173-180.

TELLER, D. N., BARNAY-SCHWARTZ, M., DEGUZMAN, T., and LAJTHA, A. 1977. Energetics of amino acid transport into brain slices: effects of glucose depletion and substitution of Krebs cycle intermediates. *Brain Res.*, 131:321-334.

THORN, W., GRIESHABER, T., and JUNGE, H. 1973. γ-Aminobuttersäure und NH_3-Gehalt in Kaninchengehirnen nach Hypoxie und Ischamie. *Pflügers Archives*, 345:347-351.

TREMBLAY, J. P., and GRENON, G. 1977. Benzodiazepines mimic the presynaptic action of GABA on a cholinergic synapse of aplysia. *Society for Neuroscience Annual Meeting Abstracts*, III:520.

TURSKY, T. 1970. Inhibition of brain glutamate decarboxylase by adenosine triphosphate. *Eur. J. Biochem.*, 12:544-549.

VAN DEN BERG, C. J., REIJNIERSE, G. L. A., BLOCKHUIS, G. G. D., KROON, M. C., RONDA, G., CLARKE, D. D., and GARFINKEL, D. 1975. A model of glutamate metabolism in brain: A biochemical analysis of a heterogeneous structure. In S. Berl, D. D. Clarke, and D. Schneider (eds.), *Metabolic Compartmentation and Neurotransmission: Relation to Structure and Function in Brain*, pp. 515-544. New York: Plenum Press.

VAN GELDER, N. M. 1969. The action *in vivo* of a structural analogue of GABA: Hydrazinoproprionic acid. *J. Neurochem.*, 16:1355-1360.

VON HUNGEN, K., ROBERTS, S., and HILL, D. F. 1975. Serotonin-sensitive adenylate cyclase activity of immature rat brain. *Brain Res.*, 84:257-267.

WALLACH, D. P. 1961. Studies on the GABA pathway. I. The inhibition of γ-aminobutyric acid-α-ketoglutaric acid transaminase in *vitro* and *in vivo* by U7524 (amino-oxyacetic acid). *Biochem. Pharmacol.*, 5:323-331.

WALKER, R. J. 1976. The action of kainic acid and quisqualic acid on the glutamate receptors of three identifiable neurones from the brain of the snail. *Helix aspersa. Comp. Biochem. Physiol.*, 55C:61-67.

WILTSE, H. E., and MENKES, J. H. 1972. Brain damage in the aminoacidurias. In A. Lajtha (ed.), *Handbook of Neurochemistry*, vol. 7, pp. 143-167. New York: Plenum Press.

WOOD, J. D., and PEESKER, S. J. 1972. A correlation between changes in GABA metabolism and isonicotinic acid hydrazide-induced seizures. *Brain Res.*, 45:489-498.

WOOD, J. D., and PEESKER, S. J. 1975. The anticonvulsant action of GABA-elevating agents: A re-evaluation. *J. Neurochem.*, 45:277-282.

WU, J-Y. 1976. Purification, characterization and kinetic studies of GAD and GABA-T from mouse brain. In E. Roberts, T. N. Chase, and D. B. Tower (eds.), *GABA in Nervous System Function*, pp. 7-55. New York: Raven Press.

WU, J-Y., and ROBERTS, E. 1974. Properties of brain L-glutamate decarboxylase: Inhibition studies. *J. Neurochem.*, 23:759-767.

YOUNG, A. B., and SNYDER, S. H. 1974. The glycine synaptic receptor: Evidence that strychnine binding is associated with the ionic conductance mechanism. *Proc. Nat. Acad. Sci. USA*, 71:4002-4005.

YOUNG, A. B., ENNA, S. J., ZUKIN, S. R., and SNYDER, S. H. 1976. Synaptic GABA receptors in mammalian CNS. In E. Roberts, T. N. Chase, and D. B. Tower (eds.), *GABA in Nervous System Function*, pp. 305-336. New York: Raven Press.

YOUNG, A. B., OSTER-GRANITE, M. L., HERNDON, R. M., and SNYDER, S. H. 1974. Glutamic acid: selective depletion by viral induced granule cell loss in hamster cerebellum. *Brain Res.*, 73:1-14.

3

RADIOIMMUNOASSAY TECHNIQUES IN KINETIC STUDIES

SYDNEY SPECTOR, PH.D.

The problem of precise determination of drugs in blood and other biological fluids has been studied by many groups in pharmacology in order to understand the pharmacodynamics of the drugs. The methods that have been developed—bioassay, colorimetry, spectrophotometry, fluorometry, mass spectroscopy—are both sensitive and reproducible.

Most of these methods, however, are time-consuming and laborious, so that one cannot do large numbers of analyses. The introduction of the immunological assay has provided a method that is sensitive, reproducible, convenient, and easy to perform in large numbers.

The immunological assays, which have proved to be of great value for the determination of proteins, hormones, and various peptides, can likewise be used for compounds of small molecular weight such as drugs. Because of the small size of drug molecules, these agents per se are not good antigens for the production of an antibody. The haptenic molecules can be made antigenic, however, by conjugating them to a larger carrier molecule, in most instances a protein. There are innumerable chemical procedures for coupling a drug to a protein. The chemistry is greatly simplified if the drug contains such reactive groups as COOH or NH_2 groups, for then one can link the haptenic moiety to the protein using a carbodiimide reagent to form amide linkages. A covalent amide linkage may also be generated by initially developing an "active ester" of a drug with p-nitrophenol and then causing a nucleophilic attack on the ester by amine groups on the protein. We have used this procedure to develop a barbiturate immunogen (Spector and Flynn, 1971). Erlanger and colleagues (1957, 1959) used the mixed-anhydride procedure for conjugating steroids to proteins. In our laboratory, we have coupled the beta-adrenergic drug propranolol to bovine serum albumin using the mixed-anhydride method (Kawashima, Levy, and Spector, 1976). Haptens con-

COMPETITION WITH ^{3}H-DIHYDROMORPHINE FOR BINDING SITE

COMPOUND	STRUCTURE	CONCENTRATION WHICH INHIBITS LABELED Ag-Ab COMPLEX 50%
	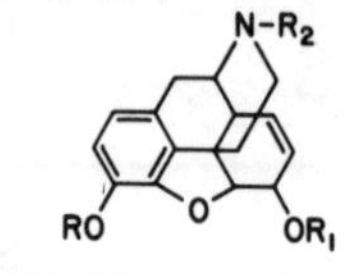	
MORPHINE	R = H R_1 = H R_2 = CH_3	30 pg
CODEINE	R = CH_3 R_1 = H R_2 = CH_3	> 50,000 pg
NORMORPHINE	R = H R_1 = H R_2 = H	30 pg
MORPHINE GLUCURONIDE	R = 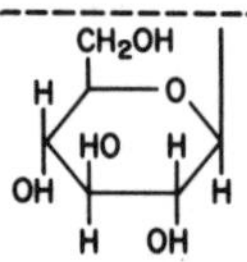 R_1 = H R_2 = CH_3	10,000 pg
NALORPHINE	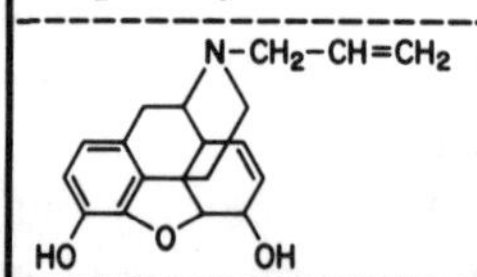	40 pg
LEVALLORPHAN	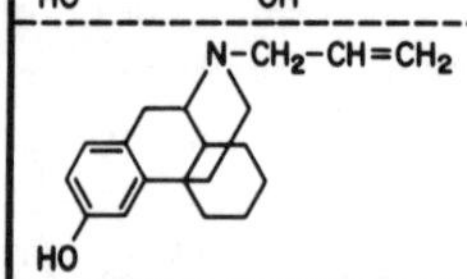	200 pg
METHADONE	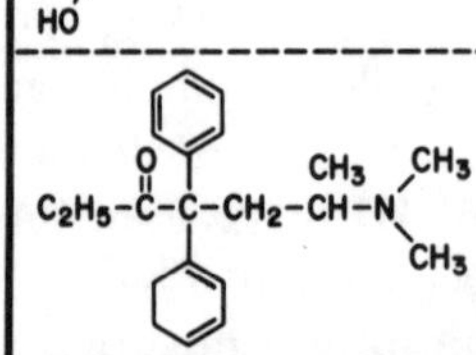	> 50,000 pg

Table 1

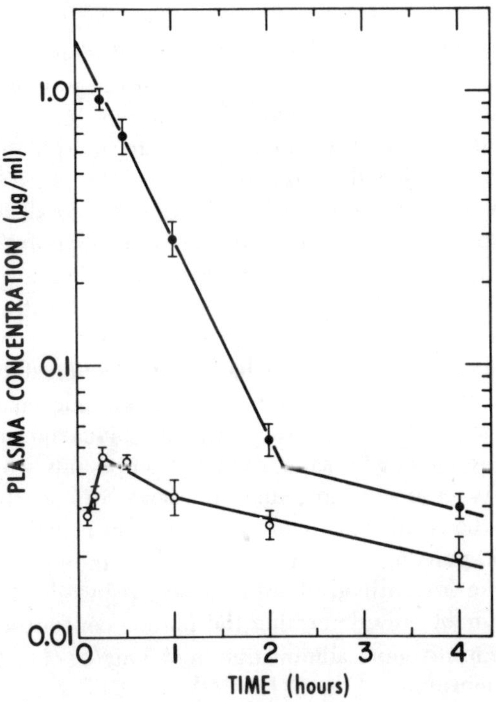

Figure 1. Plasma concentration of codeine (•) and biotransformed morphine (○) determined by radioimmunoassay after intravenous administration of 5 mg/kg of codeine. Mean ± range from three rats.

taining an aromatic amino group may be conjugated to proteins by diazotization procedures. There are many examples of coupling by diazotization beginning with the work of Landsteiner (1945). Hamburger (1966) coupled chloramphenicol through a diazo linkage; we used that technique to develop specific antibodies against serotonin (Peskar and Spector, 1973) and naloxone (Berkowitz et al., 1975). Erlanger in his review (1973) illustrates methods for preparing protein conjugates with various haptenic groups such as amines, alcohols, phenols, and sugars to develop specific antibodies.

In preparing a drug-protein conjugate, consideration must be given to the determinant group on the drug that one desires the antibody to recognize. Beiser et al. (1959) showed that specific antibodies to steroids could be developed by conjugating the carrier to different parts of the steroid molecule. We were interested in developing antibodies that could differentiate morphine from codeine. By conjugating the protein to C_3 of morphine, we developed antibodies that failed to differentiate morphine from codeine but could differentiate substitutions on the N atom (Gintzler, Mohacsi, and Spector, 1976). When the protein was conjugated through a substitution of the N atom, the immunogen stimulated the production of antibodies that could differentiate morphine from codeine. Using antibodies produced by the immunogen in which the carrier protein is conjugated to the nitrogen atom of the opiate alkaloid and the antibodies developed by protein conjugated at carbon atom 3 in the phenolic ring, gave us a sensitive method for estimating tissue levels of codeine and morphine simultaneously. Table 1 demonstrates the specificity of the radioimmunoassay for morphine using the N-carboxymethyl normorphine antiserum. Since the hapten was conjugated to the protein carrier through the nitrogen, any change in the side chain is not recognized by the antibody. Thus, the antibody binds normorphine, nalorphine, and naloxone as well as morphine. Compounds with a substitution at the 3-hydroxy group of morphine are, however, poorly bound by the antibody. One-thousand times more codeine than morphine is required to produce a 50-percent inhibition of the binding of labeled ^{3}H-dihydromorphine for antibody binding sites. Using the two different antibodies, one cannot only determine the plasma concentrations of codeine in rats after the intravenous administration of 5 mg/kg of codeine but also its conversion to morphine (Figure 1). Codeine exhibited a biphasic decay curve, the half-life of the first phase being 26 minutes. Morphine could be detected in the plasma as early as five minutes after codeine administration; it attained its highest level in about 15 to 30 minutes and declined thereafter.

The narcotic antagonist naloxone has a short duration of action. Its kinetics have not been investigated because assays are not sensitive enough to analyze the drug's very low tissue and fluid concentrations *in vivo*. We conjugated naloxone to a protein carrier by diazotizing ethyl-D-carbamylcyanomethyl-acetimidate as described previously (Berkowitz et al., 1975). Naloxone is a potent, short-acting narcotic antagonist. Figure 2 shows its rapid entry and egress from the brain of rats receiving a dose of 5 mg/kg subcutaneously. Naloxone had a higher brain-to-serum ratio than morphine during the four-hour study; in contrast to morphine, which sustained peak brain levels for up to two hours, brain levels of naloxone declined quickly within one hour. The rapid decrease in the levels of naloxone in the brain may well explain its short duration of action.

Another drug for which we developed a radioimmunoassay was the alkaloid reserpine (Levy, Kawashima, and Spector, 1976). This drug has been used in combination with other agents to treat mildly hypertensive

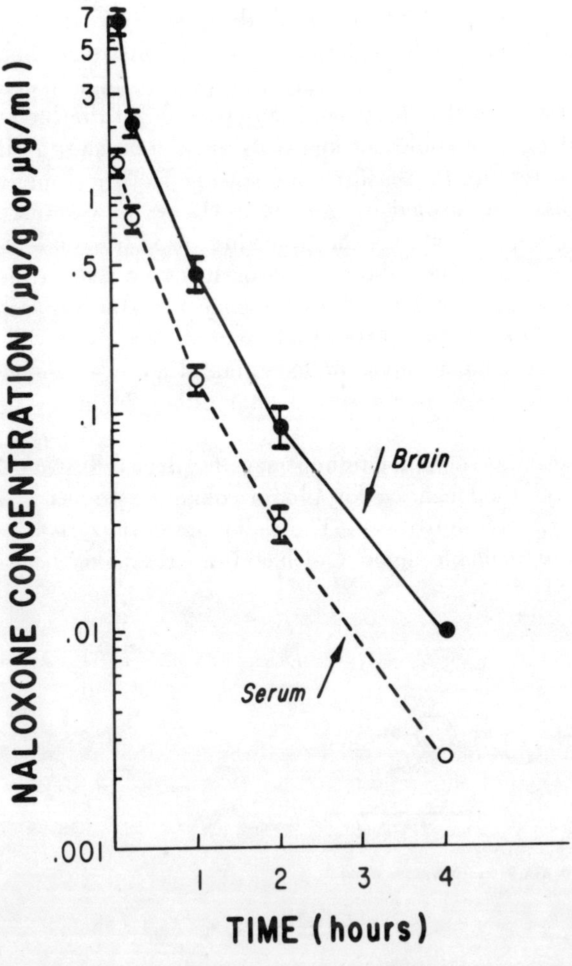

Figure 2. Serum and brain concentrations of naloxone in rats at intervals after intravenous injection, 5 mg/kg. Each point represents mean for three to five animals. Vertical bars indicate S.E. Note higher brain concentrations of naloxone and parallel decline of drug concentrations with time.

patients as well as psychotic patients who do not respond to phenothiazines. Reserpine elicits a wide variety of physiological responses, most of them attributed to the depletion of biogenic amines, but the final details of its mechanism of action have not been elucidated. Although Sheppard and collegues (1957) reported long-term residual radioactive reserpine in brain of guinea pigs and rats, the compound was always referred to as a "hit and run" drug because analytical methods were not sensitive enough to detect small amounts of it. Shore and his group (Norn and Shore, 1971), using reserpine of high specific activity, showed that levels of the drug persisted. Because of the high specific activity of the drug, one could not follow its disposition after a pharmacological dose. This required a sensitive and specific analytical method like the radioimmunoassay described by our group (Levy, Kawashima, and Spector, 1976). Figure 3 illustrates the procedure used to couple reserpine to the protein bovine serum albumin (BSA). Reserpic acid, a metabolite of reserpine, cross-reacts at 2000 times the concentration required for reserpine. The other metabolite of reserpine, methyl reserpine, will cross-react at 100 times the concentration of reserpine. Figure 4 demonstrates the disposition of reserpine in rat serum after either an intravenous or oral dose of 1 mg/kg.

These representative radioimmunoassays for drugs illustrate how useful this sensitive method can be for pharmacokinetic studies of both acute and chronic drug administration. The radioimmunoassay is especially valuable when the available amount of blood or other biological fluids such

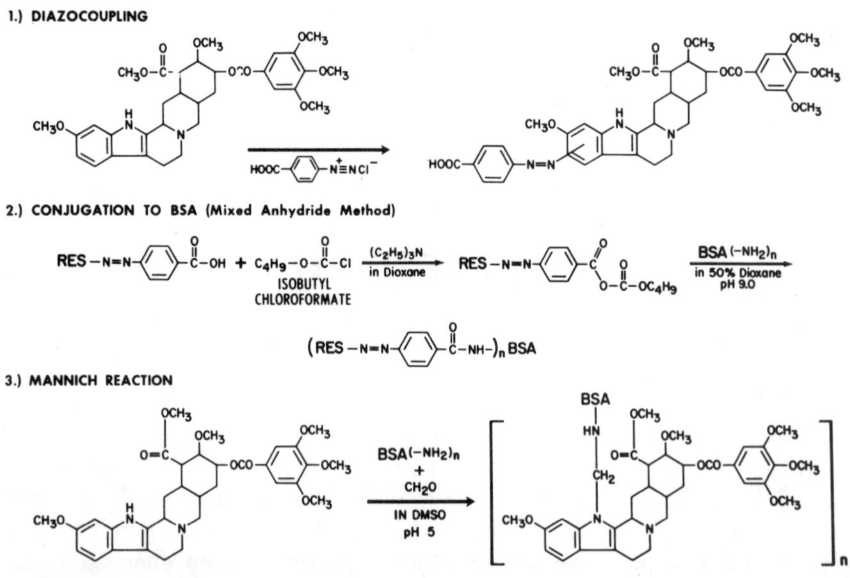

Figure 3. Procedure for preparation of reserpine-bovine serum albumin (BSA) immunogens.

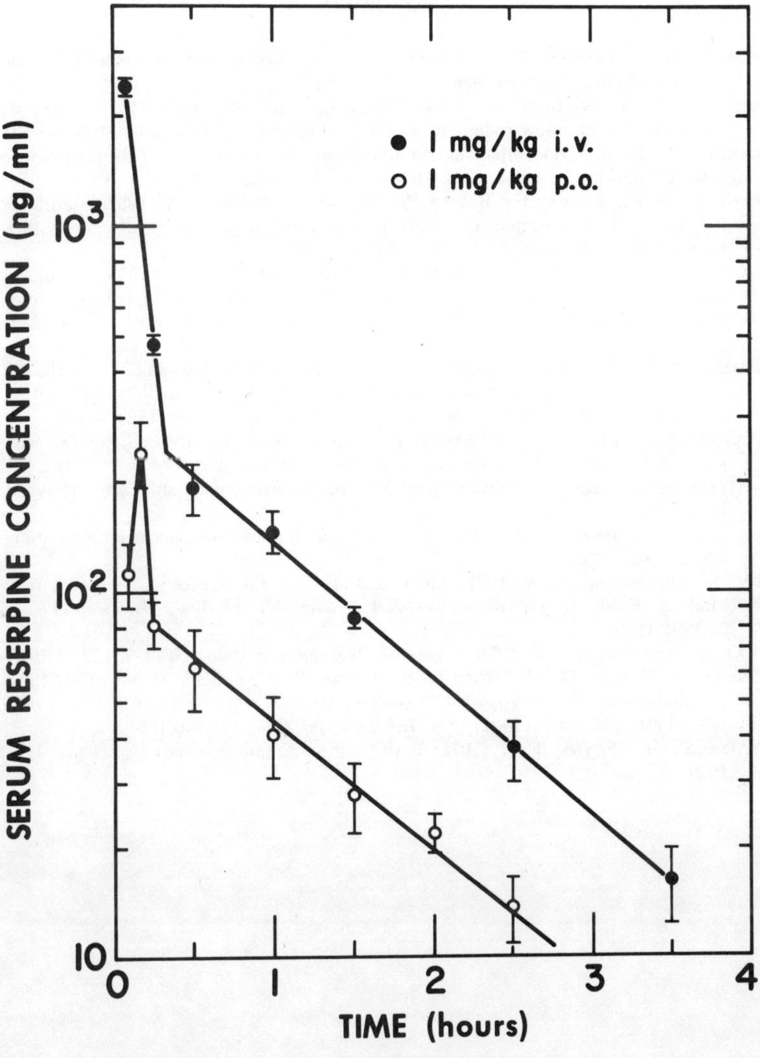

Figure 4. Disposition of reserpine in rat serum after either an intravenous (•) or oral (○) dose of 1 mg/kg.

as cerebrospinal fluid is limited, for example, in studying drug pharmacokinetics in infants. The pharmacologist is also interested in the localization of drugs. The use of the antibodies for immunofluorescent localization studies affords an attack on the question of the possible site of action of the drug.

REFERENCES

BEISER, S. M., ERLANGER, B. F., AGATE, F. G., and LIEBERMAN, S. 1959. Antigenicity of steroid-protein conjugates. *Science* 129:564-65.

BERKOWITZ, B. A., NGAI, S. H., HEMPSTEAD, J., and SPECTOR, S. 1975. Disposition of naloxone: Use of a new radioimmunoassay. *J. Pharmacol. Exp. Ther.* 195:499-504.

ERLANGER, B. F. 1973. Principles and methods for the preparation of drug protein conjugates for immunological studies. *Pharmacol. Rev.* 25:271-280.

ERLANGER, B. F., BOREX, F., BEISER, S. M., and LIEBERMAN, S. 1957. Steroid-protein conjugates. I. Preparation and characterization of bovine serum albumin with testosterone and cortisone. *J. Biol. Chem.* 228:713-727.

ERLANGER, B. F., BOREX, F., BEISER, S. M., and LIEBERMAN, S. 1959. Steroid-protein conjugates. II. Preparation and characterization of conjugates of bovine serum albumin with progesterone, deoxycorticosterone and estrone. *J. Biol. Chem.* 234:1090-1094.

GINTZLER, A. R., MOHACSI, E., and SPECTOR, S. 1976. Radioimmunoassay for the simultaneous determination of morphine and codeine. *Eur. J. Pharmacol.* 38:149-156.

HAMBURGER, R. N. 1966. Chloramphenicol-specific antibody. *Science* 152:203-205.

KAWASHIMA, K., LEVY, A., and SPECTOR, S. 1976. Stereospecific radioimmunoassay for propranolol isomers. *J. Pharmacol. Exp. Ther.* 196:517-523.

LANDSTEINER, K. 1945. *The Specificity of Serological Reaction.* Cambridge: Harvard University Press.

LEVY, A., KAWASHIMA, K., and SPECTOR, S. 1976. Radioimmunoassay for reserpine. *Life Sci.* 19:1421-1430.

NORN, S., and SHORE, P. A. 1971. Further studies on the nature of persistent reserpine binding: Evidence for reversible and irreversible binding. *Biochem. Pharmacol.* 20:1291-1295.

PESKAR, B., and SPECTOR, S. 1973. Serotonin: Radioimmunoassay. *Science* 179:1340-1341.

SHEPPARD, H., TSIEN, W. H., SIGG, E. B., LUCAS, R. A., and PLUMMER, A. J. 1957. The metabolism of C^{14} reserpine—C^{14} concentration vs. time in the brains and other tissues of rats and guinea pigs. *Arch. Int. Pharmacodyn.* 113:160-168.

SPECTOR, S., and FLYNN, E. T. 1971. Barbiturates: Radioimmunoassay. *Science* 174:1036-1039.

4

CATECHOLAMINE TRANSMITTER SYSTEMS

FLOYD E. BLOOM, M.D., G. R. SIGGINS, PH.D.,
J. E. SCHULTZ, PH.D., and S. J. HENRIKSEN, PH.D.

Neuropharmacologists assume that hormones, neurotransmitters, and most drugs produce their biological effects on the nervous system by interacting with specific receptors. Recent demonstrations that these receptors can to some degree be isolated, quantified, and localized (Creese, Burt, and Snyder, 1977) have made this working concept a practical experimental reality. When we consider the kinetic problems that underlie the mechanisms of action of psychiatric drugs with specific reference to such central neurotransmitter systems as the catecholamines, it is clear that the catecholamine receptors must constitute the central focus of our studies. In this chapter we briefly review the basis for assessing certain psychiatric drugs used to treat affective disorders in terms of the primary interactions with catecholamine synapses in the brain. In large measure, the philosophy of this approach has been followed in other recent reviews dealing with central nervous system effects of benzodiazepines (Bloom, 1977) and drugs of abuse (Bloom, 1976).

The methodologies of cellular neurobiology provide a structural and functional framework within which specific molecular interaction hypotheses of drug actions can be refined and tested. Tests of drug action at the cellular level seek to determine whether a given action is both necessary and causal in the resultant behavioral response or whether effects observed at the cellular level are simply epiphenomena of a more sensitive and essential effect at some other cellular site. With direct relevance to the kinetic effects of psychiatric drugs, these cellular tests offer a means

This work was supported by grants from the National Institute of Mental Health (MH-29466) and from the Volkswagen Foundation. We thank Nancy Callahan for preparation of the manuscript and Jesse Schulman for technical assistance.

for quantitative assessment of drug actions across several days of chronic treatment.

ORGANIZATION OF NEURON-DRUG INTERACTIONS

General drug actions. The awesome structural and functional complexity of the brain handicaps the analysis of specific drug effects. The situation is further compounded by the rapidity of cellular interactions and by the lack of knowledge of many fundamental details. One simplifying approach is to organize the possible modes of drug interaction on neurons for purposes of detecting general events for further analysis. As a first step, some psychiatric drug actions are generalizable to all nerve cells such as effects on general energy metabolism (David, Gatz, and Jones, 1971), maintenance of membrane integrity and transmembrane ionic equilibria (Ueda, Wada, and Ballinger, 1971). For the most part, actions affecting common biologic properties of all neurons occur at relatively high dose levels *in vitro* and are not the drug actions we seek now to comprehend.

Transmitter-specific drug actions. Chemical dynamics: A second category of drug actions pertains to selective effects on neurons grouped together by their specific common use of the same chemical synaptic transmitter. Here the potential molecular mechanisms for drug specificity are more easily envisioned because of the numerous points within the life cycle of transmitters that have been uncovered through biochemical pharmacology. By way of background information, the tissue content of a given transmitter within a brain region is generally held to be the result of a dynamic interplay between rates of synthesis (determined by substrate availability and by co-factor regulatory mechanisms which in part reflect functional activity of the neuron) and by rates of transmitter release (determined by neuronal firing rate coupled to transmitter secretion and conservation mechanisms such as reuptake, restorage, and catabolism).

By study of these more elemental neuronal processes, one particular transmitter molecule or one particular transmitter-related enzymatic event may be scrutinized apart from the mass of brain cells. With respect to these transmitter-specific modes of neuronal interaction, antipsychotic drugs—especially tricyclic antidepressants and lithium (Li)—have been interpreted as showing specific actions on several different transmitter systems. In the case of the catecholamine transmitters norepinephrine (NE) and dopamine (DA), most recent evidence remains compatible with earlier views that tricyclic antidepressant drugs are best characterized by their ability to inhibit the uptake of amines into peripheral and central nerve terminals (Glowinski and Axelrod, 1964; Carlsson et al., 1968). With a secondary amine in the side chains, drugs like desmethylimipramine (DMI) can have enhanced effectiveness on noradrenergic systems, while tricyclics with tertiary amine side chains like amitriptyline can have relatively greater effects on serotonin uptake (Iversen, 1965; Carlsson et al., 1968). Attaining antidepressant effects with these drugs in man requires several days of treatment (Roffman et al., 1977), whereas most animal studies on blockade of neurotransmitter reuptake deal only with acute drug exposures. It would seem more reasonable, therefore, to consider additional sites and mechanisms for antidepressant drug effects before concluding that blockade of reuptake is the necessary and sufficient explanation for antidepressant effectiveness. For example, some workers (Schubert, Nyback, and Sedvall, 1970) have interpreted the data on tricyclic drugs to indicate that the prolongation of norepinephrine in the synaptic cleft could—through unknown "feedback" mechanisms—inhibit the activity of the noradrenergic neurons. The explanation would thus be diametrically opposed to the interpretation that such drugs act to enhance the action of the noradrenergic synapses. Studies of brain catecholamine turnover, however, support the idea that acute exposure to clinically effective tricyclic antidepressants slows down norepinephrine metabolism (Nyback, Borzecki, Sedvall, 1968; Schubert, Nyback, and Sedvall, 1970); that interpretation is further supported by acute studies of firing rate of neurons in the major noradrenergic nucleus, the locus coeruleus (LC) (Nyback et al., 1975). Recently, however, it has been possible to turn the analysis of presynaptic actions of antidepressants to studies of the postsynaptic receptor (Schultz, 1976) and, in particular, to the effects of drugs on the sensitivity of norepinephrine-activated adenylate cyclase (Bloom, 1975; Nathanson, 1977).

Transmitter-specific drug actions on synaptic receptors. A third major category of drug-neuron interactions derives from studies of postsynaptic receptors and their response-generating mechanisms. The ability of a drug to alter neuronal firing (and hence influence one or more metabolic indices of function) is frequently assessed with the hypothesis that the drug can simulate or antagonize one or more of the synaptic circuits that control the selected drug-sensitive cell. Research into the mechanisms of action of amphetamine, phenothiazines, or LSD has shown by direct testing that these drugs interact with synaptic messages transmitted through secretion of catecholamines or serotonin (Cooper, Bloom, and Roth, 1978).

To clarify the way in which the central postsynaptic receptors for norepinephrine may be used as tests for the specific actions of antidepressant drug kinetics, we must first review briefly the physiological effects of identified central noradrenergic synapses and their mechanisms of action.

The ability of NE to affect the pattern and rate of eletrical activity of central neurons has been known for some time (Bloom, 1975, 1978). The majority of these data has been derived from studies that employ micro-iontophoresis to administer relatively small amounts of NE to single neurons within the intact brain and that interpret the ensuing functional changes in rate and pattern of discharge or transmembrane properties as evidence of the general role of NE in interneuronal communication.

By proper experimental controls, tests with microiontophoresis of NE (Bloom, 1974) reveal generally reproducible inhibitory effects of NE on neuronal discharge. Such responses, however, do not necessarily imply an underlying NE-mediated input to the cells being tested. Corroboration of this inference requires the demonstration that selective stimulation of the afferent NE-axons will produce the effects produced by microiontophoresis of NE. The cells of origin for the cortical NE projections have been established (Hoffer et al., 1973; Segal and Bloom, 1974 a, b), and it has been possible to establish cytochemically that the cells being tested receive NE-containing synapses (Bloom, Hoffer, and Siggins, 1971; Landis and Bloom, 1975; Koda and Bloom, 1977). In the absence of such corroborative data, iontophoretic responses simply cannot be interpreted functionally.

The varicosities of the axons demonstrated by fluorescence histochemistry indicate presumed sites of transmitter release. However, because of the limited resolution of the optical microscope relative to the very fine nature of the complexly interrelated cellular processes of the neuropil, electron microscopy is needed to determine precisely which neurons in a given region receive synaptic contact from NE-containing axons.

No single electron-microscopic histochemical method has yet achieved the consistency and selectivity of localization desired for analysis of NE-transmitting synapses. Permanganate fixation methods (Landis and Bloom, 1975; Koda and Bloom, 1977) offer the most direct approach to the successful visualization of small, granular synaptic vesicles, which seem identical morphologically and pharmacologically to the storage vesicles of NE in peripheral sympathetic nerve terminals. Using these and other cytochemical methods, NE-containing synapses have been identified ultrastructurally in two cortical regions, cerebellum and hippocampus, with defined postsynaptic target cells. In addition, presumptive NE-containing synapses have been identified cytochemically in squirrel monkey cerebral cortex (Freedman, Hoffer, and Woodward, 1975). These studies provide the structural documentation for the physiologic studies described next which are pertinent to psychiatric drug kinetics.

Norepinephrine-containing synapses in the cerebellum can be localized at the electron-microscopic level by degeneration after 6-OHDA exposure or autoradiography of sites taking up H^3-NE (Bloom, Hoffer, and Siggins, 1971), as well as by permanganate fixation (Landis and Bloom, 1975). These ultrastructural studies indicate that NE-containing fibers synapse on the Purkinje-cell dendritic tree, in the mid-to-outer molecular layer. Recent techniques for facilitating visualization of these fibers (Bloom and Battenberg, 1976) suggest that they are sufficiently dense to permit contact with each Purkinje cell.

When NE is applied to Purkinje cells from micropipettes by iontophoresis, there is a uniform and powerful depression of spontaneous discharge (Hoffer et al., 1971). Interspike interval histograms show that NE specifically augments the population of long pauses seen during normal Purkinje cell firing (Hoffer, Siggins, and Bloom, 1971). Iontophoretic administration of MJ-1999, a specific beta-adrenergic blocking agent, antagonizes NE response (Hoffer, Siggins, and Bloom, 1971). Intracellular recordings from Purkinje cells during extracellular application of NE (Siggins, Hoffer, and Bloom, 1971) results in hyperpolarization with either no change or an increase in membrane resistance.

When locus coeruleus is stimulated, Purkinje cells showed remarkably uniform inhibitory responses: cells recorded extracellularly display depression of spontaneous discharge rate (Siggins et al., 1971). With intracellular recordings, LC stimulation exactly mimicked the action of exogenous NE: both produce hyperpolarization without a decrease in membrane resistance (Siggins et al., 1971; Hoffer et al., 1973).

Next, noradrenergic effects were pursued in the hippocampal cortex, a brain region known to receive an extensive input of NE-containing fibers (Segal and Bloom, 1974a, b). We have confirmed the presence of NE terminals by both fluorescence histochemistry, 6-OHDA-induced degeneration (Bloom and Segal, unpublished) and by autoradiography after microinjection of labeled precursors into the locus coeruleus (Pickel, Segal and Bloom, 1974). The hippocampal NE projections onto pyramidal cells function in a fashion quite similar to the effects of the locus coeruleus on cerebellar Purkinje cells: LC and NE slow pyramidal cell discharge with long-latency and long-duration actions; the receptor is blocked with the beta antagonist MJ-1999 and by prostaglandins E1 or E2, and the action of the pathway is totally blocked by chronic pretreatment with 6-OHDA or acute pretreatment with reserpine and alphamethyltyrosine (Segal and Bloom, 1974b).

In both the cerebellar and hippocampal systems, cyclic 3′, 5′-adenosine monophosphate (cyclic AMP) was observed to mimic the ability of NE to depress spontaneous activity, and the NE receptor could be blocked by the MJ-1999. Partly because of the pharmacological potentiation of the inhibitory effects of NE, LC, and cyclic AMP on cerebellar Purkinje cells, we have proposed that these actions could be mediated by cyclic AMP (Hoffer, Siggins, and Bloom, 1969; Hoffer et al., 1973; Siggins, Hoffer, and Bloom, 1969; Bloom, 1975). Subsequently, the proposal has been strengthened by observations that the actions of NE on the NE-pathway and of cyclic nucleotides all hyperpolarize Purkinje cells and hippocampal pyramidal cells (Segal and Oliver, in preparation). The mechanism is believed to be a not fully explained membrane action in which membrane conductance to passive ion flow is not increased (as it is with most other known synaptic chemicals—Bloom, 1975). Even more direct confirmation of this hypothesis stems from the observation that NE and the NE pathway will selectively increase the immunocytochemical assay of Purkinje cell cyclic AMP content (Siggins et al., 1973). Such postsynaptic mediation for the NE pathways offers several possible biologic advantages, particularly the twofold advantages of (1) biochemical amplifications of the catecholamine signal and (2) the possibility of directly altering the postsynaptic cell through the ability of cyclic AMP to regulate, among other actions, protein and carbohydrate metabolism.

Direct electrophysiological tests of the presumptive behavioral function of the norepinephrine projections have been accomplished by direct electrophysiologic recording from unrestrained, unanesthetized cats (Chu and Bloom, 1974), rats (Segal and Bloom, 1976a, b) and squirrel monkey (Foote, Freedman, and Oliver, 1975). The results of these tests in behaviorally alert animals indicate that NE or locus coeruleus directly inhibits spontaneous discharge even more potently than in acute anesthetized preparations. During NE application on these test cells, however, the response to certain sensory inputs may nevertheless be increased. Thus, the relative signal: ratio of noise exhibited by a specific sensory cell in squirrel monkey auditory cortex to that of squirrel monkey vocalizations is effectively increased because NE suppresses spontaneous activity more than response to vocalizations (Foote, Freedman, and Oliver, 1975). Subsequent studies on Purkinje cell discharge in anesthetized rats also support the idea that iontophoresis of NE (Freedman et al., 1977) or stimulation of locus coeruleus (Moises and Woodward, 1977) can depress spontaneous firing while enhancing evoked synaptic inputs, and that this enhancement of responsiveness to synaptic inputs can be seen with both excitatory and inhibitory inputs. As suggested elsewhere (Bloom, 1978), these sets of electrophysiological properties attributable to the central noradrenergic circuits from the locus coeruleus may permit them to function in a manner which cannot simply be seen as analogous to "inhibition." Rather, this system may be more properly conceived as a "bias-adjusting" or "enabling" effect that can enhance "heterosynaptically" the properly timed activity of other afferent messages onto their targets in common with locus coeruleus.

These "enabling" effects of the LC pathway have also been evaluated with respect to the cellular discharge patterns of hippocampal neurons in awake rats through chronically implanted recording and stimulating electrodes (Segal and Bloom, 1976a, b). Under these conditions the coeruleo-hippocampal pathway shows a longer and more pronounced inhibition of pyramidal cells than that observed in the anesthetized rat. When biologically nonsignificant but loud auditory stimuli are presented to the rat, hippocampal units generally respond with inhibition, and preconditioning stimulation of the LC before such auditory stimuli results in greater inhibition of discharge, as might be expected by the algebraic summation of two inhibitory drives. When rats are trained to associate the same loud tone with the presentation of a food reward, however, the tone no longer inhibits hippocampal units, but instead results in poststimulus excitation of discharge. When locus coeruleus-conditioning stimuli are paired with the tone under these conditions, the locus coeruleus stimulation enhances even more the "excitatory" translation of the tone stimulus, even though, when tested against simple spontaneous discharge in the knowledgeable state, the LC pathway is by itself always inhibitory.

These data strongly suggest that the brain uses the LC pathway to attribute special arousal value to particular environmental signals. In fact, when the natural firing patterns of norepinephrine-containing neurons are related to the spontaneous behavior of unrestrained cats, most identified LC neurons appear most active in paradoxical sleep (in a phasic relation to periods of rapid eye movement) and in the earliest stages of awakening from paradoxical sleep (with rapid tonic activity) (Chu and Bloom, 1974).

Norepinephrine and Psychiatric Drug Kinetics

In searching for clues to the cellular mechanisms that underlie the actions of psychiatric drugs used in treating affective psychoses, we were struck by the seeming paradoxes between the neurochemical and electrophysiologic effects of tricyclic antidepressants and lithium. Li is a particularly puzzling drug since it seems most effective as an antidepressant for patients suffering from bipolar affective psychosis (Bunney and Murphy, 1976). In those patients, both manic and depressive episodes are improved. Tests of the cellular actions of Li are not extensive despite the simplicity of the drug and its lack of catabolism. For example, Li has been reported to depress the basal adenylate cyclase activity of brain slices and to suppress the degree to which adenylate cyclase activity can be stimulated by norepinephrine (Forn and Valdecasas, 1971; Dousa and Hechter, 1970). In support of such a view, Segal (1974) reported that acute injections or iontophoresis of Li reduce the inhibitory effects of norepinephrine and of locus coeruleus stimulation but do not impair responses to cyclic AMP. These data could be interpreted to mean that Li acts by antagonizing the degree to which the NE receptor is coupled to activation of adenylate cyclase (Bunney and Murphy, 1976).

On the other hand, as mentioned above, tricyclic antidepressants are known to inhibit presynaptic reuptake of release catecholamines which might be expected to enhance their synaptic inhibitory effects. Such effects can also be seen when both drugs are applied iontophoretically to cerebellar Purkinje cells (Hoffer et al., 1971) and to hippocampal pyramidal cells (Segal and Bloom, 1974a, b).

As is well known, however, these acute effects of the two different antidepressant drugs may not reflect the events in play when antidepressant actions take place after several days of drug treatment. In fact, as has emerged from recent studies on various types of cellular and molecular responses, an important biologic property of central synaptic receptors is their dynamic ability to regulate sensitivity. Thus, drugs or lesions that disrupt transmitter release result in supersensitive central noradrenergic receptors (Sporn et al., 1976), while administration of drugs that can prolong or otherwise enhance the effectiveness of released norepinephrine has been reported to produce subsensitive receptors (Vetulani and Sulser, 1975; deMontigny and Aghajanian, 1977).

Recent studies by Schultz (1976) prompted us to use iontophoretic tests on cerebellar Purkinje cells to evaluate the possibility that after chronic treatment with either Li or DMI a new class of effects might emerge which could better explain the drugs' therapeutic effects. Schultz had treated rats with oral doses of imipramine for one to 21 days and observed that receptor sensitivity of cortical adenylate cyclase changed with length of the treatment period. In the first few days, no differences were observed between saline-gavaged rats and drug-gavaged rats. After six days of treatment, however, basal adenylate cyclase levels fell by about 40 percent and the ability of added norepinephrine to activate cyclase *in vitro* also declined. A similar subsensitivity with almost identical time course was observed in these studies when the rats were treated with the antipsychotic drug chlorpromazine. In some tests phenothiazines have been observed to block the effects of iontophoretic norepinephrine (Skolnick et al., 1976; Siggins, Henriksen, and Landis, 1976) as well as exhibit their more agreed-upon actions as antidopaminergic drugs (Creese, Burt, and Snyder, 1976, 1977; Creese and Snyder, 1977).

We therefore repeated the earlier acute iontophoretic tests of Li on hippocampal neurons and of DMI on both cerebellar and hippocampal neurons, using oral treatment methods for chronic administration periods of 10 to 14 days, and at various times tested the effectiveness of NE electrophysiologically and biochemically. The cerebellar Purkinje cell is a good indicator for these tests since its robust, spontaneous activity and easily identifiable discharge pattern offer a homogeneously detectable group of target cells known to bear the beta-adrenergic receptors of NE synapses.

Although these studies have just begun, it does seem clear even from an initial overview of the data that chronic treatment of normal rats has so far revealed only one very general common denominator for the longer-term effects evoked by treatment with Li or DMI. Acute effects of Li (given orally, parenterally, or iontophoretically) seem in general to support the view that responsiveness to norepinephrine may be selectively antagonized as reported by Segal (1974) for hippocampal pyramidal cells. However, after 10 to 14 days of treatment with oral Li (sufficient in our animals to produce serum Li levels of 0.8 to 1.2 mM), the overall discharge rate and pattern of Purkinje cells were significantly reduced and there was no longer any apparent blockade of responses to iontophoretic NE. Neurochemical studies of cerebellar slices from these rats showed no consistent chronic subsensitivity to NE-stimulated cyclase. Thus both indices of receptor function observed acutely with Li treatment would appear to have been normalized by dynamic elements of the receptive cells, perhaps to keep the system functional while discharge rates are persistently depressed.

In confirmation of earlier studies (Hoffer, Siggins, and Bloom, 1971), DMI acutely applied iontophoretically or parenterally can enhance the responsiveness to iontophoretic NE; in normal rats, but not those treated with 6-hydroxydopamine (Hoffer et al., 1971), DMI can produce direct slowing of the Purkinje cell. After chronic oral treatment with DMI, Purkinje-cell firing rates are depressed as in the case of chronic Li treatment. Similar to the biochemical studies of the Li-treated rats, cerebellar slices of DMI-treated rats also show no subsensitivity to activation of the adenylate cyclase *in vitro*. Our preliminary results of NE receptivity in the tricyclic-treated rats suggest, however, that thresholds to NE are elevated, possibly by an induced receptor subsensitivity as Schultz reported (1976) for cortical slices. Since Purkinje cells constitute only a very small fraction of cerebellar cortical adenylate cyclase, the subsensitivity may be difficult to resolve biochemically (Skolnick et al., 1976). The present electrophysiologic data also must be taken as an indication of some dynamic reequilibration of the receptive process, such that the system maintains full effectiveness of the NE pathway despite the perturbation caused by DMI.

Tentative Conclusions

What can these studies of acute versus chronic effects of psychiatric drugs on firing rates and neurochemical receptivity tell us about the way in which the normal brain operates in response to drugs? In our view the initial message, still dimly perceived, is that the functioning brain does not tolerate the perturbations produced by even specific synaptic actions of drugs. It responds by setting into motion cellular modulatory events that attempt through various shifts in receptor sensitivity to restore the operation of the system to more normal values. Until a more precise picture emerges of the chemical and pathophysiologic details of critical synaptic changes in affective psychoses, the nature of these pathologic states as "treated" by drugs remains quite open to investigation. It is possible that some defect in molecular dynamics produces psychotogenic receptors which have for one or another reason lost their ability to be modulated back into equilibrium. At the moment this view might better fit the data on the effects of drugs in experimental animals since most signs of drug action disappear when the period of effective treatment in man has been reached. The persistence of greatly slowed target-cell discharge rates remains an important lead to be followed. An alternative open-ended hypothesis is one those devoted to catecholamine hypotheses of mental illness have long been expecting: namely, that the brain is too complicated an organ to rely on only one form of chemical neurotransmission for all important modes of information modification. Perhaps better explanations of antipsychotic drug action may, therefore, be expected to flow from the continued discovery of new families of transmitter substances. Until that state of events arrives, however, the available well-defined test systems for sites of catecholamine synaptic action in the brain permit still a third hypothesis to be tested: the effects of lithium and desmethylimipramine that are critical to the therapeutic effect may not be those revealed on cerebellar neurons, despite the ease of evaluating these test cells. It is this approach we shall be pursuing until more suitable systems for drug analysis are developed.

REFERENCES

BLOOM, F. E., 1974. To spritz or not to spritz: The doubtful value of aimless iontophoresis. *Life Sci.*, 14:1819-1834.

BLOOM, F. E. 1975. The role of cyclic nucleotides in central synaptic function. *Rev. Physiol. Biochem. Pharmacol.*, 74:1-103.

BLOOM, F. E. 1976. Possible sites in the neuron for interactions of drugs of abuse. *Ann. N.Y. Acad. Sci.*, 281:11-24.

BLOOM, F. E. 1977. Neural mechanisms of benzodiazepine actions. *Am. J. Psychiatry*, 134:6.

BLOOM, F. E. 1978. Central noradrenergic systems: physiology and pharmacology. In M. A. Lipton, A. DiMascio and K. Killam (eds.), *Psychopharmacology—A Generation of Progress*, pp. 131-142. New York: Raven Press.

BLOOM, F. E. and BATTENBERG, E. L. F. 1976. A rapid, simple and more sensitive method for the demonstration of central catecholamine-containing neurons and axons by glyoxylic acid induced fluorescence: II. A detailed description of methodology. *J. Histochem. Cytochem.*, 24:561-571.

BLOOM, F. E., HOFFER, B. J., and SIGGINS, G. R. 1971. Studies on norepinephrine-containing afferents to Purkinje cells of rat cerebellum: I. Localization of the fibers and their synapses. *Brain Res.*, 25:501-521.

BUNNY, W. E., JR. and MURPHY, D. L. 1976. The neurobiology of lithium. *Neurosci. Res. Program Bull.*, 14:111-207.

CARLSSON, A., CORRODI, H., FUXE, K., and HOKFELT, T. 1968. Effect of some antidepressant drugs on the depletion of intraneuronal brain catecholamine stores caused by 4-alpha-dimethyl-m-tyramine. *Eur. J. Pharmacol.*, 5:357-361.

CHU, N-S. and BLOOM, F. E. 1974. Activity patterns of catecholamine-containing pontine neurons in the dorso-lateral tegmentum of unrestrained cats. *J. Neurobiol.*, 5:527-544.

COOPER, J. C., BLOOM, F. E., and ROTH, R. H. 1978. *The Biochemical Basis of Neuropharmacology*. New York: Oxford University Press (in press).

CREESE, I., BURT, D. B. R., and SNYDER, S. H. 1976. Dopamine receptor binding predicts clinical and pharmacological potencies of antischizophrenic drugs. *Science*, 192:481-483.

CREESE, I., BURT, D. R., and SNYDER, S. H. 1977. Dopamine receptor binding enhancement accompanies lesion-induced behavioral supersensitivity. *Science*, 197:596-598.

CREESE, I. and SNYDER, S. H. 1977. Brain neurotransmitter and drug receptors. *Medicinal Chemistry*, 5:135-153.

DAVID, L. F., GATZ, E. E., and JONES, J. R. 1971. Effects of chlordiazepoxide and diazepam on respiration and oxidative phosphorylation in rat brain mitochondria. *Biochem. Pharmacol.*, 20:1883-1887.

DEMONTIGNY, C. and AGHAJANIAN, G. K. 1977. Sensitization of postsynaptic serotonin receptors by chronic pretreatment with tricyclic antidepressants: an iontophoretic study. *Soc. Neuroscience Abstr.*, 3:248.

DOUSA, T. and HECHTER, O. 1970. The effect of NaCl and LiCl on vasopressin-sensitive adenylate cyclase. *Life Science I*, 9:765-770.

FOOTE, S. L., FREEDMAN, R., and OLIVER, A. P. 1975. Effects of putative neurotransmitters on neuronal activity in monkey auditory cortex. *Brain Res.* 86:229-242.

FORN, J. and VALDECASAS, F. G. 1971. Effects of Li on brain adenyl cyclase activity. *Biochem. Pharmacol.*, 20:2773-2779.

FREEDMAN, R., HOFFER, B. J., and WOODWARD, D. J. 1975. A quantitative microiontophoretic analysis of the responses of central neurones to noradrenaline: interactions with cobalt, manganese, verapamil, and dichloroisoprenaline. *Br. J. Pharmacol.*, 54:529-539.

FREEDMAN, R., HOFFER, B. J., WOODWARD, D. J., and PURO, P. 1977. Interaction of norepinephrine with cerebellar activity evoked by mossy and climbing fibers. *Exp. Neurol.*, 55:269-288.

GLOWINSKI, J. and AXELROD, J. 1964. Inhibition of uptake of tritiated norepinephrine in the intact rat brain by imipramine and structurally related compounds. *Nature*, 204:1318.

HOFFER, B. J., SIGGINS, G. R., and BLOOM, F. E. 1969. Prostaglandins and E antagonize norepinephrine effects on cerebellar Purkinje-cells: Microelectrophoretic study. *Science*, 166:1418-1420.

HOFFER, B. J., SIGGINS, G. R., and BLOOM, F. E. 1971. Studies on norepinephrine-containing afferents to Purkinje-cells of rat cerebellum: II. Sensitivity of Purkinje-cells to norepinephrine and related substances administered by microiontophoresis. *Brain Res.*, 25:523-534.

HOFFER, B. J., SIGGINS, G. R., WOODWARD, D. J., and BLOOM, F. E. 1971. Spontaneous discharge of Purkinje neurons after destruction of catecholamine-containing afferents by 6-hydroxydopamine. *Brain Res.*, 30:425-430.

HOFFER, B. J., SIGGINS, G. R., OLIVER, A. P., and BLOOM, F. E. 1973. Activation of the pathway from locus coeruleus to rat cerebellar Purkinje neurons: Pharmacological evidence of noradrenergic central inhibition. *J. Pharmacol. Exp. Ther.*, 184:553-569.

IVERSEN, L. L. 1965. Inhibition of noradrenaline uptake by drugs. *J. Pharm. Pharmacol.*, 17:62-69.

KODA, L. Y. and BLOOM, F. E. 1977. A light and electron microscopic study of noradrenergic terminals in the rat dentate gyrus. *Brain Res.*, 120:327-335.

LANDIS, S. C. and BLOOM, F. E. 1975. Ultrastructural identification of noradrenergic boutons in mutant and normal mouse cerebellar cortex. *Brain Res.*, 96:299-306.

MOISES, H. J. and WOODWARD, D. J. 1977. Locus coeruleus stimulation potentiates Purkinje cell responses to iontophoretically applied gamma-aminobutyric acid. *Soc. Neuroscience Abstr.*, 3:255.

NATHANSON, J. 1977. Cyclic nucleotides and nervous system function. *Physiological Rev.*, 57:157-256.

NYBACK, H., BORZECKI, Z., and SEDVALL, G. 1968. Accumulation and disappearance of catecholamines formed from tyrosine-^{14}C in mouse brain: effect of some psychotropic drugs. *Eur. J. Pharmacol.*, 4:395-401.

NYBACK, H. V., WALTERS, J. R., AGHAJANIAN, G. K., and ROTH, R. H. 1975. Tricyclic antidepressants: effects on the firing rate of brain noradrenergic neurons. *Eur. J. Pharmacol.*, 32:302-312.

PICKEL, V. M., SEGAL, M., and BLOOM, F. E. 1974. A radioautographic study of the efferent pathways of the nucleus locus coeruleus. *J. Comp. Neurol.*, 155:15-42.

ROFFMAN, M., KLING, M. A., CASSENS, G., ORSULAK, P. J., REIGLE, T. G., and SCHILDKRAUT, J. J. 1977. The effects of acute and chronic administration of tricyclic antidepressants on MHPG-SO_4 in rat brain. *Comm. Psychopharmacol.*, 1:195-206.

SCHUBERT, J., NYBACK, H., and SEDVALL, G. 1970. Effect of antidepressant drugs on accumulation and disappearance of monoamines formed in vivo from labelled precursors in mouse brain. *J. Pharm. Pharmacol.*, 22:136-138.

SCHULTZ, J. 1976. Psychoactive drug effects on a system which generates cyclic AMP in brain. *Nature*, 261:417-418.

SEGAL, M. 1974. Lithium and the monoamine neurotransmitter in the rat hippocampus. *Nature*, 250:71-73.

SEGAL, M. and BLOOM, F. E. 1974a. The action of norepinephrine in the rat hippocampus: I. Iontophoretic studies. *Brain Res.*, 72:79-97.

SEGAL, M. and BLOOM, F. E. 1974b. The action of norepinephrine in the rat hippocampus: II. Activation of the input pathway. *Brain Res.*, 72:99-114.

SEGAL, M. and BLOOM, F. E. 1976a. The action of norepinephrine in the rat hippocampus. III. Hippocampal cellular responses to locus coeruleus stimulation in the awake rat. *Brain Res.*, 107:499-511.

SEGAL, M. and BLOOM, F. E. 1976b. The action of norepinephrine in the rat hippocampus. IV. The effects of locus coeruleus stimulation on evoked hippocampal unit activity. *Brain Res.*, 107:513-525.

Siggins, G. R., Battenberg, E. F., Hoffer, B. J., Bloom, F. E., and Steiner, A. L. 1973. Noradrenergic stimulation of cyclic adenosine monophosphate in rat Purkinje neurons: An immunocytochemical study. *Science*, 179:585-588.

Siggins, G. R., Henriksen, S. J., and Landis, S. C. 1976. Electrophysiology of Purkinje neurons in the weaver mouse: Iontophoresis of neurotransmitters and cyclic nucleotides, and stimulation of the nucleus locus coeruleus. *Brain Res.*, 114:53-65.

Siggins, G. R., Hoffer, B. J., and Bloom, F. E. 1969. Cyclic 3′5′ adenosine monophosphate: Possible mediator for the response of cerebellar Purkinje-cells to microelectrophoresis of norepinephrine. *Science*, 165:1018-1020.

Siggins, G. R., Hoffer, B. J., and Bloom, F. E. 1971. Studies on norepinephrine-containing afferents to Purkinje-cells of rat cerebellum: III. Evidence for mediation of norepinephrine effects by cyclic 3′5′-adenosine monophosphate. *Brain Res.*, 25:535-553.

Siggins, G. R., Hoffer, B. J., Oliver, A. P., and Bloom, F. E. 1971. Activation of a central noradrenergic projection to cerebellum. *Nature*, 233:481-483.

Skolnick, P., Daly, J. W., Freedman, R., and Hoffer, B. J. 1976. Interrelationship between catecholamine-stimulated formation of adenosine 3′-5′ monophosphate in cerebellar slices and inhibitory effects on cerebellar Purkinje-cells: Antagonism by neuroleptic compounds. *J. Pharmacol. Exp. Ther.*, 197:280-292.

Sporn, J. R., Harden, T. K., Wolfe, B. B., and Molinoff, P. B. 1976. Beta-adrenergic receptor involvement in 6-hydroxydopamine-induced supersensitivity in rat cerebral cortex. *Science*, 194:624-625.

Ueda, I., Wada, T., and Ballinger, C. M. 1971. Sodium potassium-activated ATPase of beef brain—effects of some tranquilizers. *Biochem. Pharmacol.*, 20:1697-1700.

Vetulani, J. and Sulser, F. 1975. Action of various antidepressant treatments reduces reactivity of noradrenergic cyclic AMP-generating system in limbic forebrain. *Nature*, 257:495-496.

5

PHARMACOLOGIC DIFFERENTIATION OF GABA-RECEPTIVE SITES

ERNEST J. PECK, JR., PH.D.

Our laboratory is interested in processes involved in chemical communication between cells. Cells use chemical signals for communication via entities termed receptors. The receptors we study include steroid receptors, which are soluble cytoplasmic proteins of steroid-responsive cells, and membrane-bound receptors located at the synapse. The latter will be the subject of this chapter.

We are interested in the isolation and physical characterization of the postsynaptic receptor for gamma-aminobutyric acid (GABA). If we have the receptor for gamma-aminobutyric acid in pure form, antibodies to it can be used to localize those neurons of the nervous system that employ GABA as a chemical signal. Purified receptors can also be used to characterize the pharmacology of the GABA synapse.

Most investigators agree that neurotransmitter receptors are macromolecules, probably multiunit complexes, which reside on or within the postsynaptic membrane and which possess, as one of their component parts, a binding or receptive site with "high" affinity and specificity for the neurotransmitter, its agonists, and perhaps its antagonists. These criteria have proven basic to the identification and isolation of the nicotinic acetylcholine receptor (Karlin, 1974; DeRobertis and Schact, 1974) as well as to studies of neurotransmitter receptors of central nervous system (CNS) origin (Snyder, 1975a; DeRobertis, 1975; Peck et al., 1976; Peck, 1977; Snyder and Bennett, 1976). In every case the binding of radiolabeled ligands was used for the study of these receptive sites. The success of this technique with the nicotinic receptor, however, was based

Thanks to Bruce Lester, Ann Miller, and James Schaeffer for their assistance and helpful comments. This work was supported by National Institutes of Health grants NS11753 and HD08389.

on two conditions not available for most receptors of central nervous system origin. First, the electroplax (cellular unit of the electric organ of some fishes and eels) represents a source enriched for acetylcholine receptive sites. Second, the snake venom toxins are extremely high-affinity ligands that are readily adapted for affinity chromatography. By contrast, central nervous structures with high densities of homogeneous innervation are rare. In addition, few ligands exist that interact with extremely high affinity at receptive sites for the amino acid transmitters.

These problems are compounded by the variety of receptive species present in central nervous tissues. Thus receptive or binding sites exist for neuronal and glial transport systems, anabolic and catabolic enzymes, and postsynaptic receptors. Each of these receptive sites possesses some, if not all, of the following properties and thus makes difficult the use of radiolabeled ligands as the assay for postsynaptic receptors:

1. Reasonably high affinity for the neurotransmitter under investigation.
2. Saturability or limited capacity with respect to neurotransmitter binding (i.e., the number of sites is not infinite).
3. Pharmaco- and stereospecificity with respect to ligand binding.
4. Tissue specificity—that is, these sites are expected to occur in great numbers in regions of the CNS rich in terminals for a given transmitter and to a lesser extent in regions poor in such terminals.

These criteria, together with a fifth, the correlation of ligand binding with biologic response, are utilized to define receptors. Although no study of neurotransmitter-receptive sites from the CNS has to date considered all five criteria, most have considered the first three and several the first four. And therein lies the difficulty—how does one distinguish between the postsynaptic receptor and the multitude of other receptive sites likely to share the same or similar properties?

The use of radiolabeled ligand binding as the assay for postsynaptic gamma-aminobutyric acid receptors is, like assays for other neurotransmitter systems, confounded by the wide variety of receptive species present in the CNS. The GABA system possesses all the receptive sites mentioned above and, in addition, may have presynaptic receptive sites regulating neurotransmitter release. Each is likely to possess high affinity, limited capacity, and stereospecificity with respect to the equilibrium binding of labeled GABA. In addition, these receptive sites may be enriched in regions of the CNS rich in GABA neurons. Thus, four of the five criteria for a postsynaptic receptor may apply to each of these receptive systems. How can one differentiate between these species?

The GABA enzymes are the most easily distinguished. L-glutamate decarboxylase (EC 4.1.1.15) or GAD, and GABA-transaminase (EC 2.6.1.19) or GABA-T, have been purified and characterized (Wu, 1976). GAD is a cytoplasmic enzyme with an extremely low affinity for the product of its enzymatic action (K_i* for GABA ~50m*M*). GAD is also very sensitive to sulfhydryl reagents (K_i for 5,5′-dithiobis 2-nitrobenzoic acid ~10 μ*M*) whereas the GABA postsynaptic receptor seems unaffected by sulfhydryl reagents (Curtis, Duggan, and Johnston, 1970). GABA-T, a mitochondrial enzyme, is also sensitive to sulfhydryl reagents (K_i for 5,5′-dithiobis 2-nitrobenzoic acid ~50 μ*M*) and has a relatively low affinity for GABA. Thus the K_m for GABA is about m*M*, at least one-thousandfold higher than that expected for a postsynaptic receptor. Thus, their affinities for GABA and their sensitivities to sulfhydryl reagents make it unlikely that GAD or GABA-T could be confused with a postsynaptic receptor.

It is more difficult to distinguish presynaptic or postsynaptic receptors from transport systems since all are membrane-bound and their affinities for GABA are relatively high. The term "affinity" is applied rather loosely to transport systems since the kinetic parameter, K_m, is derived from studies of transport velocity and, except under special conditions, this K_m is probably not equivalent to the dissociation constant (K_d) for complexes of GABA with its transport receptive site. Since the unknown K_d is the true measure of affinity, the extent to which the binding of GABA to carrier receptive sites will interfere with analyses of GABA binding to postsynaptic receptive sites is unknown. It is likely, however, that transport systems involved with the termination of GABA's influence at the synapse will have dissociation constants for GABA similar to that of the postsynaptic receptor.

GABA uptake systems exhibit an absolute requirement for sodium (Martin, 1973). The free energy for transport of GABA may arise from ionic and electrical gradients across the neuronal membrane and/or GABA may be co-transported with sodium along its electrochemical potential gradient (Martin, 1976). This transport process may involve carrier proteins whose affinity for GABA is altered by the binding of sodium. If so, the high-affinity carrier protein might be recognized by its sodium dependence for GABA binding.

Theoretically, the most useful property for the differentiation of trans-

---

*Abbreviations employed in this chapter:

IC_{50}, that concentration of inhibitor which displaces 50 percent of labeled ligand from receptive sites when both [ligand and site] are $<<<$ K_d of their complex

K_d, dissociation constant for receptor-ligand complexes derived from equilibrium studies

K_i, inhibitory constants derived from kinetic or equilibrium studies

K_m, Michaelis constant derived from initial velocity studies

port and postsynaptic receptive sites is pharmacologic specificity. This criterion has been employed by a number of investigators to study GABA-receptive sites (Peck, Schaeffer, and Clark, 1973; DeFeudis, 1974; DeFeudis et al., 1975; dePlazas and DeRobertis, 1975; Enna and Snyder, 1975; Peck, Schaeffer, and Clark, 1976; Peck et al., 1976; Snyder, 1975b). Unfortunately, pharmacologic differences between the transport of GABA and the GABA-induced generation of inhibitory postsynaptic potentials (IPSP) are not well defined. Structural analogs of GABA which are potent inhibitors of GABA transport also have postsynaptic actions similar to GABA's (Johnston, 1976). For example, the competitive inhibitor of glial GABA transport, β-alanine (Schon and Kelley, 1974), also produces inhibitory responses with a potency similar to that of GABA (Obata, Takeda, and Shinozaki, 1970). Thus, although pharmacologic agents may lend insight to the nature of these multiple receptive sites, it seems unlikely that alone they will suffice to distinguish between transport and postsynaptic receptive sites. This is especially true because dose-response relationships are difficult to establish in central nervous tissue.

Our approach to the isolation and characterization of GABA-receptive sites has been via the subcellular fractionation of discrete central nervous tissues. Cerebellar cortex and hippocampus contain high densities of interneurons that synthesize endogenous GABA, transport exogenous GABA, and use GABA as a neurotransmitter. Starting materials such as these, which are enriched for GABA interneurons, allow increased specific activities of the various GABA-receptive sites. The isolation of GABA-receptive sites proceeds from synaptosomes through synaptic plasma membranes to junctional complexes (JC) (Peck, Schaeffer, and Clark, 1973, 1976; Peck et al., 1976).

Our early attempts at such a preparation (Peck, Schaeffer, and Clark, 1973) resulted in the characterization of a sodium-independent GABA-receptive site of moderate affinity ($K_d \sim 20\ \mu M$) which shares some of the properties of the postsynaptic receptor and the glial transport receptive site. Presumptive synaptic membranes were prepared from cerebellar cortical tissue using hypertonic homogenization and density-gradient centrifugation techniques. From such preparations we solubilized a chlorpromazine-insensitive, sodium-independent GABA-receptive site. This site was competitively inhibited by bicuculline (an antagonist of transport and postsynaptic systems) and β-alanine (an analog with postsynaptic activity and high affinity for the glial transport system) but not affected by diaminobutyric acid (an inhibitor of neuronal transport). This site binds GABA with a dissociation constant of 10 to 20 μM. A receptive site with similar properties was recently solubilized by organic solvent extraction of central nervous tissue (dePlazas and DeRobertis, 1975). The identity of this site remains uncertain. Our initial claim that this represented *the* postsynaptic receptor has been tempered by the demonstration by electron microscopy that the membranes from which the site is solubilized are heavily contaminated with microsomes. Thus, this site may be derived from microsomal/glial membranes, not synaptic membranes as originally thought. At present the identity of this receptive site remains uncertain since it shares properties of the postsynaptic receptor and the glial transport system. Only purification and immunohistochemical localization will allow the unambiguous identification of this receptive site.

We have re-examined the binding of GABA to purified synaptic plasma membranes and junctional complexes isolated from cerebellar cortex, cerebral cortex, and hippocampus and confirmed the existence (as reported by Snyder and co-workers, Enna and Snyder, 1975; Enna, Kuhar, and Snyder, 1975; Zukin, Young and Snyder, 1974) of two GABA-binding sites, one with a K_d of about 0.15 μM which is Na^+-independent and a second with a K_d of 3 to 7 μM which is strictly dependent on Na^+ for binding activity. In our hands Na^+-dependent binding is competitively inhibited by nipecotic acid and diaminobutyrate with K_i values of 40 and 350 μM respectively. These compounds are potent competitive inhibitors of synaptosomal GABA transport with K_i values of 15 and 121 μM respectively (Peck, 1977). The similarity in these values, despite differences in the temperature employed for binding (O° C) and transport (22° C) studies, suggests to us that Na^+-dependent binding is associated with the neuronal transport system. The Na^+-dependent receptive site, with a K_d for GABA of 5 μM, is completely removed from synaptic plasma membrane by treatment with 0.1 percent Triton under conditions that leave junctional complexes intact (Cotman and Taylor, 1972). Na^+-independent binding, on the other hand, is not affected by nipecotic acid or diaminobutyrate but is competitively inhibited by muscimol (IC_{50} ~10 nM) and bicuculline (IC_{50} ~15 μM). These properties plus the resistance of this site to solubilization by 0.1 percent Triton suggest that it may be the postsynaptic receptor residing in, or tightly associated with, the junctional complex. We have used electron microscopy extensively to confirm our contention that synaptic plasma membranes and junctional complexes are, in fact, being employed for GABA binding. Studies are currently under way to solubilize GABA-receptive sites from the junctional complex preparation and to purify them for comparison with the previously solubilized and partially purified component of cerebellar membranes (Peck, Schaeffer, and Clark, 1973, 1976; Peck et al., 1976).

Snyder and co-workers have reported the existence of two GABA-receptive systems, both of high affinity (Enna and Snyder, 1975). One is sodium-dependent, has a K_d for GABA of about 1.2 μM and is inhibited by sulfhydryl reagents as well as by chlorpromazine and ß-alanine (K_i values of 21 and 35 μM respectively) while the other is sodium-independent, has a K_d for GABA of about 0.4 μM, is not sensitive to sulfhydryl reagents, and is inhibited by low levels of bicuculline, imidazoleacetic acid, and 3-aminopropanesulfonic acid. From these pharmacologic porperties the sodium-independent site appears to be the postsynaptic receptor while the dependent site is suggested to be the glial transport site. Unfortunately, crude membrane preparations derived from whole brain were employed and the resultant specific binding activities were low (<1 pmol of sites per gram of tissue for the Na^+-independent site). Studies employing crude membranes from discrete brain regions gave similar low levels of binding (Enna, Kuhar, and Snyder, 1975). In these studies Na^+-dependent binding ranged from about 2 to 40 pmol/gram while Na^+-independent binding ranged from 0.1 to 2.0 pmol/gram of tissue. From this and previous studies (Zukin, Young, and Snyder, 1974) came the conclusion that Na^+-independent binding reflects sites associated with the postsynaptic receptor mechanism while Na^+-dependent sites are associated with glial transport systems. Horng and Wong (1977a, b) have confirmed the existence of at least two GABA-receptive sites and suggest the existence of others. They report that Triton at low concentrations (0.01 percent) abolishes 80 percent of Na^+-dependent GABA binding without altering Na^+-independent sites. Higher concentrations of Triton (0.5 percent) abolished GABA binding but evidently not via solubilization. Multiple washing of membranes treated with 0.5 percent Triton allowed the demonstration of ultrahigh affinity components with K_d values of 4.5 and 30 nM with capacities of 1 and 4 pmole/mg of protein respectively. A similar multiplicity of high-affinity, Na^+-independent sites was reported by Enna and Snyder (1976) for mammalian retina. The binding of ^3H-GABA to these sites is inhibited by (+)-bicuculline, 3-aminopropanesulfonic acid, muscimol, imidazoleacetic acid, and adlumidine with IC_{50} values (that concentration of unlabeled analog or competitive agent required to reduce ^3H-GABA binding at subsaturating levels to 50 percent) ranging from 10 nM to 1 μM.

Several comments about these studies seem necessary. IC_{50} values are employed extensively in characterizing GABA-receptive sites, but subsaturating values of ^3H-GABA are not always used to study inhibition by analogs or drugs. In addition, the concentration of receptive sites for either IC_{50} determinations or saturation analyses are not indicated (Horng and Wong, 1977a, b; Enna and Snyder, 1976). The use of ^3H-GABA at or near its K_d (0.3 to 1 K_d) precludes the calculation of true K_d values from IC_{50} analyses. In addition, artifacts will arise if the concentration of receptive site is above its K_d. Thus these studies suggest that sites with ultrahigh affinity are receptors (since binding properties parallel the neurophysiological actions of analogs); more detailed and careful analyses of these sites are necessary, however, to insure their identification. It seems unlikely that Triton "enhances the apparent affinity of GABA agonists and antagonists"; rather, the removal of high levels of nonspecific binding by partial purification (through solubilization) probably allows the demonstration of sites previously unnoticed.

Thus three, and perhaps four, GABA-receptive sites have been reported for the central nervous system. Our original investigations of a GABA-receptive site competitively inhibited by β-alanine and bicuculline may have focused on a glial transport system within a microsomal fraction isolated from central nervous tissue. This is currently under investigation. Recent studies from our laboratory as well as those of Snyder and coworkers (Enna and Snyder, 1975; Enna, Kuhar, and Snyder, 1975; Zukin, Young, and Snyder, 1974; Horng and Wong, 1977a, b) suggest that additional GABA-receptive sites can be demonstrated in central nervous tissue. To date no GABA-receptive site has been assigned an unambiguous physiologic role. This state of confusion results from the existence of multiple classes of "high-affinity," membrane-bound GABA-receptive sites in the central nervous system. Although ligand binding, pharmacologic specificity, and regional distribution are important for characterization, these criteria alone may prove insufficient for the differentiation of these receptive sites. Alternative approaches, such as the manipulation of synaptic processes, may allow one to differentiate between receptive species. Examples of this approach include surgical or chemical deafferentation as employed for the dopamine system (Kebabian, Petzold, and Greengard, 1972; vonVoigtlander, Boukma, and Johnson, 1973; Mishra et al., 1974) and developmental or hormonal manipulation as used by us for the GABA system (Peck et al., 1976; Peck, 1977). Thus the alteration of discrete synaptic processes may allow application of the fifth criterion for receptor identification, the correlation of ligand binding with physiologic responses.

It seems reasonable at this point to discuss briefly why we wish to purify GABA-receptive sites from the mammalian CNS. Our interest from a mechanistic viewpoint derives from the fascinating differences observed for various inhibitory transmitters (as, for example, coupled to ionophore mechanisms versus coupled to cAMP- or cGMP-mediated responses) and the differences observed for the action of GABA at central versus peripheral neurons. From a pharmacologic or applied standpoint, we believe that an understanding of the action of various convulsants, anticonvulsants, anesthetics, etc. at the synaptic level, and the rational design of future drugs specific for inhibitory (or excitatory) GABA responses, will depend on a complete elucidation of the receptive sites employed by neuronal transport and receptor systems as well as glial transport systems.

Gamma-aminobutyric acid, when applied iontophoretically, depresses the firing rate of nerve cells throughout the mammalian central nervous system. The role of GABA as an inhibitory neurotransmitter in cerebral and cerebellar cortex seems well established (Curtis and Johnston, 1974; Krnjevic, 1974). Thus the commonly reported action of GABA is hyperpolarization of CNS neurons with a concomitant decrease in excitability.

In contrast, some peripheral neurons seem to respond to GABA with increases in excitability and/or depolarization. Thus dorsal-root and sympathetic-ganglion neurons *in vivo* and *in vitro* respond to applied GABA with depolarization and either increased (dorsal-root ganglion) or decreased (sympathetic ganglion) excitability (DeGroat, Lalley, and Saum, 1972; Obata, 1973; Ransom and Nelson, 1976; Adams and Brown, 1975; Lawson, Bisco, and Headley, 1976). Adams and Brown conclude that the mechanism of GABA action on rat superior cervical ganglion neurons is similar to that of central neurons, that is, an increase in Cl^- permeability, and that high intracellular Cl^- concentrations with equilibrium potentials less than resting potentials account for depolarizing responses to applied GABA. Concentrations of GABA in rat superior cervical ganglia are sufficiently high to allow speculation that it might serve as a transmitter or modulator (300 pmol/mg of protein, similar to levels of dopamine and nonepinephrine according to Bertilsson, Suria, and Costa, 1976). The latter role is suggested by the studies of Bowery et al. (1976) which show that gamma-aminobutyric acid and ß-alanine release endogenous GABA from neuroglial cells, thus depolarizing ganglion cells indirectly via the released GABA.

The role of GABA as an inhibitory neurotransmitter (Curtis and Johnston, 1974; Krnjevic, 1974) has allowed speculation that compounds that elevate GABA levels in the brain should be anticonvulsant agents (as, in reverse, those depressing GABA levels should be convulsants). Experimentation to establish this point has met with mixed success at best (Wood and Peesker, 1975). The synapse is a dynamic system and, as with any system in flux, mere levels of transmitter at the terminal are not likely to predict the efficacy of a drug. Rather, the effects of a drug on synthetic and degradative enzymes, neuronal and glial transport systems (as well as storage systems), pre- and postsynaptic receptors are apt to be involved in its convulsant or anticonvulsant properties.

Many drugs have been implicated in elevating endogenous GABA levels. These include ethanol (Chan, 1976), pargyline, desipramine, imidazoleacetic acid (Tunnicliff, 1976), ethanol-O-sulfate, di-n-propylacetate (Anlezark et al., 1976), and aminooxyacetic acid (Kuriyama, Roberts, and Rubenstein, 1966). Others, including allylglycine (Fisher and Davie, 1976), isonicotinic acid hydrazine (Tunnicliff, 1976), 6-aminonicotinamide (Bielicki and Krieglstein, 1976), ketamine, alphaxalone (Dye and Taberner, 1975), and verruculogen (Hotujac, Muftic, and Filipovie, 1976) are known to depress endogenous levels of GABA. With few exceptions, however, their pharmacologic effects are not straightforward.

Thus, these drugs, all believed to modify the metabolism of GABA, are likely to affect other sites as well, some in a compensatory manner to nullify the expected result (Chase and Walters, 1976). Combined with multiple brain targets, the multiple loci of action discussed above can produce a complex ultimate response.

In considering realistic approaches to the pharmacology of the GABA synapse, one must hope for: (1) site-directed agents (to reduce the number of CNS targets) and (2) agents directed at a single (or complementary) mechanism(s). It is our thesis that postsynaptic receptors (and perhaps other membrane-bound receptive sites) are reasonable targets for such agents. It is possible that multiple receptors or receptor mechanisms for GABA exist which subserve specific CNS pathways or regions (see discussion of central versus peripheral systems above). It is certain that postsynaptic receptors possess affinities for GABA and certain pharmacologic agents far in excess of those displayed by metabolic enzymes and greater than those of transport systems. Thus, targeting with respect to mechanisms may be feasible on the basis of the ultrahigh affinities displayed by receptors. Certainly, more definitive studies of high-affinity, limited-capacity receptors and other receptive species for GABA found on or within neuronal (and glial) membranes should allow or enhance the development of potent and specific pharmacologic agents directed at GABA-mediated processes.

We have initiated research to study the efficacy of synaptic plasma membrane (SPM) binding assays as probes of the pharmacologic specificities of drugs that interact with the GABA system. Such assays, if conducted under controlled conditions of receptive site and ligand concentration, could prove to be short-cuts in determining drug specificity and rapid methods for screening drugs prior to research at the clinical level. For example, electrophysiological investigations of others indicate that pentobarbital enhances inhibitory influences of GABA (Nicoll et al., 1975; Ransom and Barker, 1975, 1976). Receptor activation seems to be amplified and prolonged. This could result from enhanced or sustained release of GABA from presynaptic terminals, alterations in neuronal or glial uptake mechanisms, or alterations of postsynaptic GABA receptors. To test these possibilities we used intact synaptosomes, SPM, and JC to examine the effects of pentobarbital on synaptosomal ^{3}H-GABA uptake as well as binding of ^{3}H-GABA to Na^+-dependent and Na^+-independent GABA-receptive sites. Even at high concentrations of pentobarbital (greater than 1.0 m*M*) there is no appreciable effect on GABA uptake or binding (Peck, Miller, and Lester, 1976). Thus the influence of pentobarbital which is evident at 0.1 m*M* must originate from mechanisms other than GABA uptake or binding to GABA-receptive sites. The use of this simple probe may alert researchers to the need for pursuing other possible sites of action for this drug, including its effects on the presynaptic release of GABA and on ionophores coupled with postsynaptic sites.

It seems important at this point to pause and consider how these studies should *not* be done. The use of crude membrane fractions with high values for nonspecific binding precludes any substantive conclusion about pharmacologic specificity. Furthermore, conditions for receptive site assay must be carefully established. Association and dissociation rate constants as well as thermodynamic parameters are necessary to conduct careful analyses of pharmacologic interaction. Attention should be paid to the concentrations of receptive site *and* ligand employed. Finally, in the best of worlds, postsynaptic receptive sites totally separated from other GABA-receptive species should be used for specificity studies.

Recent studies with synaptic plasma membrane in the presence of Na^+ (to examine receptive sites believed to be neuronal transport sites) and junctional complexes in the absence of Na^+ (to examine the sodium-independent site considered to be the postsynaptic receptor) have examined the effects of phenobarbital, diphenylhydantoin, pentylenetetrazole, and picrotoxin. Neither picrotoxin nor phenobarbital had significant effects on the putative postsynaptic receptor. A number of research groups have reported that picrotoxin does not interact with high-affinity GABA-receptive sites (Enna and Snyder, 1975; Peck, 1977; Horng and Wong, 1977b); however, Barker (personal communication) has evidence from electrophysiologic studies on spinal-cord neurons in culture that picrotoxin blocks GABA competitively. The disparity between electrophysiologic and biochemical findings remains to be resolved.

Picrotoxin did depress slightly the Na^+-dependent binding system (from 100 to 80 percent). In this assay, Na^+-dependent binding includes both neuronal transport (Na^+-dependent, nipecotic acid-inhibited) *and* postsynaptic (Na^+-independent, nipecotic acid-insensitive) receptive sites since both reside on the SPM used for Na^+-dependent-binding. Perhaps the Na^+-independent receptive site on junctional complexes (used to assay Na^+-independent receptive sites) is inhibited by picrotoxin *when sodium is present* (as is the case for the Na^+-dependent binding assay and electrophysiologic studies). This is currently under investigation in our laboratory with the use of junctional complexes and solubilized transport receptive sites.

Interestingly, diphenylhydantoin (an anticonvulsant used in treatment of epilepsy) enhances the binding of ^{3}H-GABA to both Na^+-dependent and Na^+-independent receptive sites. Pentylenetetrazole (PTZ), a convulsant, also enhances binding of ^{3}H-GABA to transport (Na^+-dependent) sites as well as to postsynaptic (Na^+-independent) sites; however, the latter effect is marginal. At very high concentrations, PTZ displaces or inhibits GABA binding at both sites. Thus, diphenylhydantoin (5 to 100 μM) may increase the efficacy of released GABA by increasing the activity of postsynaptic receptors, but it may increase the capacity of the transport system (inactivation mechanism) as well. Pentylenetetrazole, on the other hand, seems to activate the transport mechanism (and thus decrease synaptic efficacy of GABA) without appreciably enhancing the receptor mechanism. In addition, at high concentrations PTZ blocks the binding of GABA to both receptor and transport sites.

We are currently engaged in studies to characterize these multiple effects by kinetic and thermodynamic analyses of the interactions of ^{3}H-GABA with these sites in the presence and absence of various convulsant and anticonvulsant drugs. Studies like those described above permit rapid focus on particular drugs at potentially effective concentrations. Under controlled conditions such assays provide rapid methods for initial assessment of drug specificity and efficacy.

REFERENCES

Adams, P. R. and Brown, D. A. 1975. Actions of γ-aminobutyric acid on sympathetic ganglion cells. *J. Physiol. (Lon.)*, 250:85-120.

Anlezark, G., Horton, R. W., Meldrum, B. S., Christina, M., and Sawaya, B. 1976. Anticonvulsant action of ethanolamine-O-sulphate and di-n-propylacetate and the metabolism of γ-aminobutyric acid (GABA) in mice with audiogenic seizures. *Biochem. Pharmacol.*, 25:413-417.

Bertilson, L., Suria, A., and Costa, E. 1976. γ-Aminobutyric acid in rat superior cervical ganglion. *Nature*, 260:540-541.

Bielicki, L., and Krieglstein, J. 1976. Decreased GABA and glutamate concentrations in rat brain after treatment with 6-aminonicotinamide. *Naunyn Schmiedebergs Arch. Pharmacol.*, 294:157-160.

Bowery, N. G., Brown, D. A., Collins, N. G. S., Galvan, M., Marsh, S., and Yamini, G. 1976. Indirect effects of amino-acids on sympathetic ganglion cells mediated through the release of γ-aminobutyric acid from glial cells. *Br. J. Pharmacol.*, 57:73-91.

CHAN, A. W. K. 1976. Gamma aminobutyric acid in different strains of mice. Effect of ethanol. *Life Sci.*, 19:597-604.

CHASE, T. N., and WALTERS, J. R. 1976. Pharmacologic approaches to the manipulation of GABA mediated synaptic function in man. In E. Roberts, T. N. Chase, and D. B. Tower (eds.), *GABA in Nervous System Function*, pp. 497-513. New York: Raven Press.

COTMAN, D. W., and TAYLOR, D. 1972. Isolation and structural studies on synaptic complexes from rat brain. *J. Cell Biol.*, 55:696-712.

CURTIS, D. R., DUGGAN, A. W., and JOHNSTON, G. A. R. 1970. The inactivation of extra cellularly administered amino acids in the feline spinal cord. *Exp. Brain Res.*, 10:447-462.

CURTIS, D. R., and JOHNSTON, G. A. R. 1974. Amino acid transmitters in the mammalian central nervous system. *Rev. Physiol.*, 69:97-188.

DEFEUDIS, F. V. 1974. Preferential "binding" of γ-aminobutyric acid and glycine to synaptosome enriched fractions of rat cerebral cortex and spinal cord. *Can. J. Physiol. Pharmacol.*, 52:138-147.

DEFEUDIS, F. V., BALFACON, G., DESARGARRA, M. R., MADTES, P., SOMOZA, E., and GERVAS-CAMACHO, J. 1975. Action of N-methyl-bicuculline on the binding of γ-aminobutyric acid in the rat cerebral cortex. *Exp. Neurol.*, 49:497-505.

DEGROAT, W. C., LALLEY, P. M., and SAUM, W. R. 1972. Depolarization of dorsal root ganglia in the cat by GABA and related amino acids: Antagonism by picrotoxin and bicuculline. *Brain Res.*, 44:273-277.

DEPLAZAS, S. F., and DEROBERTIS, E. 1975. Isolation of hydrophobic proteins binding amino acids: γ-aminobutyric acid binding in the rat cerebral cortex. *J. Neurochem.*, 25:547-552.

DEROBERTIS, E. 1975. Synaptic receptors: Isolation and molecular biology. *Modern Pharmacology-Toxicology*, 4:387.

DEROBERTIS, E., and SCHACT, J., eds. 1974. *Neurochemistry of Cholinergic Receptors*. New York: Raven Press.

DYE, D. J. and TABERNER, P. V. 1975. The effects of some newer anaesthetics on the *in vitro* activity of glutamate decarboxylase and GABA transaminase in crude brain extracts and on the levels of amino acids *in vivo*. *J. Neurochem.*, 24:997-1001.

ENNA, S. J., KUHAR, M. J., and SNYDER, S. H. 1975. Regional distribution of postsynaptic receptor-binding for gamma-aminobutyric acid (GABA) in monkey brain. *Brain Res.*, 93:168-174.

ENNA, S. J., and SNYDER, S. H. 1975. Properties of γ-aminobutyric acid (GABA) receptor binding in rat brain synaptic membrane fractions. *Brain Res.*, 100:81-97.

ENNA, S. J., and SNYDER, S. H. 1976. Gamma-aminobutyric (GABA) receptors binding in mammalian retina. *Brain Res.*, 115:174-179.

FISHER, S. K., and DAVIE, W. E. 1976. The effects of the convulsant allylglycine (2-amino-4-pentenoic acid) in the activity of glutamic acid decarboxylase and the concentration of GABA in different regions of guinea pig brain. *Biochem. Pharmacol.*, 25(16):1881-1885.

HORNG, J. S., and WONG, D. T. 1977a. Effects of Triton X-100 on the binding of ^{3}H-gamma-aminobutyric acid (^{3}H-GABA) to membrane of rat brain. *Fed. Proc.*, 36:801.

HORNG, J. S., and WONG, D. T. 1977b. N^+-independent binding of GABA to the Triton X-100 treated synaptic membranes from cerebellum of rat brains. *Life Sci.*, 20:445-452.

HOTUJAC, L., MUFTIC, R. H., and FILIPOVIE, N. 1976. Verruculogen: A new substance for decreasing GABA levels in CNS. *Pharmacology*, 14:(4)297-300.

JOHNSTON, G. A. R. 1976. Physiologic pharmacology of GABA and its antagonists in the vertebrate nervous system. In E. Roberts, T. N. Chase, and D. B. Tower (eds.), *GABA in Nervous System Function*, pp. 395-411. New York: Raven Press.

KARLIN, A. 1974. Acetylcholine-receptor: Progress report. *Life Sci.*, 14:1385-1415.

KEBABIAN, J. W., PETZOLD, G., and GREENGARD, P. 1972. Dopamine-sensitive adenylate cyclase in caudate nucleus of rat brain and its similarity to the "dopamine receptor." *Proc. Natl. Acad. Sci. U.S.A.*, 69:2145-2149.

KRNJEVIC, K. 1974. Chemical nature of synaptic transmission in vertebrates. *Physiol. Rev.*, 54:418-540.

KURIYAMA, K. ROBERTS, E., and RUBENSTEIN, M. K. 1966. Elevation of γ-aminobutyric acid in brain with amino-oxyacetic acid and susceptibility to convulsive seizures in mice: A quantitative re-evaluation. *Biochem. Pharmacol.*, 15:221-236.

LAWSON, S. N., BISCO, T. J., and HEADLEY, P. M. 1976. The effect of electrophoretically applied GABA on cultured dissociated spinal cord and sensory ganglion neurons of the rat. *Brain Res.*, 117(3):493-497.

MARTIN, D. L. 1973. Kinetics of the sodium-dependent transport of gamma-aminobutyric acid by synaptosomes. *J. Neurochem.*, 21:345-356.

MARTIN, D. L. 1976. Carrier-mediated transport and removal of GABA from synaptic regions. In E. Roberts, T. N. Chase, and D. B. Tower (eds.), *GABA in Nervous System Function*, pp. 347-386. New York: Raven Press.

MISHRA, R. K., GARDNER, E. L., KATZMAN, R., and MAKMAN, M. H. 1974, Enhancement of dopamine-stimulated adenylate cyclase activity in rat caudate after lesions in substantia nigra: Evidence for denervation supersensitivity. *Proc. Natl. Acad. Sci. U.S.A.*, 71:3883-3887.

NICOLL, R. A., ECCLES, J. C., OSHIMA, T., and RUBIA, F. 1975. Prolongation of hippocampal inhibitory postsynaptic potentials by barbiturates. *Nature*, 258:625-627.

OBATA, K. 1973. Transmitter sensitivities of some nerve and muscle cells in culture. *Brain Res.*, 73:71-88.

OBATA, K., TAKEDA, K., and SHINOZAKI, H. 1970. Further study on pharmacological properties of cerebellar-induced inhibition of Deiter's neurones. *Exp. Brain Res.*, 11:327-342.

PECK, E. J., JR. 1977. GABA receptive sites in the mammalian central nervous system. In W. Fields (ed.), *Neurotransmitter Function*, pp. 105-114. New York: Straton Intercontinental Medical Books.

PECK, E. J., JR., MILLER, A. L., and LESTER, B. R. 1976. Pentobarbital and synaptic high-affinity receptive sites for gamma-aminobutyric acid. *Brain Res. Bull.*, 1:595-597.

PECK, E. J., JR., SCHAEFFER, J. M., and CLARK, J. H. 1973. γ-Aminobutyric acid, bicuculline and post-synaptic binding sites. *Biochem. Biophys. Res. Commun.*, 52:394-400.

PECK, E. J., JR., SCHAEFFER, J. M., and CLARK, J. H. 1976. In pursuit of the GABA receptor. In E. Roberts, T. N. Chase, and D. B. Tower (eds.), *GABA in Nervous System Function*, pp. 319-336. New York: Raven Press.

PECK, E. J., JR., SCHAEFFER, J. M., MILLER, A. L., and CLARK, J. H. 1976. Analysis of receptive sites in synaptosomal fractions. *Neuroscience Symposium*, 1:1-27.

RANSOM, B. R., and BARKER, J. L. 1975. New theory for receptor mechanism of carotid body chemoreceptors. *Nature*, 254:703-705.

RANSOM, B. R., and BARKER, J. L. 1976. Pentobarbital selectively enhances GABA-mediated postsynaptic inhibition in tissue cultured mouse spinal neurons. *Brain Res.*, 114(3):530-535.

RANSOM, B., and NELSON, P. G. 1976. Neuropharmacological responses from nerve cells in tissue culture. In L. L. Iversen, S. D. Iversen, and S. H. Snyder (eds.), *Handbook of Psychopharmacology*, vol. 2, pp. 101-127. New York: Plenum Press.

SCHON, F., and KELLEY, J. S. 1974. Characterization of [^{3}H] GABA uptake into satellite glial cells of rat sensory ganglia. *Brain Res.*, 66:289-300.

SNYDER, S. H. 1975a. Amino acid neurotransmitters: Biochemical pharmacology. In D. B. Tower (ed.), *The Nervous System*, vol. 1, pp. 355-361. New York: Raven Press.

SNYDER, S. H. 1975b. Glycine synaptic receptor in the mammalian central nervous system. *Brit. J. Pharmacol.*, 53:473-484.

SNYDER, S. H., and BENNETT, J. P., JR. 1976. Neurotransmitter receptors in the brain: Biochemical identification. *Ann. Rev. Physiol.*, 38:153-175.

TUNNICLIFF, G. 1976. Centrally-acting drugs and the formation of brain γ-aminobutyric acid. *Gen. Pharmacol.*, 7:259-262.

VONVOIGTLANDER, P. F., BOUKMA, S. J., and JOHNSON, G. A. 1973. Dopaminergic denervation supersensitivity and dopamine stimulated adenyl cyclase activity. *Neuropharmacology*, 12:1081-1086.

WOOD, J. D., and PEESKER, S. J. 1975. The anticonvulsant action of GABA-elevating agents: A re-evaluation. *J. Neurochem.*, 25:277-282.

WU, J.-Y. 1976. Purification characterization and kinetic studies of GAD and GABA-T from mouse brain. In E. Roberts, T. N. Chase, and D. B. Tower (eds.), *GABA in Nervous System Function*, pp. 7-55. New York: Raven Press.

ZUKIN, S. R. YOUNG, A. B., and SNYDER, S. H. 1974. Gamma-aminobutyric binding to receptor sites in the rat central nervous system. *Proc. Natl. Acad. Sci. U.S.A.*, 71:4802-4807.

6

NEUROENDOCRINOLOGY AND PSYCHIATRIC DRUGS

J. MARK ORDY, PH.D.

Rationale for "Neuroendocrine-Window" Strategy in Evaluation of Affective Disorders and Psychotropic Drugs

The basic aims of this chapter are to review and evaluate the evidence obtained by the "neuroendocrine-window" strategy on: (1) a possible association between neuroendocrine dysfunction and some affective disorders, and (2) psychotropic drug modification of neurotransmitters, neuropeptides, hormones and behavior. As a starting point, it appears desirable to provide a very brief description of: (1) the essential developments that have led to the emergence of the "neuroendocrine-window" strategy, (2) recent views concerning the intricate structure-function relations of the neuroendocrine system, and (3) psychotropic drug modification of the neuroendocrine system, with particular emphasis on limbic-hypothalamic neurotransmitters, transducer cell neuropeptide-releasing or -inhibiting factors, pituitary adrenocorticotropic hormone (ACTH), growth hormone (GH), prolactin (PRL), thyrotropin (TSH), the target-endocrine hormones, stress, emotional behavior, and psychopathology.

The limbic (L) system and the hypothalamic-pituitary-adrenal (HPA) axis are critically involved in homeostatic adaptation and emotional behavior (Mason, 1975; Siegel and Eisenman, 1976; Ganong, 1970, 1974, 1977). Components of the limbic (L) system play an important role in the regulation of the hypothalamic-pituitary-adrenal axis (LHPA), and in consolidation of learning and memory through neuroendocrine modulation of motivation, emotions, or reward properties of environmental stimuli (de Wied, 1977a, b). Until recently, it has been very difficult to develop indices

Sincere thanks to T. Beavers and L. Williams for their dedicated efforts in preparation of this chapter.

of disturbed LHPA functioning, or to determine the specific interaction effects of stress, drugs, and psychopathology in the LHPA system.

The "neuroendocrine-window" strategy proposes that changes in patterns of circulating hormones may be used as a "window" to draw inferences concerning central neuroregulator abnormalities in some psychiatric disorders (Sachar, 1975, 1977; Usdin et al., 1977). Putative neurotransmitters and neuropeptides of the neuroendocrine system cannot be measured directly in the intact human brain; the assessment of LHPA function in man is always indirect, and is critically dependent on the development of sensitive and specific radioimmunoassays for pituitary and target-endocrine hormones. Virtually all psychotropic drugs appear to modify particular hormones (Wurtman and Fernstrom, 1976). An association has also been noted between some emotional disturbances and diseases of the LHPA system (Locke and Schally, 1972; Liddle, 1974; Brown, 1975; Gwinup and Johnson, 1975; Whybrow and Hurwitz, 1976).

More provocative evidence in support of the results obtained from the neuroendocrine-window strategy comes from animal studies of neurotransmitter and neuropeptide localization in the limbic system, and the neuropharmacological modification of the neuroendocrine system and behavior. The specific features in the neuroendocrine-window strategy include: (1) development of sensitive and specific radioimmunoassays for different hormones in small samples of blood, (2) use of a variety of challenging drugs for the activation of the LHPA system in differential diagnosis of psychopathology, (3) an association between emotional disturbances and such endocrinopathies or disorders of the LHPA system as Addison's disease and Cushing's syndrome, (4) significant physiological, neurochemical, and anatomical relationships that have been established between brain regions implicated in learning, motivation, emotion and in neuroendocrine regulation of the LHPA system, (5) immunohistochemical identification and localization of neurotransmitters and neuropeptides in the hypothalamus involved in regulation of pituitary and target-endocrine hormones, and (6) recognition that hypothalamic neuropeptides, pituitary ACTH, and adrenal corticosteroid hormones appear to influence learning and memory independently of their better known "classical" hormone effects on target organs.

The neuroendocrine system is broadly defined as those structures of the limbic system, particularly the hypothalamus, that are implicated in the regulation of the pituitary and the target endocrines. The components of the limbic system include the hippocampus, amygdala, septal area, cingulate gyrus, fornix, mammillary bodies, and the hypothalamus (Nauta, 1963; Raisman, 1966; Livingston and Escobar, 1971). Although the hypothalamus is part of the limbic system, its singular importance in neuroendocrinology has rated it separate treatment as the "final common pathway" for regulating the pituitary and endocrine target organs. Neurons in the hypothalamus have been identified as neuroendocrine transducer cells. These peptidergic neuroendocrine cells transduce neural inputs to neurohormones or neuropeptide outputs. The neuropeptide releasing or inhibitory factors regulate pituitary hormones. Neurons of the limbic system, particularly those of the hypothalamus, are in turn sensitive to hormones and form part of complex "feedback loops" involving the brain, pituitary and endocrine-target organs (Gibbs, 1969; McEwen, 1975). The neuroendocrine components of the LHPA system can be activated by various inputs, ranging from such subtle psychological factors as anticipated, noxious, or aversive stimuli, the metabolic factors involved in gluconeogenesis and electrolyte balance, to the more direct effects of physical trauma and stress. The LHPA system is by far the most intensively studied unit in psychoendocrinology. Figure 1 illustrates the wide range of influences that may activate the LHPA system, including the ACTH and corticosteroid inhibition of hypothalamic peptidergic (CRF) factor.

The hypothalamus is the structural and functional focal point at which neurotransmitters converge on peptidergic releasing or inhibiting factors, including corticotropin-releasing factor (CRF), to regulate ACTH, and all other pituitary hormones. Since CRF has not been characterized chemically, ACTH and corticosteroids have been used for assaying CRF release in response to neurotransmitters. Acetylcholine (ACh) and serotonin (5-HT) stimulate CRF release, whereas norepinephrine (NE), γ-aminobutyric acid (GABA), and melatonin inhibit CRF secretion (Brownstein et al., 1976; Jones et al., 1976). Dopamine (DA) has not been implicated in CRF release (Fuxe and Hoekfelt, 1970). Figure 2 illustrates schematically the proposed model of neurotransmitter regulation of hypothalamic CRF into the portal capillaries of the pituitary.

Earlier clinical research efforts on a possible association between neuroendocrine dysfunction and some affective disorders have been summarized (Sachar, 1976; Carroll and Mendels, 1976; Rubin, 1977; Carroll, 1977; Sachar, 1977). Several reviews have also dealt with neuropharmacological effects on neuroendocrine functions in man (de Wied and de Jong, 1974; Frohman, 1975; Frohman and Stachura, 1975; Givant and Sulman, 1976). Hypothalamic neurotransmitter, neuropeptide and hormone effects on learning, motivation and emotion have also been reviewed (Lipton et al., 1977; de Wied et al., 1976; de Wied, 1977 a, b).

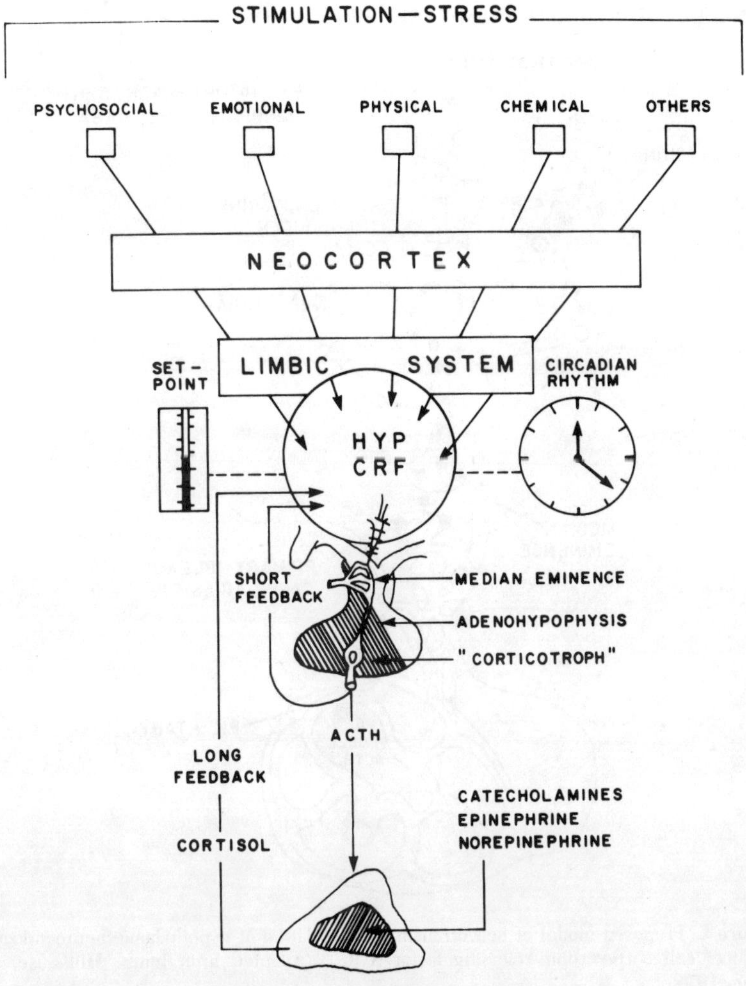

Figure 1. Effects of various influences on limbic-hypothalamic-pituitary-adrenal (LHPA) system. (Adapted from Gwinup and Johnson, 1975)

The Limbic-Hypothalamic-Pituitary-Adrenal System in Psychopathology

Assessment of LHPA function in psychiatric disorders has been focused predominantly on the primary affective disorders. This emphasis is based on (1) clinical observations that have linked LHPA impairment with mood

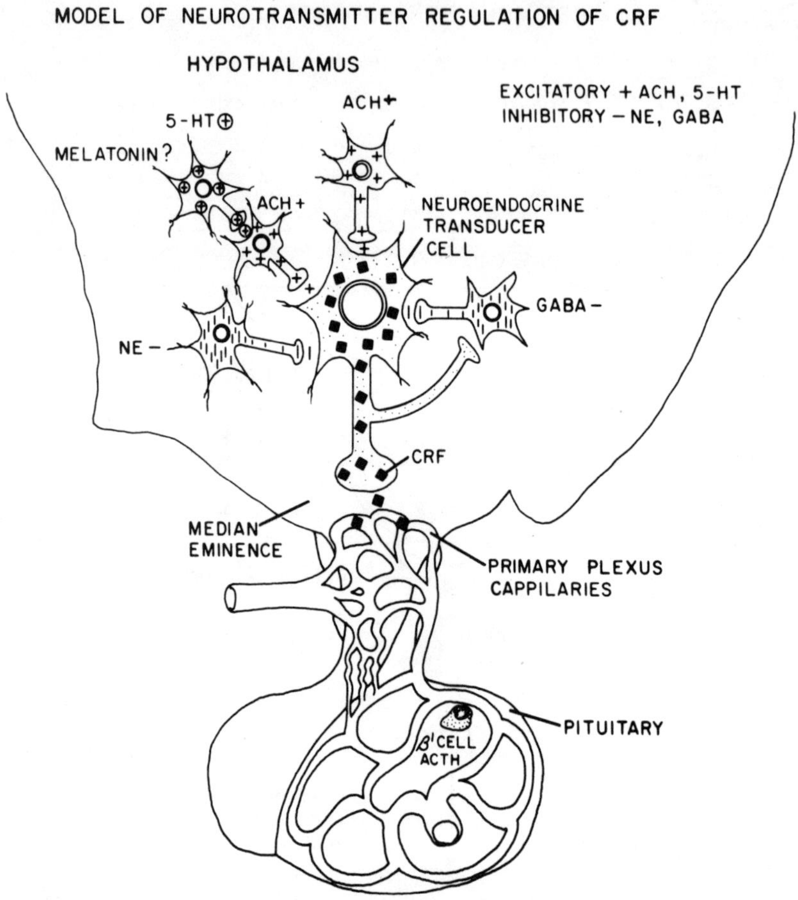

Figure 2. Proposed model of neurotransmitter regulation of hypothalamic neuroendocrine transducer cell corticotropin-releasing factor (CRF). (Adapted from Jones, Hillhouse, and Burden, 1976).

disorders, (2) behavioral symptoms of hypothalamic pathology—for example, loss of appetite, altered sex drive, aggression, sleep disturbances, impairment in autonomic nervous system arousal, and marked diurnal variations in mood—which are frequently also observed in patients with some primary affective disorders; (3) assessment of deviations in blood ACTH and cortisol, which makes it possible to make inferences concerning impairments in limbic neurotransmitters; and (4) abnormalities in some of these putative neurotransmitters or neuroregulators of hypothalamic CRF, which have also been implicated in the etiology of some affective disorders.

The standard clinical procedures for testing the hypothalamic-pituitary-adrenal axis (HPA) in various endocrine disorders have been summarized in detail (Locke and Schally, 1975; Liddle, 1974; Gwinup and Johnson, 1975). Many of these endocrine tests have been applied in psychiatric disorders and the results of these tests have also been reviewed from 1970 to 1976 (Carpenter and Bunney, 1971; Carroll and Mendels, 1976). In summary, the two major approaches to the study of the LHPA function in psychopathological states include: (1) tests of possible functional differences in such central neuronal regulatory mechanisms as ACh, DA, NE, 5-HT, GABA, and CRF; and (2) tests of tissue exposure to ACTH and/or cortisol. Table 1 summarizes briefly the two major approaches for studying the functional capacity of the LHPA system in psychopathological states.

Dysfunction in Affective Disorders

Any attempt to evaluate the evidence for neuroendocrine dysfunction in some affective disorders must first include such important methodological issues as: (1) operational definitions of and objective criteria for psychopathology, (2) sensitivity and specificity of bioassay and radioimmunoassay of CRF, ACTH, and cortisol, and (3) statistical evaluation of a

Table 1

Approaches to Evaluating the Human Limbic-Hypothalamic-Pituitary-Adrenal (LHPA) System

Regulatory Mechanisms

1. Neurotransmitters: ACh, DA, NE, 5-HT, GABA
2. Neuroendocrine transducer cell releasing factor-inhibiting factor (RF-IF) peptides
   A. Corticotropin-releasing factor—CRF
3. Circadian rhythm profile:
   A. Corticotropin (ACTH) B. Cortisol
4. Dexamethasone suppression
5. Metyrapone
6. Insulin hypoglycemia
7. Lysine vasopressin
8. Pyrogen

Tissue Concentration of ACTH, Cortisol

1. Plasma ACTH, cortisol
2. Plasma CBG capacity
3. Free cortisol:
   A. Plasma B. CSF C. Urine D. Tissue
4. Cortisol metabolism:
   A. Production rate B. Metabolic Clearance C. Biological Half-life D. Excretion of metabolites

(Adapted from Carroll and Mendels, 1976)

sufficient number of subjects tested over appropriate time intervals to provide reliable generalizations at specified levels of confidence. There is considerable uncertainty regarding most of these methodological issues. CRF has not been characterized chemically and a specific and reliable method for CRF assay is not yet available. ACTH has been estimated by a number of different bioassay procedures, making comparisons among different studies difficult. Although ACTH can now be determined by radioimmunoassay, the relatively complex laboratory procedures are not widely used for clinical evaluations (Berson and Yalow, 1968). Radioimmunoassay of cortisol is now readily available for clinical testing, but because only a small fraction of plasma cortisol that is not protein-bound is responsible for tissue effects, clear-cut interpretations of changes in levels are difficult (Carroll and Mendels, 1976). Such endocrine drug-challenge tests as insulin tolerance, dexamethasone suppression, etc. were not designed to detect the more subtle neuroendocrine dysfunctions that may be present in psychopathology. Finally, an important but neglected aspect of methodology is the absence of statistical evaluations of the data. Single case studies are basic in clinical evaluations, but the results can serve only as starting points for making scientific generalizations based on an adequate number of cases. For testing specific hypotheses, at least six to eight subjects are essential, with repeated sampling of ACTH, cortisol, etc. over four to six or other appropriate 24-hour time intervals. These statistical sampling criteria are needed to strengthen specific hypotheses concerning neuroendocrine dysfunction and psychopathology at statistically significant levels of confidence (Rubin, 1977). The above statistical criteria were used to evaluate the results of most of the studies cited here.

Regulation of ACTH and Cortisol in Psychopathology

Since the circadian rhythm profiles or patterns of both ACTH and cortisol reflect fundamental central nervous system (CNS) regulatory mechanisms, many researchers have proposed that this highly predictable, circadian pulsatile rhythm may be disrupted in some affective disorders (Sachar, 1975). Patients with lesions of the hypothalamus but an intact pituitary experience a disruption of circadian rhythms of both ACTH and cortisol (Locke and Schally, 1973). In hypophysectomized rats, circadian rhythm of hypothalamic CRF is maintained (Gwinup and Johnson, 1975). Based partly on this type of information on CNS control mechanisms for circadian profiles, many studies have attempted to show disturbances in the temporal diurnal cortisol profile of psychiatric patients. This type of evidence has been proposed as an index of CNS circadian control dysfunction of the LHPA system in psychopathology (Sachar, 1975). To interpret the evidence, it seems desirable to investigate diurnal ACTH and cortisol profiles in normal subjects. Two studies have examined concurrently the diurnal secretory patterns of both ACTH and cortisol (17-OHCS) with radioimmunoassays, in the same normal human subjects (Berson and Yalow, 1968; Gallagher et al., 1973). In the 1968 study, plasma ACTH and 17-OHCS were determined in eight normal subjects at 1200, 1600, 2000, 2400, 0400, and 0800 hours. A diurnal temporal relationship between ACTH and 17-OHCS across the six time periods covering 24 hours was noted, but the correlation between the ACTH and cortisol diurnal profiles was not a major focus of the study and was not evaluated statistically. From the individual values of eight subjects reported in the study, I computed a correlation coefficient for ACTH and 17-OHCS over the six time intervals covering the 24 hours. This correlation coefficient is significant statistically ($r = 0.89$, $n = 6$, $p < .02$). Since the results are critical for interpreting subsequent studies, the statistically evaluated results of the Berson and Yalow (1968) study of ACTH and cortisol diurnal profiles are presented in Figure 3 (top). It would be interesting to determine whether the significant diurnal correlation profiles of ACTH and cortisol observed in the normal subjects (Figure 3, top) are altered or dissassociated in some affective disorders.

Another research group (Sachar, 1975, 1976) has proposed that the number of secretory "episodes" of cortisol varies significantly in some affective disorders. This has also been examined in normal subjects. In an important and relevant study (Gallagher et al., 1973), plasma concentrations of ACTH and cortisol were determined at five- and 20-minute intervals in one normal subject to estimate the number, frequency, and distribution time of ACTH and cortisol secretory episodes, their half-life, as well as the amounts and secretion rates of ACTH and cortisol per unit time. From these critical results concerning 24 hour temporal relations in ACTH and cortisol secretory episodes, Gallagher's group concluded that the superimposed diurnal rhythm profiles of ACTH and cortisol of the pituitary-adrenal axis were definitely programmed by CNS regulators, rather than by simple negative feedback control of pituitary ACTH by adrenal cortisol.

Although simple feedback regulation of ACTH by cortisol represents only one aspect of a complex CNS regulatory mechanism, secretory episodes of cortisol do occur consistently five to ten minutes after ACTH secretory episodes in normal human subjects (Gallagher et al., 1973). Since significant increases in cortisol are such a characteristic adrenal re-

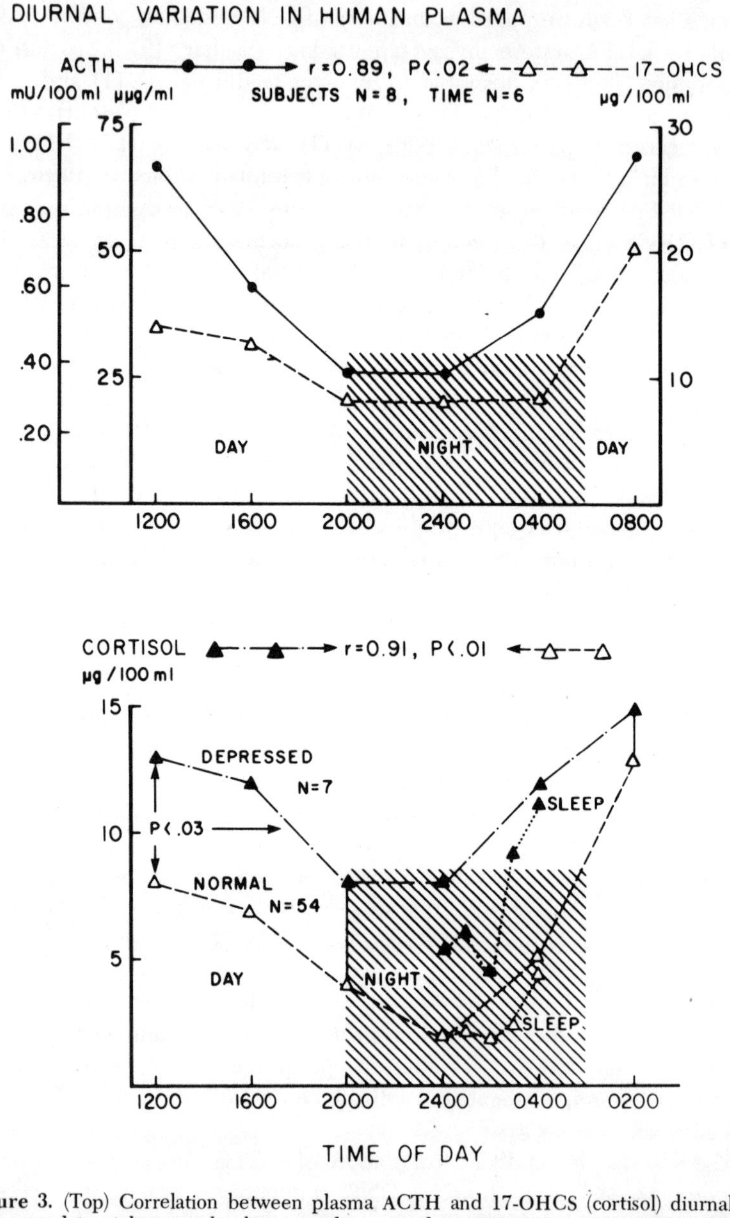

Figure 3. (Top) Correlation between plasma ACTH and 17-OHCS (cortisol) diurnal profiles reported in eight normal subjects as determined at 1200, 1000, 2000, 2400, 0400, and 0800 hours (Berson and Yalow, 1968). (Bottom) Diurnal cortisol profiles for seven depressed and 54 normal subjects determined across the above 24-hour time intervals (Sachar, 1975).

sponse to ACTH in stress, numerous attempts have been made to establish cortisol levels, including diurnal profiles, in affective disorders. In one of the more widely cited studies, cortisol levels were determined in seven depressed patients at two-hour intervals, over a 24-hour period, and then compared with those of 54 normal subjects (Sachar, 1975, 1977). The results of this and similar studies led to the conclusion that diurnal cortisol secretory patterns of depressed subjects differed from those of normals in the following respects: (1) the 24-hour cortisol levels in depressed patients were higher, (2) their diurnal temporal profile was not comparable to that of normals, (3) the 24-hour pattern of depressed patients was characterized by more secretory episodes, and (4) these differences in 24-hour secretory patterns of cortisol in affective disorders were not due simply to differences in stress reactivity. To examine the evidence for some of these hypotheses, the cortisol levels reported in the widely cited Sachar (1975) study were plotted for the seven depressed and 54 normal subjects across the same 1200, 1600, 2000, 2400, 0400, and 0800 hour intervals as those for ACTH and cortisol of eight normals (Berson and Yalow, 1968) illustrated in Figure 3. The statistical analyses showed that the cortisol levels of the seven depressed patients were, in fact, significantly higher across the six time intervals covering the 24 hours than those of the 54 normal controls ($p < .03$). A significant correlation coefficient of $r = 0.91$, $p < .01$, indicated, however, that the diurnal temporal cortisol patterns over 24 hours were essentially the same in the depressed and normal subjects, with the important difference of cortisol levels being higher in the depressed group, but showing the same 24-hour temporal profile. The statistically evaluated results of the Sachar (1975) study are illustrated in Figure 3 (bottom).

Although many other studies have reported alterations of cortisol levels in affective disorders, many inconsistencies in this relationship have also been reported in the clinical literature (Carpenter and Bunney, 1971; Carroll and Mendels, 1976). These discrepancies have been attributed to: (1) differences in psychotic turmoil and ego defense or coping mechanisms of different subjects at the time of testing, (2) differences between states of acute and chronic reactivity to stress in psychopathology, (3) differences in methods and time intervals of cortisol evaluation, and (4) possible differences in cortisol turnover in affective disorders rather than in plasma cortisol concentrations (Carroll and Mendels, 1976).

Several other potentially valuable approaches have also been used to study possible correlations between psychopathology and dysfunction of CNS regulatory mechanism of ACTH and cortisol. Such compounds as dexamethasone, metyrapone, insulin, lysine-vasopressin, and pyrogen have all been used to evaluate dysfunction in neuroendocrine regulatory mechanisms (Table 1). Results from the dexamethasone and insulin tolerance tests, in conjunction with the cited possible differences in circadian rhythm profiles of cortisol, suggest that there may in fact be significant differences in LHPA activity in some affective disorders, particularly in some depressive states (Carroll and Mendels, 1976).

Because of the great lability of the LHPA axis in response to environmental influences, the problems of sensitivity and specificity of ACTH bioassay and of appropriate statistical evaluations pose formidable difficulties for testing the LHPA system under baseline and stress conditions. However, several studies have attempted to establish differences between normal subjects and psychiatric patients in pituitary ACTH secretion under baseline and stress, or drug-challenge and activation conditions. In a control study, baseline plasma ACTH levels were reported to range between 12 and 55 pg/ml in 36 young normal subjects (Landon and Greenwood, 1968). In the study by Berson and Yalow (1968), the mean plasma ACTH value of nine depressed patients was 75 pg/ml, significantly higher than the baseline mean of 22 pg/ml of 70 normal controls ($p < .05$) and the 45 pg/ml mean for 223 nonpsychiatric patients ($p < .05$). In the nine depressed patients who were first sedated and then exposed for 30 seconds to electroconvulsive therapy (ECT), mean plasma ACTH increased very significantly to 300 pg/ml by five to ten minutes after ECT. It remained significantly higher at 15 minutes ($p < .08$) and was significantly lower than the baseline mean of 75 pg/ml by two hours after ECT ($p < .05$). Because of their great relevance, the results from the Berson and Yalow (1968) study were also evaluated statistically for this review and are presented in Figure 4 (top).

Some researchers have proposed that ACTH responses to different categories of stress may be mediated either through CNS neurogenic pathways' converging on hypothalamic CRF, or through systemic circulation, involving stress-induced neural impulses from the brainstem to the adrenal medulla, and the "triggering" of pituitary ACTH by increased circulating epinephrine from the adrenal medulla (Vernikos-Danellis, 1965; Harris and George, 1969). Increases in blood ACTH concentrations after an epinephrine infusion have been reported in the rat (Farrell and McCann, 1952) and in human subjects (Vernikos-Danellis and Marks, 1962). In other human studies, however, increases in blood ACTH were not observed (Vance and Shioda, 1964). These conflicting findings suggest that the role of circulating epinephrine in the release of ACTH in man remains questionable. The extensive use of tranquilizers in neuropsychiatric disorders has also prompted considerable interest in their possible role

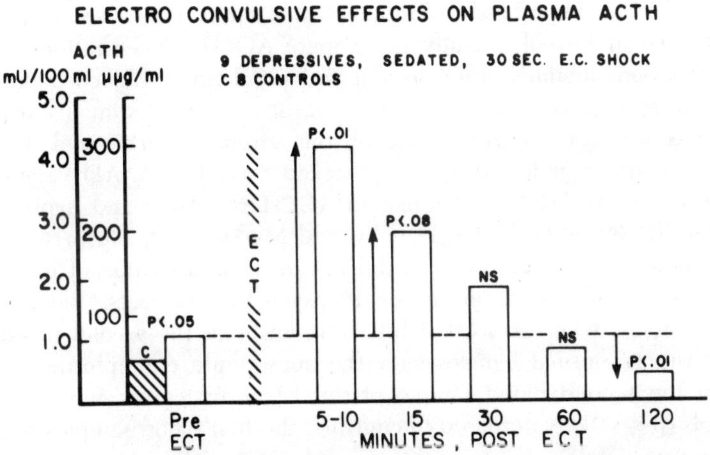

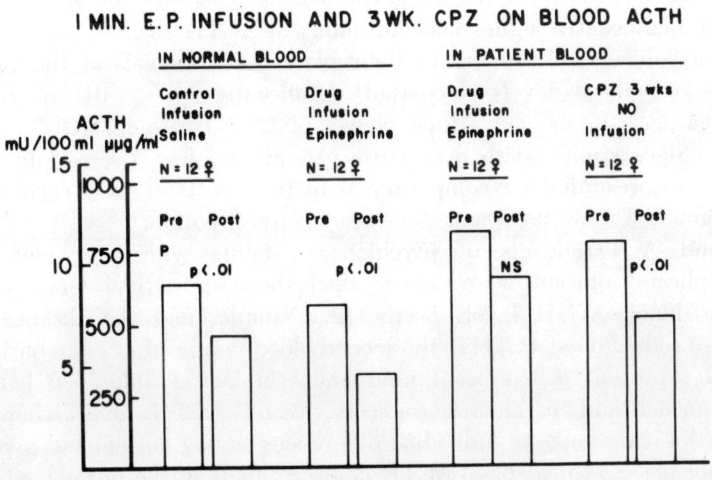

Figure 4. (Top) Plasma ACTH baseline levels in normal controls, general hospital patients, and nine depressed patients (and in the nine depressed patients after electroconvulsive (ECT) therapy) (Berson and Yalow, 1968). (Bottom) Blood ACTH levels pre- and post-saline, and after one-minute epinephrine infusion in normal and psychiatric female patients, and the effects of three weeks of chlorpromazine (CPZ) treatment in psychiatric patients (Ordy et al., 1976).

as hypothalamic neurotransmitter- and/or CRF-blocking agents for inhibiting the pituitary output of ACTH in response to stress (Marks, Hall, and Bhattacharya, 1970; de Wied and de Jong, 1974; Frohman and Stachura, 1975) and in psychopathology (Ordy et al., 1976).

To test the hypotheses of epinephrine-induced release of pituitary ACTH, we undertook a study to compare ACTH concentrations in samples of blood obtained from normal and psychiatric subjects before and after an epinephrine infusion (Ordy et al., 1976). Estimates of blood ACTH concentrations were made by the adrenal ascorbic-acid depletion (AAAD) method in hydrocortisone-blocked rats. The AAAD values were converted to ACTH by reference to ACTH standards and expressed as mU ACTH/100 ml (Vernikos-Danellis and Marks, 1962). Surprisingly, the one-minute epinephrine infusion did not result in a significant increase in blood ACTH of the 12 normal or 12 psychiatric subjects. Blood ACTH concentrations were, in fact, significantly lower in the second blood sample of the 12 normal females after the one-minute epinephrine infusion, and in the second blood sample of the 12 normal saline-infused female controls ($p < .01$). Compared to controls, the first blood samples of the 12 female psychiatric patients in the epinephrine infusion group and also the 12 patients in the three-week chlorpromazine (CPZ) treatment group contained significantly higher concentrations of ACTH than those of the 24 normal subjects. Compared to their blood ACTH levels at the time of admission, these levels decreased significantly ($p < .01$) in the 12 psychiatric patients after three weeks of CPZ treatment (Ordy et al., 1976). Since studies with psychiatric patients are few, the results of our study are presented for comparison with the effects of ECT reported by Berson and Yalow (1968) and shown in Figure 4 (bottom).

Blood ACTH levels of psychiatric patients with pre- and post-epinephrine infusion were higher than those of normal females. The higher blood ACTH levels in the first sample, and the absence of a prompt reduction of ACTH in the second blood sample after epinephrine infusion represent a significant neuroendocrinological difference between the normal and psychiatric subjects. Blood ACTH levels, however, showed a wide range of individual differences among normal and psychiatric subjects. So-called basal ACTH concentrations in the normal subjects, as determined by bioassay, were also higher than those reported in the earlier studies using radioimmunoassay (Berson and Yalow, 1968; Gallagher et al., 1973). Similarly, wide individual differences have been reported in levels of circulating catecholamines in response to different test conditions and various forms of stress in normal human subjects (von Euler, 1964). According to the "epinephrine-release hypothesis," stress-induced systemic circulation of epinephrine triggers the release of pituitary ACTH. Obviously, conflicting findings on epinephrine-induced release of ACTH have been reported with human subjects. Animal studies have also failed to confirm this hypothesis. Adrenal denervated, medullectomized, sympathectomized, and completely adrenalectomized animals still respond to a variety of stresses with pituitary ACTH secretions (Harris and George, 1969). The significantly lower ACTH levels in our second blood sample also represent paradoxical findings (Figure 4, bottom).

More recent studies, however, have established that (1) epinephrine-secreting ascending neurons from the medulla oblongata project back to the hypothalamus (Hoekfelt et al., 1974); (2) central catecholamine neural pathways may regulate ACTH in response to hemodynamic changes; and (3) not only ACTH, but cortisol, growth hormone, vasopressin, and prolactin may all respond to catecholamine-induced hemodynamic changes (Gann et al., 1977). Concerning the paradoxical findings cited, these more recent studies suggest that bursts of significant increases in circulating catecholamines may inhibit rather than trigger ACTH by their direct effects on CRF, or by reduging the amount of CRF in portal vessels of the median eminence by constricting these portal blood vessels (Ganong, 1977). According to other recent studies, the median eminence and the pituitary have fenestrated capillaries which, by escaping the blood-brain barrier system, make them permeable to some substances in general circulation. Circulating epinephrine and norepinephrine, however, do not seem to influence pituitary ACTH directly (Ganong, 1977). The significant decreases in plasma ACTH reported in psychiatric patients two hours after ECT (Berson and Yalow, 1968), and two minutes after a one-minute epinephrine infusion (Ordy et al., 1976) seem consistent with rapid depletion or a possible inhibitory effect by very rapid bursts of significant increases in circulating catecholamines on pituitary ACTH secretions (Figure 3, top and bottom). However, such other factors as ACTH secretory episodes, the half-life of ACTH and epinephrine, as well as the amounts and secretion rates of ACTH, must also be considered as important factors (Gallagher et al., 1973; Ordy et al., 1976).

Differences in cortisol secretions have led to the proposal that there may be differences in LHPA activity between normal individuals and psychiatric patients, and that these differences are independent of possible variations in stress reactivity (Sachar, 1977). However, since most studies have compared baseline values, stress response, or drug modification of ACTH and cortisol, it is not clear how such a theory could be tested experimentally, even though many clinical observations support the hypothesis (Sachar, 1977).

Changes in Neuroendocrine Regulation of Growth Hormone, Prolactin, and Thyrotropin in Psychopathology

The effects of stress and drugs on the hypothalamic-pituitary-adrenal axis are well known (Mason, 1975). Recent studies have shown that such other pituitary hormones as growth hormone (GH), prolactin (PRL), and thyrotropin (TSH), as well as such target-gland hormones as testosterone, are highly responsive to stress. Since these hormones have widespread effects on biochemical, physiological, and behavioral processes, differences in basal conditions, or in stress reactivity of the hormones between normal and psychiatric subjects, may also provide important clues on neuroendocrine dysfunction in psychopathological states (Sachar, 1975). Consequently, evaluation of diurnal profiles of these hormones and their response to stress and drugs in normal persons and psychiatric patients has also become important in the neuroendocrine-window strategy. As in the case of ACTH, the secretion of GH, PRL, and TSH is regulated by complex limbic, hypothalamic, and extralimbic neurotransmitter interactions, involving both stimulatory and inhibitory factors (RF-IF) designated as hormones (H) when the hypothalamic factors (F) become characterized chemically. Although regulated by different hypothalamic neurotransmitter interactions, GH and PRL have similar polypeptide chemical structures and both hormones may share in a diversity of physiological functions in man (Frantz, 1973). Phylogenetic studies have indicated a common evolutionary ancestral polypeptide origin for the GH-PRL super family (Fellows et al., 1976). There is now considerable evidence on neurotransmitter identity in hypothalamic control of pituitary GH (Martin, 1976), PRL (MacLeod, 1976) and TRH (Lipton et al., 1977). Hypothalamic TRH and pituitary TSH have received considerable attention in drug treatment for depressive disorders (Hollister, Davis, and Berger, 1977) and in reference to the possible changes in endocrine regulation of energy metabolism in these disorders (Heninger, Mueller, and Davis, 1976). An extensive review of the literature concerning hypothalamic neurotransmitters, TRH, pituitary TSH, and the thyroid hormones thyroxine (T4) and triiodothyronine (T3) in depressive illness and in the responses to the antidepressant drug imipramine has been published (Prange et al., 1976). A considerably greater number of recent studies, however, has examined drug-stress interaction effects on hypothalamic regulation of GH and PRL in normal subjects, patients with affective disorders, and laboratory animals (Sachar, 1976). Regarding possible differences in neuronal regulatory mechanisms for GH and PRL in psychopathology, it seems pertinent to note that GH and PRL daily secretions also occur in episodic bursts, within a broader diurnal profile (Sassin et al., 1972). This secretory pattern may also occur in LH but not in TSH (Willoughby and Martin, 1976).

Until the recent great emphasis on the "dopamine-prolactin probe" in the neuroendocrine-window strategy of biological psychiatry, the second major neuroendocrine system to be studied in affective disorders, after LHPA, was the hypothalamic-pituitary-growth hormone system (Carroll and Mendels, 1976). The earlier emphasis on GH in psychopathology was based on the findings that GH is one of the more stress-responsive hormones and that it reacts very promptly to a variety of psychological, physiological, and chemical influences (Pecile and Muller, 1976). The increased interest in GH also resulted, in part, from (1) the development of a sensitive radioimmunoassay for GH, (2) its regulation by hypothalamic catecholamines, and (3) the proposal that abnormalities in brain catecholamines may be major neurochemical factors in mental illness. As is the case for ACTH, GH levels are affected by a large number of psychological, neural, metabolic, and pharmacological factors. The factors used to investigate GH in psychopathology, particularly in depressed patients, included evaluation of GH and PRL in relation to slow-wave REM sleep (Sassin et al., 1972) and in response to tests with l-dopa, l-5-hydroxytryptophan, apomorphine, ACTH 1-24, and insulin hypoglycemia (Carroll and Mendels, 1976). Since GH levels are related to diurnal sleep-wake cycles, several studies have attempted to evaluate possible differences in the GH diurnal profile between normal subjects and psychiatric patients. In contrast to ACTH and cortisol which appear elevated in depressed patients, GH levels are extremely low, less than 2 ng/ml, in both normals and patients, under baseline conditions. These levels do not appear to increase significantly in depressed patients. In normal subjects, a significant increase in plasma GH levels has been reported soon after sleep onset, especially after appearance of the slow-wave REM stage (Sassin et al., 1972). The Sassin study showed (1) that basal prolactin levels were significantly higher than GH levels in the same normal subjects, (2) that both GH and prolactin increased significantly during sleep, and (3) that they had the same diurnal pattern in human plasma, across the six selected time intervals of 1200, 1600, 2000, 2400, 0400, and 0800 hours (Sassin et al., 1972). Figure 5 (top) illustrates diurnal variations in human plasma PRL in relation to GH as observed in the same six normal subjects by Sassin's group (1972). Although the correlation of $r = 0.52$, $n = 6$, $p > .29$, between diurnal variations in PRL and GH was not significant statistically, it is apparent that the diurnal profiles for PRL and GH are strikingly similar (Figure 5, top).

There is an extensive clinical literature on GH responses in affective disorders and of modification of these responses by drugs (Carroll and Mendels, 1976). The test most widely used for GH in affective disorders has been insulin hypoglycemia. The hypoglycemic responses of GH to insulin in various depressive conditions have been reported to be impaired

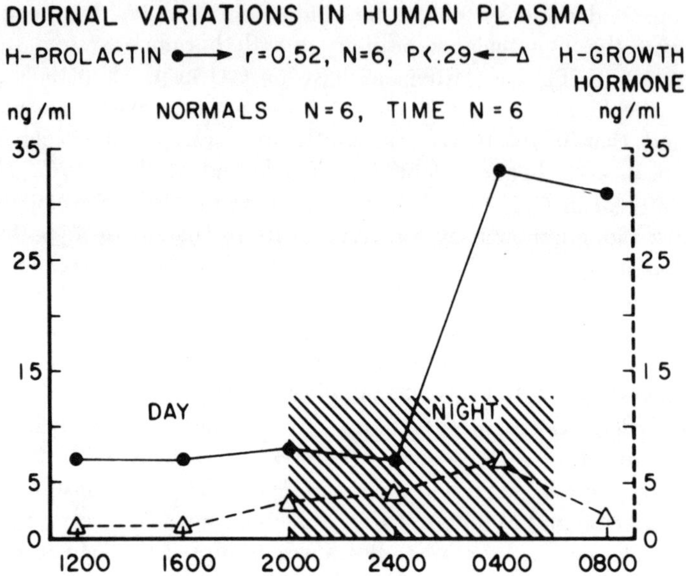

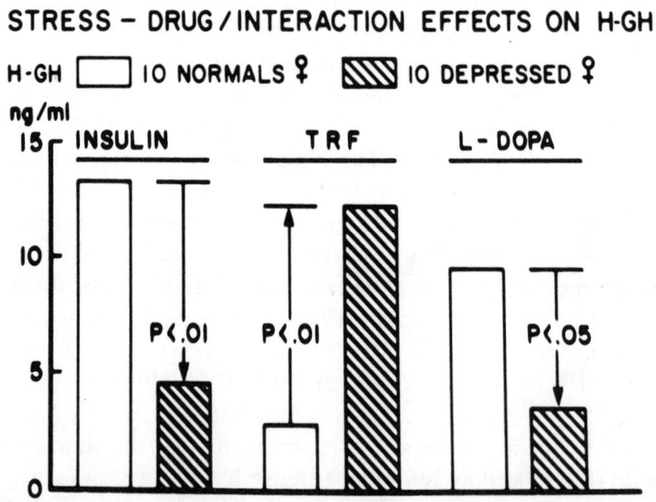

Figure 5. (Top) Diurnal variations in human plasma prolactin (PRL) in relation to growth hormone (GH) reported in six normal subjects (Sassin et al., 1972). (Bottom) Effects of insulin, thyrotropin-releasing factor (TRF), and l-dopa on growth hormone (GH) levels in normals and in depressed patients (Gruen et al., 1975; Prange et al., 1976; Sachar et al., 1972; Maeda et al., 1975).

(Mueller, Heninger, and MacDonald, 1969). Many other conflicting results concerning GH in affective disorders have been reported (Carroll and Mendels, 1976). Statistically reliable differences in GH levels between normal females and depressed females in response to insulin hypoglycemia (Gruen et al., 1975), TRF (Maeda et al., 1975) and l-dopa (Sachar et al., 1972) have been reported. Drug effects on GH levels, as reported in the three studies cited above, were also statistically evaluated for this review. The GH levels in normal and depressed females were significantly lower after insulin hypoglycemia ($p < .01$), significantly higher after TRF ($p < .01$), and also significantly lower after l-dopa ($p < .05$), compared to appropriate controls. The effects of insulin, TRF, and l-dopa on GH levels in normal subjects and in depressed patients, as reported in the three studies, are illustrated in Figure 5 (bottom).

There is little doubt that, like ACTH, GH and PRL are quite responsive to a wide range of emotional stimuli. These pituitary hormones are also part of the more labile and very rapidly responding psychoendocrine systems in human (Mason, 1975; Sachar, 1976) and nonhuman primates (Brown, Schalch, and Reichlin, 1971; Ordy et al., 1976). Many of the complex hypothalamic neurotransmitter and neuroendocrine transducer mechanisms for regulating pituitary GH (Martin, 1976) and PRL secretions (MacLeod, 1976) seem to differ in identity but be analogous in principle to those for CRF regulation of ACTH (Jones, Hillhouse, and Burden, 1976). The important difference is, however, that the two hormones lack specific peripheral target organs for partial regulation by negative feedback, as is the case for pituitary ACTH, TSH, and the gonadotropins LH and FSH (follicle-stimulating hormone). Evidence from clinical studies of possible abnormalities of GH secretion in depression has suggested that the insulin-hypoglycemia differences in GH responses between normal and depressed patients may represent an important aspect of neuroendocrine dysfunction (Gruen et al., 1975). The results presented in Figure 5 (bottom) also indicate significant differences in response of GH to TRF and l-dopa in depressed patients. At this stage, however, clinical findings must be interpreted with considerable caution until more specific tests and controls for GH assessment are standardized (Carroll and Mendells, 1976).

Psychotropic Drug Effects on Neuroendocrine Regulation in Psychopathology

There is now considerable evidence that abnormalities in such neuroregulators as neurotransmitters and in neuropeptides may be involved in maladaptive behavior and psychiatric disorders (Usdin, Hamburg, and Barchas, 1977) and that hormones play an important role in the regulation of emotional behavior and in psychopathology (Sachar, 1976). Since virtually all psychotropic drugs seem to modify brain neurotransmitters and concentrations of hormones in the blood of man and experimental animals, it is apparent that they exert this effect through the neuroendocrine system (Wurtman and Fernstrom, 1976). Until recently, the primary interest in psychotropic drugs was in their antipsychotic properties in relation to blockade of brain DA and NE receptors. Psychotropic drug effects on neuroendocrines and on hormone concentrations in the blood were of minor clinical interest because they seemed to represent only undesirable side effects. Recent studies suggest, however, that a common property of all psychotropic drugs may be based on the blockade of dopamine receptors in the brain (Iversen, 1975). One of the dramatic psychotropic drug effects on the neuroendocrine system may be the significant increases in prolactin secretion produced by drug interactions with dopamine receptors in the hypothalamus (Wurtman and Fernstrom, 1976).

Earlier reviews have examined the effects of drugs on hypothalamic-anterior pituitary function (de Wied and de Jong, 1974) and of neuropharmacological control of neuroendocrine function in human beings (Frohman and Stachura, 1975). Many recent studies have also examined a wide range of endocrine effects of psychotropic drugs. On the basis of an extensive review of the literature, "mediator," "tropin-balance," and "steroid receptor" theories have been proposed for interpreting the neuropharmacological effects of psychotherapeutic drugs on the endocrines (Givant and Sulman, 1976). Earlier reviews have summarized psychotropic drug effects on the LHPA system (Shader, Giller, and DiMascio, 1970). From a survey of the more recent literature it is apparent that psychotropic drugs affect the LHPA system primarily through their effects on neurotransmitters, neuropeptides, and hormones (Wurtman and Fernstrom, 1976). Although extensive information has been accumulated on psychotropic drug effects on emotion and behavior (Iversen and Iversen, 1975), the clinical effects of high-dose, chronic administration of psychotropic drugs in the human remain to be evaluated (Sachar, 1976).

Human studies of psychotropic drug effects on the LHPA system are quite limited and provide only fragmentary evidence concerning specific limbic neurotransmitter regulation of hypothalamic CRF, pituitary ACTH, and adrenal cortisol. Since the LHPA system is critically involved in the regulation of emotions, it is apparent that the so-called tranquilizing properties of such antipsychotic drugs as the phenothiazines and butyrophenones must occur predominantly through the LHPA system. A great deal of research has been devoted to determine whether and how dopamine receptor blockade is related to the antipsychotic actions of neuroleptic drugs and to their motor side effects in man (Matthysse, 1977). Regarding the major neuroendocrine effects of psychotropic drug effects, considerable evidence indicates that the neuroendocrine transducer-hormone secreting cells appear to be controlled by the same neurotransmitter pathways that react to the psychotropic drugs (Wurtman and Fernstrom, 1976). More specifically, the CNS neurotransmitters acetycholine, dopamine, norepinephrine, serotonin, and GABA mediate the actions of most psychotropic drugs; the same neurotransmitters seem to be involved in the regulation of the secretory activity of neuroendocrine transducer cells. However, most of the evidence concerning psychotropic drug effects on the LHPA system is based on animal studies. The interpretation of psychotropic drug effects on the LHPA system in man poses formidable difficulties since these drug effects are generally confounded with psychological drug expectancy, novel test experience, and such other factors as diet, smoking, ethanol, and physical fitness. In addition to these complex factors in human beings, there is also the general ambiguity in the diagnostic classification of many psychiatric patients. Consequently, more direct evidence on the psychotropic drug-stress interaction effects on hypothalamic neurotransmitters, pituitary ACTH and adrenal corticosteroids in nonhuman primates and other animals will be presented in a subsequent section.

In numerous clinical observations the most widely cited neuroendocrine side effects of psychotropic drugs seem to be the changes in mammary gland function after acute or chronic administration of the phenothiazines, butyrophenones, and almost all other antipsychotic compounds. It is now also widely accepted that the acute and/or chronic administration of the psychotropic drugs decreases psychotic symptoms, blocks dopamine receptors in the brain, and produces significantly increased serum PRL levels. Animal studies indicate that dopamine may control a PRL-inhibitory factor (PIF), or that dopamine itself may be the hypothalamic hormone that inhibits PRL release after it is secreted into the pituitary portal system (Wurtman and Fernstrom, 1976). Much recent work has been devoted to the possibility that the hypothalamic-dopamine prolactin responses to psychotropic drugs may represent a key approach to clarifying the role of brain dopamine in psychopathology (Meltzer and Fang, 1976; Sachar et al., 1976, 1977; Langer et al., 1977). The demonstrated role of hypothalamic dopamine in inhibiting PRL secretion, either directly or indirectly, may provide a unique opportunity for studying the "functional involvement of a single neurohormone in hypothalamic regulation" (Langer et al., 1977). Single small doses of various psychotropic drugs seem to block hypothalamic DA and produce significant increases in human PRL secretion, without affecting plasma levels of other pituitary hormones (Rubin et al., 1976). The effects of various psychotropic drugs on PRL have been tested on normal human subjects as well as patients suffering from several different psychiatric disorders. Figure 6 (top) illustrates the rapid time course of serum prolactin responses to 25 mg of CPZ in a schizophrenic patient, and also the rapid effects of 1 mg of haloperidol (HPD) and of 500 mg of l-dopa in a normal subject (Sachar et al., 1976). Figure 6 (bottom) illustrates the more extended time course of the PRL response in a normal male to 50 mg of thioridazine, 50 mg of CPZ, and 1 mg of HPD (Sachar et al., 1976, 1977).

In a very recent study, the effects of single doses of haloperidol, perchlorperazine, and thiothixene, representing three major chemical classes of psychotropic drugs, were examined on dose-PRL response curves in 19 normal young males in a comprehensive series of weekly tests (Langer et al., 1977). It would be interesting to determine if the drug dose-PRL response curves of psychiatric patients would differ significantly from those reported for normal controls in Langer's study. In one of the more comprehensive clinical studies, Meltzer and Fang (1976) examined serum PRL levels in a large number of newly admitted psychiatric patients, as well as in patients treated with chlorpromazine, thioridazine, and trifluoperazine with trihexyphenidyl, over a period of several months. Serum PRL levels were examined at 0800 in 60 normal males and 48 normal females. Basal serum PRL levels were examined in 15 male and 16 female newly admitted, drug-untreated schizophrenic patients. Whereas serum PRL levels appeared higher in females than in males, the baseline PRL levels of schizophrenic patients were not significantly higher than those of controls. It is interesting that neither serum PRL nor cortisol levels in single samples collected at 0800 reflected the psychological turmoil of the psychotic patients. The statistical evaluation of the Meltzer and Fang (1976) study is illustrated in Figure 7 (top). Following several weeks' administration of thioridazine, chlorpromazine, and trifluoperazine with trihexyphenidyl, serum PRL levels increased significantly in response to all three drugs. The PRL increase was also significantly higher in females (Figure 7, top). In the same study, serum PRL levels were correlated statistically with psychotic behavior, which was evaluated on a rating scale for schizophrenic symptoms in relation to thioridazine medication over a three-month period. The statistical evaluations of the Meltzer and Fang (1976)

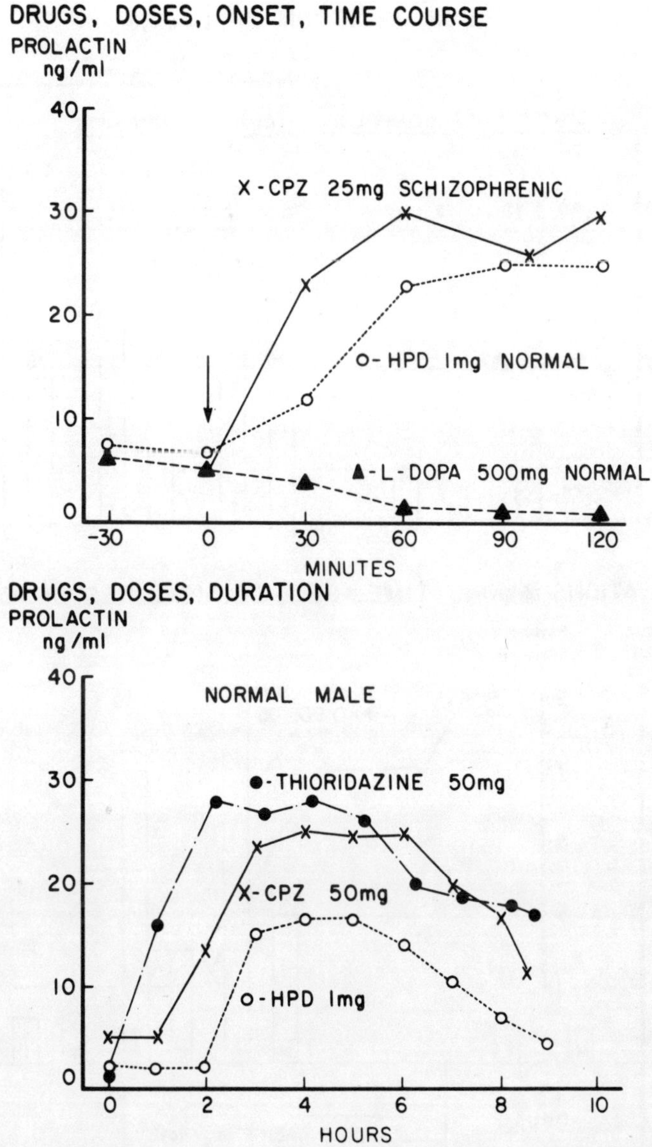

Figure 6. (Top) Rapid time course of serum prolactin responses (PRL) to 25 mg of chlorpromazine (CPZ) in schizophrenic patient, to 1 mg of haloperidol (HPD) and 500 mg of l-dopa in normal subject (Sachar et al., 1976). (Bottom) Extended time course of PRL response in a normal male to 50 mg of thioridazine, 50 mg of chlorpromazine (CPZ), and 1 mg of haloperidol (HPD) (Sachar et al., 1977).

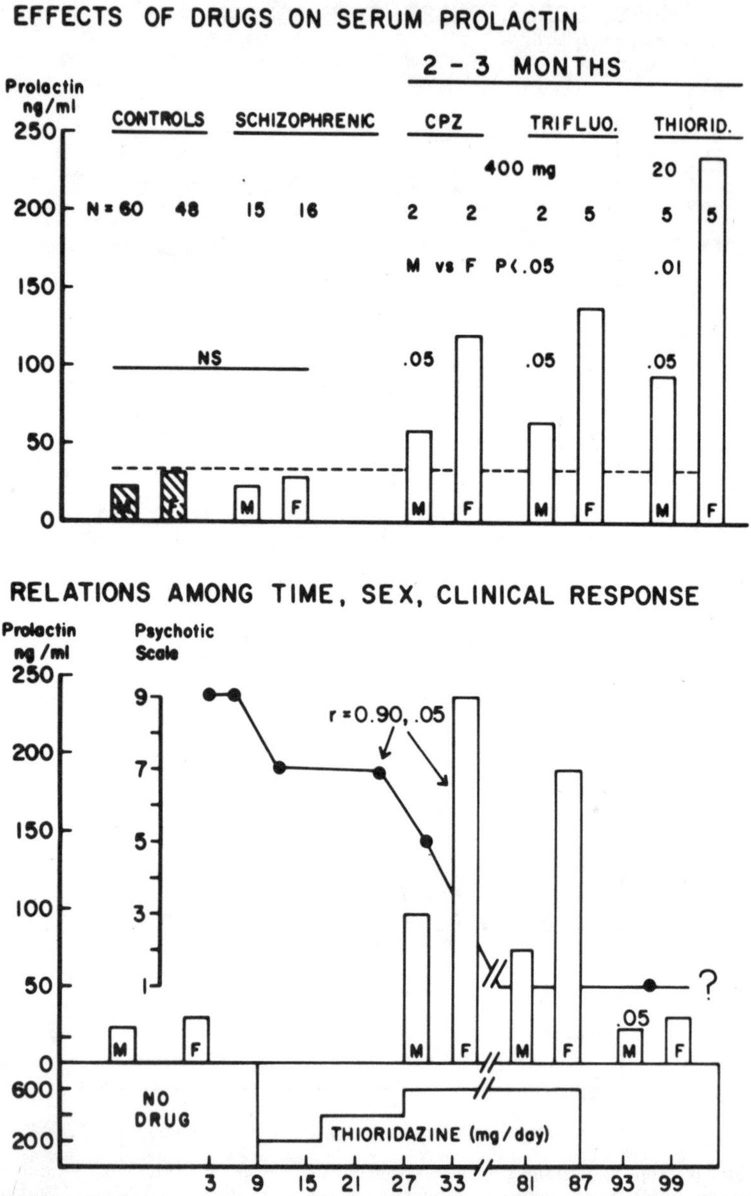

Figure 7. (Top) Serum prolactin (PRL) levels in normal controls, newly admitted psychiatric patients, and in patients treated with chlorpromazine (CPZ), thioridazine (thiorid.), and trifluoperazine (trifluo.) with trihexyphenidyl (Meltzer and Fang, 1976). (Bottom) Serum PRL levels correlated with psychotic symptoms as rated on behavior scale in relation to thioridazine over a three-month period. Note disassociation among psychotic symptoms, serum PRL levels, and cessation of thioridazine medication (?) at end of three months (Meltzer and Fang, 1976).

study show a significant negative correlation, $r = -0.53$, $p < .05$, between decreases in daily ratings of psychotic behavior and increases in serum PRL levels over a three-month period. The drug effects were significant in males ($p < .05$) but not quite significant in females ($p > .25$). CPZ treatment administered for two to three months was discontinued in nine patients. Serum PRL levels decreased promptly from 77 ng/ml in four males and from 190 ng/ml in four females to the normal range of 25 to 50 ng/ml. In these eight patients, serum PRL levels decreased significantly to baseline levels within 48 to 72 hours. Only one of the eight patients showed a significant increase in psychotic symptoms as the drug was discontinued temporarily. The other seven patients retained their improvements as reflected in the reduced psychotic symptoms evaluated on the rating scale (Meltzer and Fang, 1976). The relations among clinical response on the psychotic scale, the serum PRL levels, the dosage and time course of thioridazine treatment, as well as the important observations concerning the disassociation among these variables following cessation of drug treatment are illustrated in Figure 7 (bottom).

There is now convincing evidence concerning the effects of psychotropic drugs on the dopamine-prolactin interaction effects in normal human subjects and in various categories of psychiatric patients (Sachar, 1976). Numerous important issues remain to be clarified, however, before the "dopamine-prolactin probe" can be used as a fundamental tool in the neuroendocrine-window strategy in biological psychiatry. Regarding psychotropic drug effects on hypothalamic dopamine, it is true that earlier studies indicated that dopamine from the tuberoinfundibular (TI) tract controls the release of a prolactin-inhibiting factor (PIF), which inhibits prolactin secretion (McCann et al., 1972). There is now some evidence that TI dopamine may directly inhibit PRL by being released into the pituitary-portal circulation (Wurtman and Fernstrom, 1976). Despite this recent evidence, it seems unlikely that the hypothalamic-pituitary regulation of PRL can be associated with a single neurohormone (see Figure 2 for a model of neurotransmitter regulation of CRF). A second major point to be clarified is the disassociation between the psychological turmoil of newly admitted schizophrenic patients and their serum PRL levels (Figure 7, top). Similarly, no correlation exists between psychotic behavior and serum PRL levels after termination of drug treatment (Figure 7, bottom) (Meltzer and Fang, 1976). Finally, it should be emphasized that the physiological role of PRL in man has not been established (Frantz, 1973). In its responses to various kinds of stress, PRL seems to resemble the responses of GH and ACTH. However, PRL also differs from these hormones since its mode of CNS regulation appears to be entirely inhibitory. In addition, the stress-induced release of PRL does not seem to have specific metabolic effects (Frantz, 1973). Drug studies have also shown that chlorpromazine and l-dopa have opposite effects on PRL compared to GH. Clarification of these issues requires additional studies.

Psychotropic Drug-Stress Interaction Effects on Hypothalamic Catecholamines, Pituitary ACTH, and Adrenal Corticosteroids in Nonhuman Primates and the Rat

Some studies of the effects of drugs on the LHPA system have shown that the phenothiazines, butyrophenones, and many other compounds may inhibit stress-induced pituitary ACTH through their effects on hypothalamic neurotransmitters, particularly the catecholamines (de Wied and de Jong, 1974; Frohman and Stachura, 1975). However, extensive animal studies have shown significant increases in ACTH and corticosteroids after CPZ and reserpine (Marks, Hall, and Bhattacharya, 1970). Pretreatment with MAO inhibitors prevented reserpine-induced release of ACTH by some unknown effect on CRF. Based on these studies, it has been proposed that the psychotropic drugs may remove hypothalamic catecholamine inhibitory control over CRF and ACTH. Since CRF regulation of ACTH seems to be stimulatory (Ganong, 1977), it is not clear how psychotropic drugs affect CRF. CRF has not been characterized chemically. The direct responses of CRF to psychotropic drugs have not been determined as yet (Jones, Hillhouse, and Burden, 1976). It is also possible that psychotropic drugs may have some effects on ACTH and cortisol independent of their effects on hypothalamic catecholamines and CRF. Only these types of fundamental studies can clarify the effects of psychotropic drugs on CRF control over ACTH and cortisol. Studies with human subjects are not feasible. As a result, human studies provide only fragmentary, indirect and inconclusive evidence concerning psychotropic drug modification of hypothalamic neurotransmitter control over CRF and stress induced changes in pituitary ACTH and adrenal cortisol secretions. Studies with diurnal primates are also few. Most of the evidence on drug-stress interaction in the LHPA system is based on studies with rats. In one study with nonhuman primates , acute and chronic psychotropic drug-stress interaction effects were examined in hypothalamic norepinephrine and serotonin, pituitary ACTH and adrenal ascorbic acid in the squirrel monkey (Ordy, Samorajski, and Schroeder, 1966). In this and subsequent studies (Ordy et al., 1976), we undertook some acute experiments to examine the effects of social isolation, one-hour electric shock, a single dose of chlorpromazine (15 mg/kg intraperitoneally [i.p.]), haloperidol (1.0 mg), and reserpine (10 mg/kg i.p.) on hypothalamic norepinephrine and serotonin. Since previous experiments had shown stress decreases in hypothalamic NE, the effects of pretreatment with a single dose of CPZ and HPD on the inhibition of electric shock-induced decreases in hypothalamic NE were also examined. In these acute experiments, 12 hours of social isolation resulted in significant ventromedial hypothalamic (VMH) NE depletion to 0.60 mg/g, compared to basal levels of 1.60 mg/g in nonhandled controls. A single injection of CPZ had no effect two hours after injection on VMH norepinephrine levels. A single injection of reserpine reduced NE levels significantly to 0.20 mg/g after 12 hours. Pretreatment with a single dose of CPZ (15 mg/kg i.p.), or HPD (2.5 mg/kg i.p.) one hour before a one-hour electric shock exposure, effectively inhibited the electric shock depletion of hypothalamic (VMH) NE. One hour of electric shock also resulted in a decrease of 5-HT in the dorsomedial hypothalamic (DMH) region. The results of these acute experiments are illustrated in Figure 8 (top). The concentrations of ACTH in pituitary tissue and of adrenal ascorbic acid were also examined in controls and in one-hour electric-shock-treated monkeys. Pituitary ACTH levels increased from a mean of 17.3 in controls to 25.0 mU of ACTH/mg of pituitary tissue in the electric-shock-treated monkeys. The results of these acute experiments are illustrated in Figure 8 (bottom). The critical acute and chronic experiments on drug-stress interaction effects on the HPA axis remain to be done to determine whether or not pretreatment with CPZ or HPD would inhibit hypothalamic NE, 5-HT, pituitary ACTH, and adrenal cortisol (Figure 8, bottom-middle).

Although studies of drug-stress interaction effects on the LHPA system in nonhuman primates are fragmentary, several other studies have used lesion techniques, drugs, and stress to examine hypothalamic mediation of GH and adrenal cortisol responses in the squirrel monkey (Brown, Schalch, and Reichlin, 1971). Other studies have used stress and drugs to evaluate plasma cortisol, GH, and circulating catecholamines to study emotional arousal by a variety of stimuli as reflected in patterns of endocrine hormones in the rhesus monkey (Mason, 1975).

Recently, other animal studies have clarified considerably the role of hypothalamic NE and DA in the tonic inhibition of hypothalamic CRF, pituitary ACTH, and adrenal corticosteroids (Scapagnini and Preziosi, 1973; van Loon, 1973; Brownstein et al., 1976; Jones, Hillhouse, and Burden, 1976; Ganong, 1977; Palkovits, 1977). Although both DA and 5-HT have been shown to decrease significantly in response to stress in some hypothalamic nuclei, studies using selective blockers of dopamine-ß-hydroxylase (DBH) for decreasing NE without affecting DA, and drug studies using apomorphine to stimulate dopamine receptors, have shown

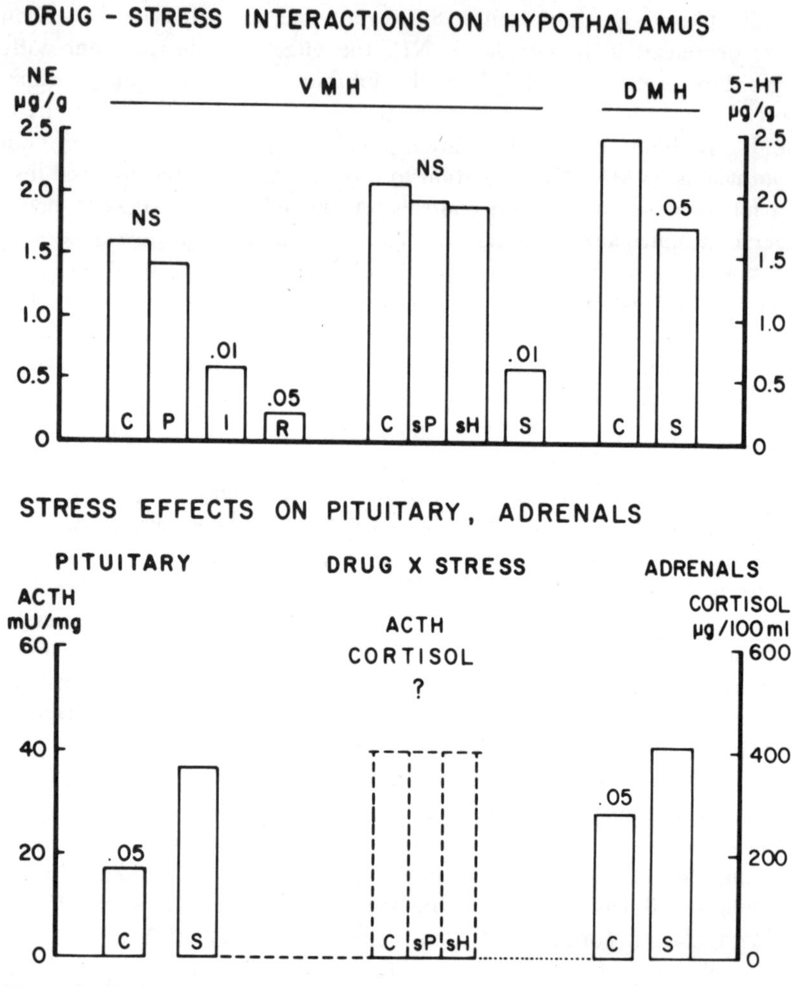

Figure 8. (Top) Drug-stress interaction effects on hypothalamic norepinephrine (NE) in ventromedial area (VMH) and serotonin (5-HT) in dorsomedial area (DMH). Control (C), phenothiazine (P), social isolation (I), reserpine (R), electric shock (S); pretreatment with phenothiazine before shock (sP) and with haloperidol (sH). (Bottom) Stress (S) effects alone on pituitary ACTH and adrenal cortisol. Drug-stress interaction effects on ACTH and cortisol remain to be determined for correlation with hypothalamic NE and corticotropin-releasing factor.

that hypothalamic NE inhibits CRF and ACTH, and that DA exerts no significant effect on CRF and ACTH regulation. It is also possible, however, that NE and GABA have no direct effect on CRF but only inhibit the stimulatory effects of ACh and/or 5-HT (Ganong, 1977). A hypothetical model of hypothalamic neurotransmitter regulation of hypothalamic CRF (Jones, Hillhouse, and Burden, 1976) and of pituitary ACTH is presented in Figure 2. More recent studies based on immunohistochemical and microchemical evidence provide more details, including possible alternative models of hypothalamic neurotransmitter regulation of CRF and pituitary ACTH (Palkovits, 1977; Ganong, 1977).

Effects of Neuropeptides, Hormones and Catecholamines on Learning, Memory, Motivation, Emotion

Learning has generally been associated with the neocortex, whereas arousal, motivation and emotion have been related to changes in the autonomic nervous system, and the secretions of the endocrine organs. In many recent studies, learning, motivation and emotion have been linked conceptually as an integrated adaptive process through the various components of the limbic system. However, the exact roles of the various limbic system components in the regulation of learning, motivation and emotion remain to be clarified. It is apparent that neuropeptides, neurotransmitters, and hormones have widespread effects not only as regulators of coordinated physiological activity throughout the body, but that they are also intimately involved in learning, motivation, and emotion. Physiologically, it is known that ACTH and corticosteroids of the LHPA system influence enzymes involved in the metabolism of catecholamines. Catecholamines in turn influence adenylate cyclase activity, which is involved in the regulation of cellular, including neuronal, metabolism. Recent studies have shown that analogs, or fragments, of ACTH $^{4-10}$, melanocyde-stimulating hormone (β-MSH), and of lipotropin-stimulating hormone (ß-LPH) may also exert effects on learning and memory in hypophysectomized rats independent of their "classical endocrine" effects (de Wied et al., 1976; de Wied, 1977a). Peptides related to ACTH appear to have short-term behavioral effects, those related to vasopressin long-term ones. It has been reported that a single injection of ACTH $^{4-10}$ delays extinction of a pole-jumping avoidance response in intact rats for several hours, one of vasopressin delays it for several days. The short-term effect of ACTH and related peptides has been related to a temporary increase in arousal and/or motivation. By altering states of arousal and/or motivation, neuropeptides may modify reward properties of environmental stimuli during learning and memory. Impaired avoidance acquisition of hypophysectomized rats in the shuttle box can be restored by treatment with ACTHα- and ß-MSH, ACTH $^{4-10}$, and vasopressin. ACTH $^{4-10}$ is closely related to ß-LPH $^{47-53}$, also to ß-MSH and to α-MSH $^{4-10}$. Which one acts as the precursor molecule of neuropeptides modulating adaptive behavior has not been determined (de Wied, 1977a, b). In addition to the studies cited above, many other experiments have shown modulating influences of catecholamines, ACTH, and other hormones on short-term memory consolidation (McGaugh et al., 1975). Table 2 illustrates the common amino acid sequences of a number of ACTH analogs that have been implicated in learning and memory.

Another interesting and probably related observation concerning the effects of peptides on the brain and on behavior is the demonstration that fragments of neurohypophyseal hormones facilitate the development of both resistance to the analgesic effect of and physical dependence on narcotic analgesics. Recent reports have shown that endogenous peptides with opiate-like activity seem to exist in the brain and in the pituitary. One of the brain peptides reported is a pentapeptide (met-enkephalin), whose structure appears identical to ß-LPH $^{61-65}$ (de Wied, 1977a, b). A related opiate-like peptide recently isolated from hypothalamic neurohypophyseal tissue, α-endorphin, has been reported to be identical to ß-LPH, of which met-enkephalin is the N-terminal pentapeptide (de Wied, 1977a, b). Peptides that affect sleep have also been detected in the brain. Their structures have not been established, but it is known that the hypothalamic-pituitary complex is the source of these peptides, and that hormones from this complex are involved in regulating sleep-waking patterns. It is becoming clear that the hypothalamic-pituitary complex produces large numbers of neuropeptides, which seem to carry specific information to appropriate limbic structures involved in regulation of learning, motivation, and emotion. There are (1) neuropeptides that affect learning, mem-

Table 2

Common Amino Acid Sequences in Corticotropin-Related Peptides

	1	8	9	10	11	12	13	14	15	16	17	18	19	20	21	22	
ß-MSH	ALA . . .	PRO-	TYR-	ARG—	MET-	GLU-	HIS-	PHE-	ARG-	TRY-	GLY—	SER-	PRO-	PRO-	LYS-	AS	
		1	2	3	4	5	6	7	8	9	10	11	12	13			
α-MSH		SER-	TYR-	SER—	MET-	GLU-	HIS-	PHE-	ARG-	TRY-	GLY—	LYS-	PRO-	VAL-NH_2			
		1	2	3	4	5	6	7	8	9	10	11	12	13			39
ACTH		SER-	TYR-	SER—	MET-	GLU-	HIS-	PHE-	ARG-	TRY-	GLY—	LYS-	PRO-	VAL			PHI

ACTH$^{4-10}$ = α-MSH$^{4-10}$ = ß-MSH$^{11-12}$; ACTH$^{1-13}$ = α-MSH$^{1-13}$.
(Adapted from Daughaday, 1974).

ory, motivation, drinking, feeding, and aggression; (2) neuropeptides with opiate-like activity; (3) neuropeptides that affect sleep; and (4) peptides that are involved in the development of tolerance and physical dependence on narcotic drugs (de Wied, 1977a, b).

Although most studies of the effects of neuropeptides and hormones on the brain and on behavior have been conducted with animals, preliminary attempts have also been made to examine the effects of fragments of ACTH, MSH, and related peptides on the behavior of normal human subjects and some psychiatric patients. In one study, daily treatments with 3 to 6 mg of ACTH $^{1-10}$ for five to seven days have been reported to reduce depression, increase communication and elevate mood in extremely depressed schizophrenic patients (Endroczi, 1972). The effects of ACTH$^{1-24}$, ACTH $^{4-10}$, and MSH $^{4-10}$ (Table 2) have been evaluated in 20 normal young males on a battery of electroencephalographic (EEG) and behavioral measures. Although ACTH $^{1-24}$ seemed to have no effects, the ACTH $^{4-10}$ and α-MSH $^{4-10}$ fragments were reported to increase EEG patterns characteristic of attention, improve visual discrimination and memory, and decrease anxiety (Kastin et al., 1975). These human studies appear consistent with some findings reported in animal studies, but they must be considered preliminary and only suggestive.

Summary and Conclusions

In view of the great intricacy of the limbic-hypothalamic-pituitary-adrenal system (LHPA), and the neuroendocrine regulation of the third motor or effector system, as well as recent explosive progress in basic and clinical research, broad generalizations and conclusions are difficult to provide in a brief summary. It may be helpful, however, to recapitulate some of the basic aims, methods, recent results, and possible future directions as major points of reference for the neuroendocrine-window strategy in biological psychiatry.

Basic Aims of Psychoendocrinology

In historical perspective, the aims of psychoendocrinology are specified most succinctly by two researchers who have devoted a lifetime to this new field. As W. B. Cannon wrote in 1922, "Probably before many years have passed we shall have satisfactory tests for the internal secretions, and then shall know better the total expression of an emotional storm in our own bodies."

J. W. Mason (1975), in his extensive review of basic and clinical studies, proposed that ". . . the hormonal trend is a resultant of a balance of opposing and cooperating forces and can be predicted with increasing accuracy as the multiple factors involved, including affective state, defensive organization, social setting, prior experiential or developmental factors, and current activities, can all be evaluated in psychodynamic perspective, for each individual subject" (p. 149).

Development of Microchemical, Immunohistochemical Techniques, Radioimmunoassays

Progress in basic and clinical research on the role of the neuroendocrine system in learning, motivation, and emotion was critically dependent upon development of microchemical and immunohistochemical techniques to identify and localize neurotransmitters and neuropeptides in the brain, and on the concurrent development of sensitive and specific radioimmunoassays of hormones in small samples of blood, urine, and other tissues.

Evidence on Neuroendocrine Dysfunction in Psychopathology

The new techniques have resulted in considerable basic and clinical evidence for an association between neuroendocrine dysfunction and some affective disorders. The more reliable evidence for such an association is that (1) neurochemical studies have implicated alterations in brain catecholamines and serotonin in depressive illness; (2) some of these CNS neurotransmitters also play a critical role in neuroendocrine regulation; (3) a common neuropharmacological property of all psychotropic drugs seems to be a blockade of dopamine and norepinephrine receptors; (4) in depressive illness, drugs that increase brain norepinephrine are effective antidepressants, whereas those that decrease it aggravate symptoms of depression; (5) some depressive illness is accompanied by abnormalities of ACTH and/or cortisol secretions of the LHPA system; major findings include hypersecretion and diurnal variations of cortisol, and escape from dexamethasone suppression; (6) other prominent neuroendocrine dysfunctions reported in depressive illness include decreased growth hormone responses to insulin and l-dopa, increased growth hormone responses to thyrotropin-releasing hormone (TRH), and decreased TSH responses to TRH; however, animal models of depression are not readily available and most human studies are generally descriptive, preliminary, and controversial, since they lack appropriate controls; (7) of the three hormone "probes" of cortisol, growth hormone, and prolactin currently used for diagnostic and therapeutic evaluations, the most clearly demonstrable involvement of hypothalamic catecholamines in pituitary regulation is represented by the dopamine prolactin interaction effects in human beings.

Role of Neurotransmitters, Neuropeptides, Hormones, Catecholamines in Learning, Memory, Motivation, Emotion

Regarding drug-stress interaction effects on the limbic-hypothalamic-pituitary-adrenal axis in animal studies, the evidence indicates that acetylcholine, norepinephrine, serotonin, and γ-aminobutyric acid all play a role in the regulation of corticotropin-releasing factor (CRF), but that norepinephrine is involved in tonic inhibitory regulation of CRF, ACTH and cortisol, and that this norepinephrine inhibition can be modified by such major tranquilizers as chlorpromazine and haloperidol.

Hypothalamic neuropeptides and pituitary hormones seem to exert effects on the brain and consequently on learning, memory, motivation, and emotion independent of their classical endocrine effects. However, the direct effects of a hormone or analog on the brain as a target organ and on behavior are in concordance with the peripheral target-organ secretion effects on tissue, that is, ACTH seems to exert central nervous system effects observable in fear-motivated avoidance learning and also to regulate the release of adrenal corticosteroids, that play a critical role in metabolic adaptation to stress.

Possible Future Neuroendocrine Research Directions in Psychopathology

The provocative dopamine-prolactin interaction has been proposed as a unique opportunity for studying a single neurohormone in normal human subjects, those with affective disorders, and in drug evaluation. When corticotropin-releasing factor is characterized chemically, however, concurrent examination of alterations in neuropeptides (CRF), ACTH, and cortisol of the LHPA system may be more illuminating than concentration on one single component, for example, cortisol in response to stress and drugs.

Also, most studies tend to identify the hypothalamic-pituitary-adrenal axis with stress, the hypothalamic-pituitary-thyroid axis with metabolism, and the hypothalamic-pituitary-gonadal axis with reproduction. Some recent studies suggest that the segregation of the third effector or motor system into three distinct axes may be more apparent than real. In future studies, multivariate designs may be essential to evaluate drug modification of emotions as they are reflected in patterns of hormone secretions in health and disease.

REFERENCES

BERSON, S. A., and YALOW, R. S. 1968. Radioimmunoassay of ACTH in plasma. *J. Clin. Invest.*, 47:2725-2751.

BROWN, G. M. 1975. Psychiatric and neurologic aspects of endocrine disease. *Hosp. Practice*, 10:71-79.

BROWN, G. M., SCHALCH, D. S., and REICHLIN, S. 1971. Hypothalamic mediation of growth hormone and adrenal stress response in the squirrel monkey. *Endocrinology*, 89:694-703.

BROWNSTEIN, M. J., PALKOVITS, M., SAAVEDRA, J. M., and KIZER, J. S. 1976. Distribution of hypothalamic hormones and neurotransmitters within the diencephalon. In L. Martini and W. F. Ganong (eds.), *Frontiers in Neuroendocrinology*, pp. 1-23. New York: Raven Press.

CANNON, W. B. 1922. New evidence for sympathetic control of some internal secretions. *Am. J. Psychiatry*, 2:15-30.

CARPENTER, W. T., and BUNNEY, W. E. 1971. Adrenal cortical activity in depressive illness. *Am. J. Psychiatry*, 128:31-40.

CARROLL, B. J. 1977. Psychiatric disorders and steroids. In E. Usdin, D. A. Hamburg, and J. D. Barchas (eds.), *Neuroregulators and Psychiatric Disorders*, pp. 276-283. New York: Oxford University Press.

CARROLL, B. J., and MENDELS, J. 1976. Neuroendocrine regulation in affective disorders. In E. J. Sachar (ed.), *Hormones, Behavior, and Psychopathology*, pp. 193-244. New York: Raven Press.

DAUGHADAY, W. H. 1974. The adenohypophysis. In R. H. Williams (ed.), *Textbook of Endocrinology*, pp. 31-79. Philadelphia: Saunders.

ENDROCZI, E. 1972. Pavlovian conditioning and adaptive hormones. In S. Levine (ed.), *Hormones and Behavior*, pp. 173-208. New York: Academic Press.

FARRELL, G., and MCCANN, S. M. 1952. Detectable amounts of adrenocorticotropic hormone in blood following epinephrine. *Endocrinology*, 50:274.

FELLOWS, R. E., BOLANDER, F. F., HURLEY, T. W., and HANDWERGER, S. 1976. Isolation and characterization of bovine and ovine placental lactogen. In A. Pecile and E. E. Muller (eds.), *Growth Hormone and Related Peptides*, pp. 315-326. New York: American Elsevier.

FRANTZ, A. G. 1973. The regulation of prolactin secretion in humans. In W. F. Ganong and L. Martin (eds.), *Frontiers in Neuroendocrinology*, pp. 337-374. New York: Oxford University Press.

FROHMAN, L. A. 1975. Neurotransmitters as regulators of endocrine function. *Hosp. Pract.*, April:54-67.

FROHMAN, L. A., and STACHURA, M. E. 1975. Neuropharmacologic control of neuroendocrine function in man, *Metabolism*, 24:211-234.

FUXE, K., and HOEKFELT, T. 1970. Central monoaminergic systems and hypothalamic function. In L. Martini, M. Motta, and F. Fraschini (eds.), *The Hypothalamus*, pp. 123-138. New York: Academic Press.

GALLAGHER, T. F., YOSHIDA, K., ROFFWARG, H. D., FUKUSHIMA, D. K., WEITZMAN, E. D., and HELLMAN, L. 1973. ACTH and cortisol secretory patterns in man. *J. Clin. Endocrinol. Metab.*, 36:1058-1073.

GANN, D. S., WARD, D. G., BAERTSCHI, A. J., CARLSON, D. E., and MARAN, J. W. 1977. Neural control of ACTH release in response to hemorrhage. *Ann. N.Y. Acad. Sci.*, 297:477-497.

GANONG, W. F. 1970. Control of adrenocorticotropin and melanocyte-stimulating hormone secretion. In L. Martini, M. Motta, and F. Fraschini (eds.), *The Hypothalamus*, pp. 313-333. New York: Academic Press.

GANONG, W. F. 1974. Brain mechanisms regulating the secretion of the pituitary gland. In F. O. Schmitt and F. G. Worden (eds.), *The Neurosciences: Third Study Program*, pp. 549-564. Cambridge: MIT Press.

GANONG, W. F. 1977. Neurotransmitters involved in ACTH secretion: Catecholamines. *Ann. N.Y. Acad. Sci.*, 297:509-517.

GIBBS, F. P. 1969. Area of pons necessary for traumatic stress-induced ACTH release under pentobarbital anaesthesia. *Am. J. Physiol.*, 217:84-88.

GIVANT, Y., and SULMAN, F. G. 1976. Endocrine effects of psychotherapeutic drugs. In E. Usdin and I. S. Forrest (eds.), *Psychotherapeutic Drugs*, pp. 387-435. New York: Marcel Dekker.

GRUEN, P. H., SACHAR, E. J., ALTMAN, N., and SASSIN, J. 1975. Growth hormone responses to hypoglycemia in post-menopausal depressed women. *Arch. Gen. Psychiatry*, 32:31-33.

GWINUP, G., and JOHNSON, B. 1975. Clinical testing of the hypothalamic-pituitary-adrenocortical system in states of hypo- and hypercortisolism. *Metabolism*, 24:777-791.

HARRIS, G. W., and GEORGE, R. 1969. Neurohumoral control of the adenohypophysis and the regulation of the secretion of TSH, ACTH, and growth hormone. In W. Haymaker, E. Anderson, and W. J. H. Nauta (eds.), *The Hypothalamus*, pp. 326-388. Springfield: Charles C. Thomas.

HENINGER, G. R., MUELLER, P. S., and DAVIS, L. S. 1976. Responsiveness of endocrine-energy metabolism systems in depression and schizophrenia: Relationships to symptomatology. In E. J. Sachar (ed.), *Hormones, Behavior and Psychopathology*, pp. 237-242. New York: Raven Press.

HOEKFELT, T., FUXE, K., GOLDSTEIN, M., and JOHANSSON, D. 1974. Immunohistochemical evidence for the existence of adrenalin neurons in the rat brain. *Brain Res.*, 66:235-251.

HOLLISTER, L. E., DAVIS, K. L., and BERGER, P. A. 1977. Thyrofropin-releasing hormone and psychiatric disorders. In E. Usdin, D. A. Hamburg, and J. D. Barchas (eds.), *Neuroregulators and Psychiatric Disorders*, pp. 250-257. New York: Oxford University Press.

IVERSEN, L. L. 1975. Dopamine receptors in brain. *Science*, 188:1084-1089.

IVERSEN, S. D., and IVERSEN, L. L. 1975. *Behavioral Pharmacology*. New York: Oxford University Press.

JONES, M. T., HILLHOUSE, E., and BURDEN, J. 1976. Secretion of corticotropin-releasing hormone *in vitro*. In L. Martini and W. F. Ganong (eds.), *Frontiers in Neuroendocrinology*, vol. 4, pp. 195-226. New York: Raven Press.

KASTIN, A. J., SANDMAN, C. A., STRATTON, L. O., SCHALLY, A. V., and MILLER, L. H. 1975. Behavioral and electrographic changes in rat and man after MSH. In W. H. Gispen, Tj. B. van Wimersma Greidanus, B. Bohus, and D. de Wied (eds.), *Prog. Brain Res.*, vol. 42, *Hormones, Homeostasis and the Brain*, pp. 143-150. Amsterdam: Elsevier.

LANDON, J., and GREENWOOD, F. C. 1968. Homologous radioimmunoassay for plasma-levels of corticotrophin in man. *Lancet*, 1:273-276.

LANGER, G., SACHAR, E. J., HALPERN, F. S., GRUEN, P. H., and SOLOMON, M. 1977. The prolactin response to neuroleptic drugs. A test of dopaminergic blockade: neuroendocrine studies in normal men. *J. Clin. Endocrinol. Metab.*, 45:996-1002.

LIDDLE, G. W. 1974. The adrenals. In R. H. Williams (ed.), *Textbook of Endocrinology*, pp. 233-283. New York: W. B Saunders.

LIPTON, M. A., PRANGE, A. J., NEMEROFF, C. B., BREESE, G. R., and WILSON, I. C. 1977. Thyrotropin-releasing hormone: Central effects in man and animals. In E. Usdin, D. A. Hamburg, and J. D. Barchas (eds.), *Neuroregulators and Psychiatric Disorders*, pp. 258-266. New York: Oxford University Press.

LIVINGSTON, K. E., and ESCOBAR, A. 1971. Anatomical basis of the limbic system concept. *Arch. Neurol.*, 24:17-21.

LOCKE, W., and SCHALLY, A. V. 1975. *The Hypothalamus and Pituitary in Health and Disease*. Springfield, Ill.: Charles C. Thomas.

MACLEOD, R. M. 1976. Regulation of prolactin secretion. In L. Martini and W. F. Ganong (eds.), *Frontiers in Neuroendocrinology*, vol. 4, pp. 169-194. New York: Raven Press.

MAEDA, K., KATO, Y., OHGO, S., CHIHARA, K., YOSHIMOTO, Y., YAMAGUSHI, N., KUROMARA, S. and IMURA, H. 1975. Growth hormone and prolactin release after injection of thyrotropin-releasing hormone in patients. *J. Clin. Endocrinol. Metab.* 40:501.

MARKS, B. H., HALL, M. M., and BHATTACHARYA, A. N. 1970. Psychopharmacological effects and pituitary-adrenal activity. In D. de Wied and J. A. W. M. Weijnen (eds.), *Prog. Brain Res.*, vol. 32. *Pituitary, Adrenal and the Brain*, pp. 57-70. Amsterdam: Elsevier.

MARTIN, J. B. 1976. Brain regulation of growth hormone secretion. In L. Martini and W. F. Ganong (eds.), *Frontiers in Neuroendocrinology*, vol. 4, pp. 129-168. New York: Raven Press.

MASON, J. W. 1975. Emotion as reflected in patterns of endocrine regulation. In L. Levi (ed.), *Emotions—Their Parameters and Measurement*, pp. 143-181. New York: Raven Press.

MATTHYSSE, S. W. 1977. The role of dopamine in schizophrenia. In E. Usdin, D. A. Hamburg, and J. D. Barchas (eds.), *Neuroregulators and Psychiatric Disorders*, pp. 3-13. New York: Oxford University Press.

MCCANN, S. M., KALRA, P. S., DONOSO, A. P., BISHOP, W., SCHNEIDER, H. P. G., FAWCETT, C. P., and KRULICH, L. 1972. The role of monoamines in the control of gonadotropin and prolactin secretion. In K. M. Krugge, D. F. Scott, and A. Weindl (eds.), *Median Eminence: Structure and Function*, pp. 224-235. Basel: Karger.

MCEWEN, B. S. 1975. The brain as a target organ of endocrine hormones. *Hospital Practice*, 10:95-104.

MCGAUGH, J. L., GOLD, P. E., VAN BUSKIRK, R., and HAYROCK, J. 1975. Modulating influences of hormones and catecholamines on memory storage processes. In W. H. Gispen, Tj. B. van Wimersma Greidanus, B. Bohus, and D. de Wied (eds.), *Progress in Brain Research*, vol. 42, *Hormones, Homeostasis and the Brain*, pp. 151-162. Amsterdam: Elsevier.

MELTZER, H. Y., and FANG, V. S. 1976. Serum prolactin levels in schizophrenia—effect of antipsychotic drugs: a preliminary report. In E. J. Sachar (ed.), *Hormones, Behavior, and Psychopathology*, pp. 177-192. New York: Raven Press.

MUELLER, P. S., HENINGER, G. R., and MACDONALD, R. K. 1969. Insulin tolerance test in depression. *Arch. Gen. Psychiatry*, 21:587-594.

NAUTA, W. J. H. 1963. Central nervous system organization and the endocrine motor system. In A. V. Nalbandov (ed.), *Advances in Neuroendocrinology*, pp. 5-21. Urbana: University of Illinois Press.

ORDY, J. M., BRIZZEE, K. R., KAACK, M. B., and CLAGHORN, J. L. 1976. Psychotropic drug-stress interaction on the hypothalamic-pituitary-adrenal axis in man and a nonhuman primate. In D. H. Ford and D. H. Clouet (eds.), *Tissue Responses to Addictive Drugs*, pp. 555-588. New York: Spectrum.

ORDY, J. M., SAMORAJSKI, T., and SCHROEDER, D. 1966. Concurrent changes in hypothalamic and cardiac catecholamine levels after anesthetics, tranquilizers and stress in a subhuman primate. *J. Pharmacol. Exp. Ther.*, 152:445-457.

PALKOVITS, M. 1977. Neural pathways involved in ACTH regulation. *Ann. N.Y. Acad. Sci.*, 297:455-476.

PECILE, A., and MULLER, E. E. 1976. *Growth Hormone and Related Peptides*. New York: American Elsevier.

PRANGE, A. J., WILSON, I. C., BREESE, G. R., and LIPTON, M. A. 1976. Hormonal alteration of imipramine response: A review. In E. J. Sachar (ed.), *Hormones, Behavior, and Psychopathology*, pp. 41-68. New York: Raven Press.

RAISMAN, G. 1966. Neural connexions of the hypothalamus. *Br. Med. Bull.*, 22:196-201.

RUBIN, R. T. 1977. Strategies of neuroendocrine research in psychiatry. In E. Usdin, D. A. Hamburg, and J. D. Barchas (eds.), *Neuroregulators and Psychiatric Disorders*, pp. 233-241. New York: Oxford University Press.

RUBIN, R. T., POLAND, R. E., O'CONNOR, D., GOUIN, P. R., and TOWER, B. B. 1976.

Selective neuroendocrine effects of low-dose haloperidol in normal adult man. *Psychopharmacology*, 47:135.

SACHAR, E. J. 1975. Hormonal changes in stress and mental illness. *Hospital Practice*, July:49-55.

SACHAR, E. J. (ed.). 1976. *Hormones, Behavior, and Psychopathology*. New York: Raven Press.

SACHAR, E. J. 1977. ACTH and cortisol secretion in psychiatric disease. *Ann. N.Y. Acad. Sci.*, 297:621-627.

SACHAR, E. J., GRUEN, P. H., ALTMAN, N., HALPERN, F. S., and FRANTZ, A. G. 1976. Use of neuroendocrine techniques in psychopharmacological research. In E. J. Sachar (ed.), *Hormones, Behavior, and Psychopathology*, pp. 161-176. New York: Raven Press.

SACHAR, E. J., GRUEN, P. H., ALTMAN, N., LANGER, G., HALPERN, F. S., and LIEFER, M. 1977. Prolactin responses to neuroleptic drugs: An approach to the study of brain dopamine blockade in humans. In E. Usdin, D. A. Hamburg, and J. D. Barchas (eds.), *Neuroregulators and Psychiatric Disorders*, pp. 242-249. New York: Oxford University Press.

SACHAR, E. J., MUSHRUSH, G., PERLOW, M., WEITZMAN, E. D., and SASSIN, J. 1972. Growth hormone responses to L Dopa in depressed patients. *Science*, 178:1304-1305.

SASSIN, J. F., FRANTZ, A. G., WEITZMAN, E. D., and KAPEN, S. 1972. Human prolactin: 24-hour pattern with increased release during sleep. *Science*, 177:1205-1207.

SCAPAGNINI, U., and PREZIOSI, P. 1973. Role of brain noradrenaline in the tonic regulation of hypothalamic hypophyseal adrenal axis. *Prog. Brain Res.*, 39:171-184.

SHADER, R. I., GILLER, D. R., and DIMASCIO, A. 1970. Hypothalamic-pituitary-adrenal axis. In R. I. Shader and A. DiMascio (eds.), *Psychotropic Drug Side Effects*, pp. 16-25. Baltimore: Williams and Wilkins.

SIEGEL, G. J., and EISENMAN, J. S. 1976. Hypothalamic-pituitary regulation. In G. J. Siegel, R. W. Albers, R. Katzman, and B. W. Agranoff (eds.), *Basic Neurochemistry*, pp. 445-470. Boston: Little, Brown.

USDIN, E., HAMBURG, D. A., and BARCHAS, J. D. 1977. *Neuroregulators and Psychiatric Disorders*. New York: Oxford University Press.

VANCE, V. K., and SHIODA, Y. 1964. Effect of intravenous epinephrine on blood ACTH concentration as measured by steroidogenesis in the hypophysectomized rat. *Endocrinology*, 74:807.

VAN LOON, G. R. 1973. Brain catecholamines and ACTH secretion. In W. F. Ganong and L. Martini (eds.), *Frontiers in Neuroendocrinology*, pp. 209-247. New York: Oxford University Press.

VERNIKOS-DANELLIS, J. 1965. The regulation of the synthesis and release of ACTH. *Vitamins and Hormones*. New York: Academic Press.

VERNIKOS-DANELLIS, J., and MARKS, B. H. 1962. Epinephrine-induced release of ACTH in normal human subjects. *Endocrinology*, 70:525.

VON EULER, U. S. 1964. Quantitation of stress by catecholamine analysis. *Clin. Pharmacol. Ther.*, 5:398.

WHYBROW, P. C., and HURWITZ, T., 1976. Psychological disturbances associated with endocrine disease and hormone therapy. In E. J. Sachar (ed.), *Hormones, Behavior, and Psychopathology*, pp. 125-144. New York: Raven Press.

DE WIED, D. 1977a. Behavioral effects of neuropeptides related to ACTH, MSH, and BLPH. *Ann. N.Y. Acad. Sci.*, 297:263-274.

DE WIED, D. 1977b. Peptides and behavior. *Life Sci.*, 20:195-204.

DE WIED, D., BOHUS, B., GISPEN, W. H., URBAN, I., and VAN WIMERSMA GRIEDANUS, TJ. B. 1976. Hormonal influences on motivational, learning, and memory processes. In E. J. Sachar (ed.), *Hormones, Behavior, and Psychopathology*, pp. 1-14. New York: Raven Press.

DE WIED, D., and DE JONG, W. 1974. Drug effects and hypothalamic-anterior pituitary function. *Annu. Rev. Pharmacol. Toxicol.*, 14:389-412.

WILLOUGHBY, J. O., and MARTIN, J. B. 1976. Episodic GH secretion: Evidence for a hypothalamic dopaminergic mechanism. In F. Labrie, J. Meites, and G. Pelletier (eds.), *Hypothalamus and Endocrine Functions*, pp. 303-320. New York: Plenum.

WURTMAN, R. J., and FERNSTROM, J. D. 1976. Neuroendocrine effects of psychotropic drugs. In E. J. Sachar (ed.), *Hormones, Behavior, and Psychopathology*, pp. 145-152. New York: Raven Press.

III.
CLINICAL STUDIES

7

PLASMA, RED BLOOD CELL PHENOTHIAZINE LEVELS, AND CLINICAL RESPONSE

CARL KINARD, M.D., JOHN M. DAVIS, M.D.,
DAVID GARVER, M.D., SIDNEY CHANG, M.D.,
HAROUTUNE DEKIRMENJIAN, PH.D.,
and
ROBERT C. SMITH, M.D., PH.D.

Blood levels of drugs are clearly of value in the management of treatment for a variety of medical problems. They are of special use in psychiatry for the determination of safe and effective dosages of lithium carbonate. The treatment of psychotic conditions, particularly of chronic schizophrenia, remains a great challenge to psychiatry. It is therefore important to attempt to optimize the efficacy of antipsychotic drugs by adjusting blood levels to empirically determined therapeutic ranges. Assuming that blood levels for an antipsychotic drug reflect drug availability at the receptor site, there would be a reliable relationship between blood level of the drug and clinical response. This paper will review the methodological problems in establishing such relationships, empirical evidence relevant to blood-level response relationships for chlorpromazine and butaperazine, and other findings of clinical interest from research on blood levels.

One may expect to find two types of relationships between the blood levels of a drug: a sigmoid relationship or a curvilinear relationship. A sigmoid blood-level response relationship is one in which low levels of a drug have produced little or no effect on the patient. After a minimum therapeutic level is reached, there may be a steady increase in response with increasing blood levels until the maximum response to the drug is reached; at this point the curve will flatten out (Figure 1, top). A curvilinear blood-level response curve will show, on the other hand, that, after the maximum response is reached, increasing plasma levels are associated with a worsening of the patient. In other words, there may be a "therapeutic window" with both upper and lower limits for drug response (Figure 1, bottom). The upper limit may reflect either a paradoxical pharmacological effect of the drug, where at higher doses the pharmacological effect is the reverse of what happens at lower doses, or increasing side effects may cancel out the therapeutic effect of the drug. In the instance of the neuroleptics, such signs of behavioral toxicity as sedation, akinesia, or akathesia may contribute to a patient's worsening and may, in fact, be difficult to distinguish from the original symptoms. If one subtracts the blood-level response curves for side effects (Figure 1, center) from the sigmoid clinical response curve in Figure 1, top, one obtains a therapeutic window as in Figure 1, bottom.

One must have a wide range of blood levels to demonstrate both ends of the therapeutic window. This may require the use of more than one dosage of the medication. Another important methodological consideration is the need for comprehensive measurements of drug side effects to determine the nature of the upper limit, if one exists. If the upper limit for the therapeutic effect is set by side effects, several issues must be considered. First, the threshold for the side effect varies from patient to patient, and perhaps only a subgroup of patients will show a therapeutic window over a clinically important range of blood levels. Second, astute clinicians may be able to differentiate between undermedicated and overmedicated nonresponders by careful observation of side effects.

Another methodological issue concerns the use of flexible dosages. Consider a hypothetical study of 60 patients of whom 20 remit spontaneously soon after admission, 20 require adequate medication to achieve remission, and 20 neither remit spontaneously nor respond to medication for reasons unrelated to blood levels. Given that the study uses a flexible dosing strategy and that clinicians follow the usual practice of starting with a low or moderate dosage and increasing it until the patient responds or has intolerable side effects, then all three groups of patients may show artifacts that will obscure the true blood-level response curve. Spontaneous remitters or responders to the hospital milieu will always tend to mask the true relationship. Since they improve rapidly, these patients will also tend to have low blood levels because they respond while on the first or lowest dosage; this would particularly obscure the lower limit of a blood-level response curve. A washout period of several weeks before drug treatment helps to screen out spontaneous remitters and patients who respond to hospital treatment in general. The second group, those who respond to adequate medication, will not show the lower limit of a

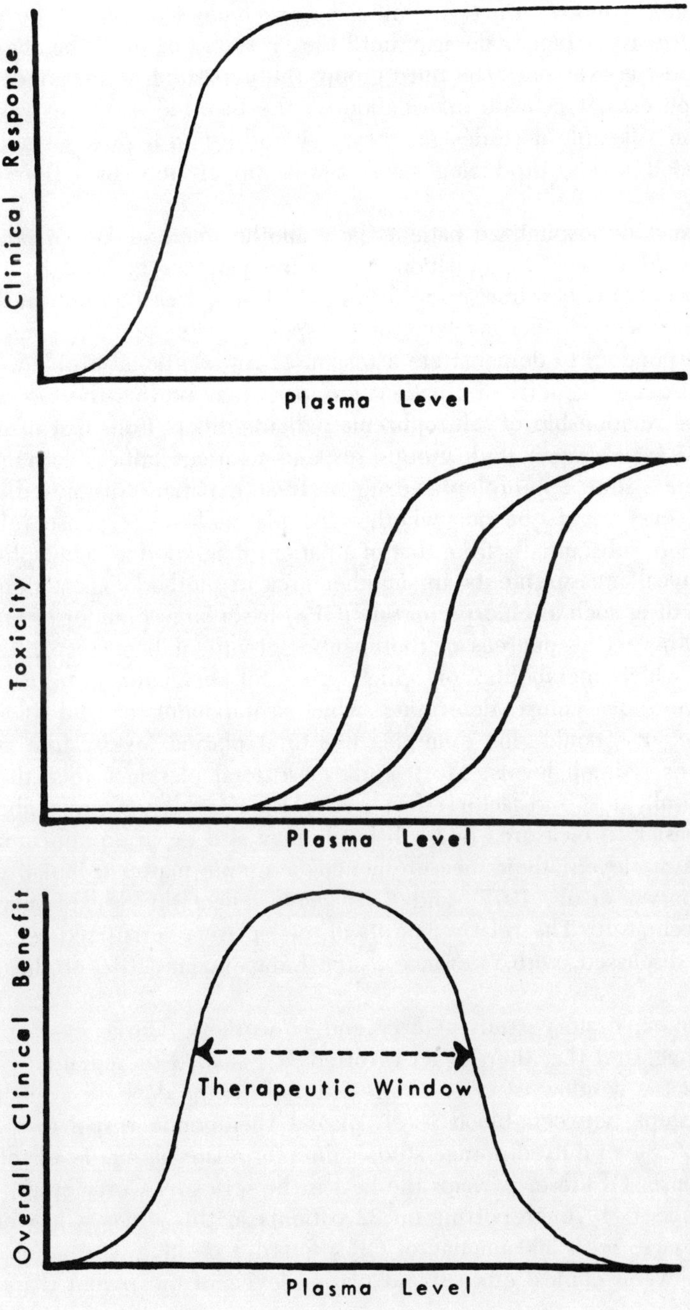

Figure 1. Theoretical concept of therapeutic window.

therapeutic window, since, as initial nonresponders, they will be placed on progressively higher dosages until they respond or until the therapeutic window is overshot. The third group, the persistent nonresponders, by definition cannot provide information on the blood-level versus response curve; in a flexible dose design, they may end up on high doses and with high blood levels, producing an artifactual upper limit to a therapeutic window.

Chronically hospitalized patients pose another methodological problem. One would expect a population of chronic patients to include a large number of patients refractory to drugs, which might easily obscure the relationship between plasma level and response. After all, one must have drug responders to demonstrate a response. An additional problem is the diagnostic homogeneity of a patient group. It may be that the blood-level response relationship of schizophrenic patients differs from that of manic-depressives, although both groups respond to neuroleptics. Certainly, if one were using a neuroleptic drug to treat a patient diagnosed as alcoholic, one might question whether the plasma-level response relationship differs substantially from that of a patient diagnosed as schizophrenic.

Chemical measurements are another area of methodological difficulty. Since a drug such as chlorpromazine (CPZ) has a large number of metabolites with varying degrees of therapeutic activity, it becomes difficult to decide which metabolite, or which group of metabolites, to measure. Moreover, one must determine which component of the blood to examine: one could, for example, use total plasma levels, free plasma levels, or red-cell levels. Most studies use total plasma levels; they are theoretically less satisfactory than free plasma levels yet are technically much easier to measure. Red-cell levels may also be in equilibrium with free plasma levels; their measurement is a simple matter (Manian et al., 1974; Garver et al., 1977), and RBC levels reflect the free plasma level more accurately. The relative merits of total plasma versus red-cell levels will be discussed, with relevance to the butaperazine (BPZ) studies cited below.

In an exploratory study, Curry and co-workers (Curry et al., 1968, 1970) suggested that there is an inverted "U"-shaped therapeutic window and that the window is wide. At present, substantial data are available on relationships between blood levels of and therapeutic response to CPZ and BPZ. Several fixed-dosage studies directly relate plasma levels of CPZ to response. Of these, perhaps the best is the series by Curry et al. (1968, 1970). Lader (1976), reporting on 32 patients in this series who were on fixed dosage, with 300 mg/day of CPZ, found a positive correlation (*r*) of +.32 between clinical efficacy and plasma levels of the parent drug. The correlation was marginally significant ($p < .04$, one-tailed). However, since most of the lower plasma levels in this study approached the lower limits of normal values, the fact that some of the patients who had these lower plasma levels did not respond adds some support to the blood-level versus clinical response relationship. Furthermore, since this study used a fairly low fixed dosage of CPZ, it is doubtful that the patients could have achieved high plasma levels. The results are therefore more relevant to the lower end of the blood-level clinical response curve.

Butaperazine is a much simpler drug to study than chlorpromazine since it has no known active metabolites. Our laboratory has conducted a series of studies with this drug, examining both plasma and red blood cell (RBC) levels. We used homogeneous diagnostic groups consisting of schizophrenic patients diagnosed by the Research Diagnostic Criteria. Acute and subacute schizoaffective patients were excluded, since such patients may represent an atypical form of affective illness. Only patients recently admitted (i.e., those suffering their first psychotic break or relapsing into schizophrenia) were selected, so that we avoided the inclusion of chronically hospitalized patients who might be preselected for nonresponse to drugs. The dosage was fixed and patients were randomly assigned to 20 mg twice daily (b.i.d.) or 40 mg b.i.d. of BPZ in an effort to secure enough patients with both high and low blood levels to define lower and upper limits of the therapeutic window. A two-week drug washout period was scheduled in an attempt to rule out spontaneous responders or responders to nonspecific hospital treatment effects.

In our first BPZ study we used ten schizophrenic patients to assess drug blood levels and clinical response during the first 12 days of treatment. Clinical response was assessed by interviews using a modification of the New Haven Schizophrenia Index (NHSI). We found that (a) a curvilinear relationship existed between both plasma and red-cell BPZ levels and therapeutic response (percentage of improvement on the NHSI psychosis score) and (b) that BPZ bound to RBCs correlated more strongly with therapeutic response than did plasma BPZ. Since the relationship between blood levels of BPZ and therapeutic response was curvilinear, this suggested a therapeutic window for the drug. A replication study with 24 patients showed no significant correlation between plasma BPZ and therapeutic response, but it did reveal a clear curvilinear relationship between BPZ bound to RBC and therapeutic response. In the replication, the mean improvement of patients whose steady-state RBC levels were within the therapeutic window for red cells (i.e., about 32 to 62 ng/ml) at 14 days was 55 percent ($N = 10$). Patients below 31 ng/ml showed a mean improvement of 17 percent ($N = 11$); and patients with levels above 62 ng/ml showed only 9 percent improvement (N = 3). These results are significant at $p < .01$. At the end of 28 days, patients whose blood levels remained continuously in the therapeutic window had a mean 89-percent improvement (N = 6); those continually below (N = 4) and above (N = 2) the therapeutic window had a mean improvement of 40 percent and 52 percent respectively. These differences are of sufficient magnitude to be clinically important.

Anecdotal data collected after the fixed-dosage protocol was completed, when dosages were adjusted for some patients for clinical reasons, provide further evidence for the therapeutic window. Several patients who had had high RBC levels of BPZ (above the therapeutic window) when they were on the fixed dosage had reduced red blood-cell BPZ levels that fell within the therapeutic window when their dosage was reduced, and they then showed a better therapeutic response. For example, one paranoid schizophrenic patient initially responded well to BPZ but later showed deterioration. Careful evaluations of his symptoms during the phase of deterioration suggested that the increased anxiety levels he manifested might have been caused, at least in part, by drug-induced akathesia. Treated with an anticholinergic drug for these possible extrapyramidal side effects, however, this patient's symptoms worsened rather than improved. This treatment effect called into question the clinical impression of akathesia. When the patient's BPZ blood-level data were analyzed, they showed that during the early phase, when the patient was clinically improving on the fixed dosage of BPZ, his red blood-cell BPZ levels were within the therapeutic window but then overshot the upper limit of the RBC therapeutic window, which correlated with his period of clinical deterioration. Subsequently, when we reduced his dosage and his blood level adjusted back into the therapeutic window, as shown by his butaperazine, the patient's anxiety and akathesia remitted, and he was discharged from the hospital.

Since our study indicated clearly that red blood-cell BPZ correlates better than plasma BPZ with response, our laboratory conducted a series of *in vitro* studies to explore this relationship in animals. Rats killed at one-half, one, two, four, and eight hours after a single intraperitoneal injection of BPZ showed whole-brain levels that correlated better with red cell (r = .90, N = 14) than with plasma levels of BPZ (r = .69, N = 15) at the time of sacrifice.

Since BPZ is 94-percent protein-bound in plasma, and since the quantity of binding sites in a given volume of plasma is more variable between patients than the quantity of binding sites in 1 ml of packed red cells, it may be argued that RBC BPZ is a more accurate measure of the free unbound BPZ that is available to reach equilibrium with other tissues such as the brain. Dilution studies, in which 1 ml of packed human red cells was incubated with 2 mg of BPZ and 1 ml of varying dilutions of human plasma, indicate that with decreasing concentrations of plasma, BPZ linearly increases in the RBC fraction rather than in the supernatant. Since dilution of the plasma results in less BPZ bound to plasma proteins, increased free BPZ is then available for binding to the red cells. These studies may be interpreted as indicating that the quantity of BPZ bound to the red cells is in equilibrium with the free (i.e., non-protein-bound), nonionized BPZ in the incubation mixture. Other work by our group indicates that there is no energy-dependent reuptake of BPZ into the red cells, and that the BPZ is bound primarily to such intercellular components as hemoglobin and not to membrane structures. In sum, several lines of research from our *in vivo* and *in vitro* studies with butaperazine support the hypothesis that a therapeutic window exists for RBC butaperazine. Our investigations also suggest that RBC butaperazine may be a fairly accurate predictor of free (non-protein-bound) plasma BPZ, and therefore a better correlate of brain BPZ levels than total plasma BPZ.

This paper has reviewed several methodological issues in blood level studies of neuroleptic medication. Particularly stressed have been the issues of a fixed dosage, a wide enough range of plasma or red-cell levels to adequately define both a possible upper and lower therapeutic limit, and avoiding the use of chronic populations that may be preselected for drug nonresponse. There seems to be a tendency in the current literature to demonstrate a curvilinear relationship between blood levels and therapeutic response. These studies and related work suggest that RBC neuroleptic levels may be a more accurate measure of free plasma levels than the more usually measured total plasma levels of the drug. Since only a small sample of patients has been studied, our conclusions should be considered preliminary, and they are presented primarily to raise questions and suggest hypotheses to be tested and confirmed in future work. Quantitatively, the evidence suggests that there is a wide therapeutic window for chlorpromazine and a moderately wide window for butaperazine. When the window is wide and when many other variables determine clinical response, blood levels are often less useful as predictors or determinants of clinical response than when a narrow window exists.

REFERENCES

Curry, S. H., Davis, J. M., Janowsky, D., and Marshall, J. H. 1968. Inpatient variation in physiological availability of chlorpromazine as a complicating factor in correlation studies of drug metabolism and clinical effect. In A. Cerletti and F. J. Bove (eds.), *The Present Status of Psychotropic Drugs*, vol. 6, pp. 72-76. Amsterdam: Excerpta Medica Foundation.

CURRY, S. H., MARSHALL, J. H. L., DAVIS, J. M., and JANOWSKY, D. S. 1970. Chlorpromazine plasma level and effects. *Arch. Gen. Psychiatry*, 22:289-296.

GARVER, D. L., DEKIRMENJIAN, H., DAVIS, J. M., CASPER, R., and ERICKSEN, S. 1977. Neuroleptic drug levels and therapeutic response: Preliminary observations with red blood cell bound butaperazine. *Am. J. Psychiatry*, 134:304-307.

LADER, M. 1976. Monitoring plasma concentrations of neuroleptics. *Pharmacopsychiatry*, 9:170-177.

MANIAN, A. A., PIETTE, L. H., HOLLAND, D., GROVER, T., and LETERRIER, F. 1974. Red blood cell drug binding as a possible mechanism for tranquilization. In I. S. Forrest, C. J. Carr, and E. Usdin (eds.), *Advances in Biochemical Psychopharmacology*, vol. 9, pp. 149-161. New York: Raven Press.

8

BLOOD LEVELS OF NEUROLEPTIC DRUGS, CLINICAL RESPONSE, AND PLASMA PROLACTIN IN CHRONIC NONRESPONDING SCHIZOPHRENIC PATIENTS

ROBERT C. SMITH, M.D., PH.D., JOHN W. CRAYTON, M.D.,
CAROL TAMMINGA, M.D., HAROUTUNE DEKIRMENJIAN, PH.D.,
JOSEPH C. SCHOOLAR, PH.D., M.D.,
and
JOHN M. DAVIS, M.D.

Blood levels of neuroleptic drugs may be one important factor in the degree of clinical improvement of schizophrenic patients treated with antipsychotic drugs, as recent research has shown. Many patients newly admitted to short-term hospitals who respond poorly to antipsychotic medication have been found to have low blood levels of butaperazine or chlorpromazine, and a few such patients have an equally poor response if their blood levels of these drugs are abnormally high (Rivera-Calimlim et al., 1976; Garver et al., 1977a, b). In acute or short-term hospitals, most patients eventually improve enough in a few weeks or a few months to be discharged and returned to their families or community, although some signs of their illness may remain. Many long-term mental hospitals, however, retain a sizeable number of patients who improve very little even with long-term neuroleptic treatment. These patients remain chronically psychotic, never reaching even the level of partial remission that would allow their reintegration into the community. With the recent attempt to empty some of the state hospitals, some of these patients are now found in nursing homes, boarding homes, or vagrant-care facilities.

Do these nonresponding schizophrenic patients have abnormal (very low or very high) blood levels of neuroleptic drugs, and are these drug levels related to the patients' poor clinical response to treatment with antipsychotic medication? To begin to answer these questions, we have initiated studies of blood levels of neuroleptic drugs in nonresponding schizophrenic patients. We are investigating the pharmacokinetics of neuroleptics after a single acute dose as well as their steady-state levels during regular treatment with a fixed dosage, correlating these blood levels with rating-scale measures of clinical response and serum prolactin levels.

Method

Four groups of patients were studied, two groups of nonresponding patients and two groups who showed better clinical response. The first group, chronic schizophrenic nonresponders (CNR) were patients hospitalized three to 17 years in long-term facilities of the Illinois state mental hospital system. These patients had received a wide variety of drugs but had improved minimally, and often were known as special problems to doctors and nurses on their wards. The patients were transferred to the clinical investigation units at Manteno State Hospital and/or Illinois State Psychiatric Institute for a two- to three-week drug-free period and then studied as specified below. The second group of nonresponding patients, acute nonresponders (ANR), were patients referred from a variety of acute treatment facilities after they had shown no clinical response during several months of treatment. These patients were referred to one of us (J.M.D.) for plasma level studies.

For comparison we used two other samples of patients (whom we call *relative responders*, RR) who were hospitalized at either the Illinois State Psychiatric Institute (ISPI-RR) or Central Tennessee Neuropsychiatric Institute (TNI-RR), and who had shown a better clinical response to neuroleptics. Diagnostically these patients were either acute or subacute schizophrenics, or chronic schizophrenics in remission but who had suffered an acute relapse. Although the extent of remission of psychotic symptoms in these patients varied considerably, they demonstrated enough clinical improvement after treatment with neuroleptics to be discharged from the hospital after several months; hence the term relative responders.

Age and Gender

The age and gender of the nonresponding sample at Manteno (mean ± s.e.m. = 31.8 ± 1.9 years) and of the relative responders at ISPI (27.9 ±

2.9 years) were not substantially different. Both groups consisted of about 30 to 40 percent men and 60 to 70 percent women.

Diagnosis

The Manteno and ISPI patients were evaluated according to the Research Diagnostic Criteria (RDC) of Spitzer et al. (1975). This diagnostic evaluation was independent of any results of the pharmacokinetic studies. Patients in the other samples were diagnosed as schizophrenic, using standard clinical evaluations based on clinical data and rating scales. All patients in this report were schizophrenic (including RDC diagnosis of schizophrenia or one of the subtypes of schizoaffective disorder), unless specifically noted otherwise.

General Design

Patients underwent a washout drug-free period of one to three weeks before beginning neuroleptic medication. Studies were performed after acute and/or chronic administration of oral butaperazine, haloperidol, thioridazine, or mesoridazine. A subsample of patients in the nonresponder groups who received butaperazine were later treated with another neuroleptic, so that comparisons of blood levels could be made in the same patient receiving two neuroleptic drugs.

To obtain data for the acute pharmacokinetic curve, a single dose of oral butaperazine (40 mg for most patients) was administered to patients who had fasted for about six hours. For nonresponders at Manteno State Hospital, blood samples were drawn after the single oral administration at 0, 2, 4, 8, 15, 25, 33, and 49 hours. Blood was drawn at similar times after the acute dose in other samples, as detailed in previous publications (Davis et al., 1974; Garver et al., 1976).

For the steady-state studies, patients received a fixed dose of butaperazine (40 mg twice daily, b.i.d.) or thioridazine (200 mg four times daily, q.i.d.) except as otherwise noted. Blood samples to determine steady-state levels were drawn after a patient had been on a standard dosage of neuroleptic medication for one to three weeks. Blood was drawn on several days 12 or 16 hours after the last dose and before that morning's dose. Steady-state drug levels reported here are the average values from separate determinations of drug levels drawn on two to five different days.

Informed Consent

The purposes and procedures of the study were explained to the patients and written informed consent for participation was obtained from them.

Blood Level Assays

Butaperazine levels were determined by a modification of the method of Davis et al. (1974 and Garver et al., 1976). The specificity of this method was further checked by: (a) measuring the excitation and emission spectra of patients' blood in patients receiving at least three weeks of butaperazine (40 mg b.i.d.), (b) testing the extracted material obtained by this method for metabolites on three solvent systems by thin-layer chromatography, and (c) comparing plasma and red blood cell (RBC) butaperazine levels measured in the same patient's blood by this fluorometric method with levels obtained using a gas-liquid chromatographic (GLC) method utilizing a nitrogen detector. Mean (± s.e.m.) plasma butaperazine levels of ten patients analyzed by the fluorometric methods were 127 ± 21 ng/ml and the corresponding GLC determinations on the same samples averaged 137 ± 26 ng/ml, with a Pearson correlation coefficient (r) of 0.95 between values from the same blood sample measured by the two different methods. Fluorometric values in RBC samples from ten patients were 90 ± 20 ng/ml and GLC values were 111 ± 23 ng/ml, with a Pearson r of 0.98 for the same sample analyzed by the two different methods.

Haloperidol levels were determined by a modification of the Forsman et al. method (1974). The initial extraction procedure was the same as above, but at the end the samples were dissolved in 0.1 ml of benzene, a volume about 33 times larger than the above method; this was done to assure complete solubilization. Because of higher sensitivity of the ^{3}H-scandium 1 mc detector that was used for these samples, the larger volume could be used effectively without loss of sensitivity. We increased the sensitivity of the method recently by using a nitrogen detector. Twenty-four patients' plasma samples, after three weeks of administration of 15 mg of haloperidol, were assayed by the two GLC methods; the GLC-electron capture detector yielded 7.9 ± 1.1 ng/ml; and the GLC-nitrogen detector gave 7.6 ± 1.1 ng/ml with a Pearson r of 0.96.

Plasma thioridazine and mesoridazine were measured by the spectrofluorometric method of Pacha (1969) with minor modifications. Both thioridazine and mesoridazine standards gave maximum fluorescence at the same wave lengths; excitation 350 mμ and emission 440 mμ. Also at these wave lengths, the extinction coefficients were identical. This spectrofluorometric method is believed to be nonspecific and measures both the parent drug and some of its metabolites.

Ingestion of Medication

To guard against patients' noncompliance in ingesting their medication, thus causing low blood levels of the drug, several precautions were taken, especially in the chronic nonresponding patients:

1. For patients who were judged to be poor risks for taking their medication, butaperazine tablets were ground up and given in applesauce.
2. Mouth checks after drug administration were made periodically in many patients, and more frequently in patients who were thought to resist medication.
3. Thioridazine was administered as an elixir.
4. A second acute butaperazine curve was run for six patients after they completed the regular protocol and a new washout period. For these repeat acute curves, one physician of the research group was always present to make sure the patient fully ingested the drug. The blood-level results of these repeated acute curves were similar to the patients' blood levels on the initial curve.

Half-Life

Butaperazine curves after single-dose administration indicated a reasonable fit with a two-compartment open model. ß-Phase half-life (T½), which is related to the rate of metabolism and elimination of the drug, was calculated after acute dosage for patients with sufficient blood-level data. Assuming a two-pool kinetic system, ß-phase T½s were calculated using slope values determined from a linear regression of semilog plots of the terminal exponential portion of the graph of blood levels versus time, using methods and equations described by Ritschel (1976) for oral drug administration with a two-compartment open system. A few of the chronic nonresponders had plasma and/or RBC levels so low at 12 to 25 hours after drug ingestion that the drug levels were unmeasurable by our method (i.e., < 8 mg/ml); hence ß-phase T½ could not be measured for these patients.

Drug History

The amount of each neuroleptic drug given to the Manteno chronic nonresponder sample for each month during the patients' total hospital course was calculated from the medical records. For some analyses drug

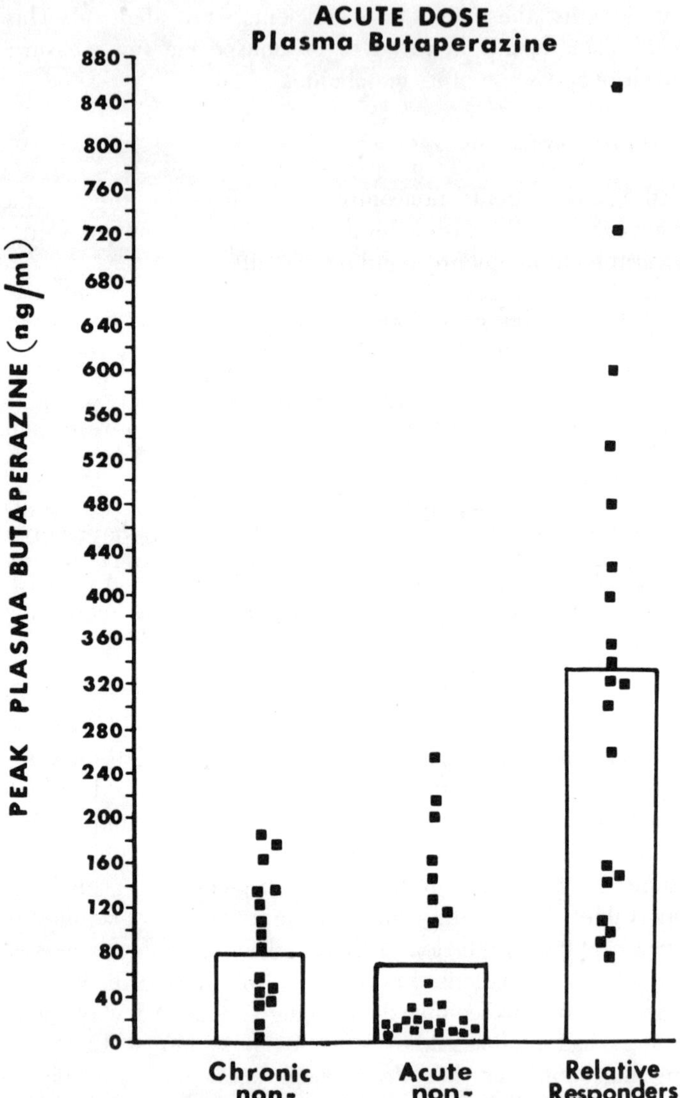

Figure 1. Peak levels of butaperazine after a single acute 40-mg oral dose in chronic nonresponders, acute nonresponders, and relative responders. (a) ■ plasma, (b) • red blood cells (RBC). Bar graphs indicate mean of group.

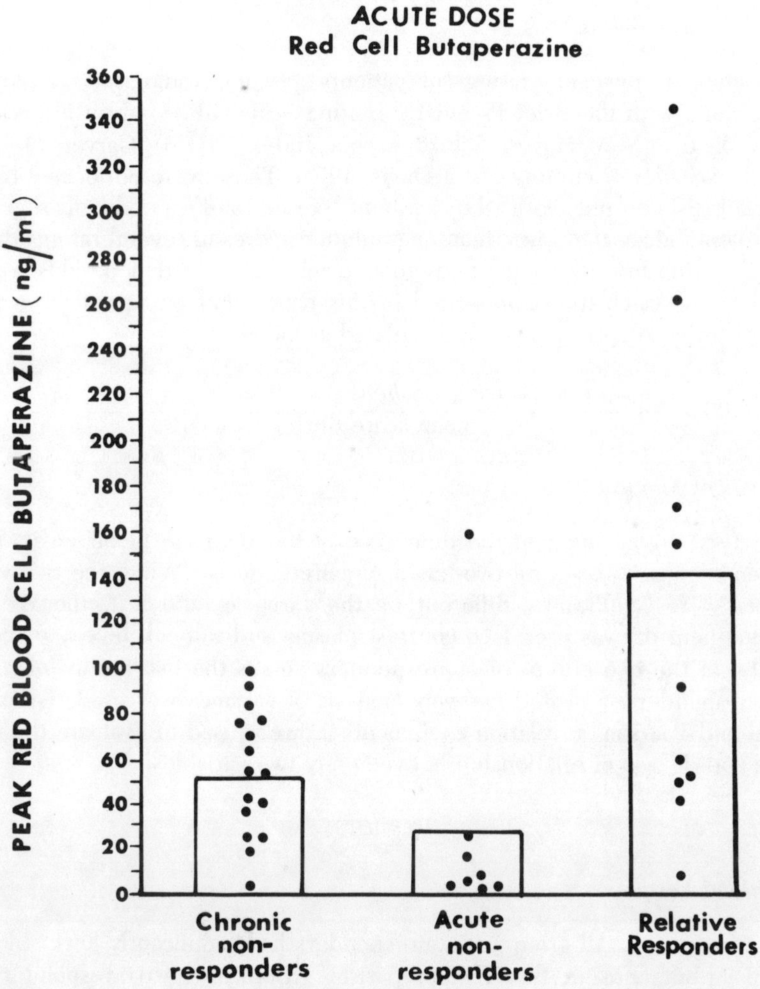

Figure 1 (Continued)

dosages were converted to chlorpromazine (CPZ) equivalents using the conversion ratios of Davis (1974).

Prolactin

Plasma prolactin was measured by one of us (C.T.) using double antibody radioimmunoassay materials and procedures provided by the NIAMDD.

Psychological Ratings

Weekly or biweekly ratings of patients' psychopathological symptoms were done with the Brief Psychiatric Rating Scale (BPRS) or an interview form of the New Haven Schizophrenia Index (NHSI) Garver et al., 1977b; Schaffer, Tamminga, and Davis, 1977). These were performed by a psychologist during both the washout period and periods of regular neuroleptic drug therapy. Mean or minimum scores of several ratings during the drug-free (washout) or regular drug administration periods were used in the calculations presented in this paper. Percentage of improvement on neuroleptic drugs was calculated as follows:

$$100 \times \frac{(\textit{mean score during washout} - \textit{mean score on neuroleptics})}{\text{mean score during washout}}$$

Statistical Analysis

Statistical evaluation of the difference of butaperazine blood levels between groups is based on two-tailed unpaired t-tests. (When the two variances were significantly different by the variance ratio test, the Welch t-value (and df) was used.) To contrast plasma and red cell levels, respectively, in the two groups of nonresponders versus the two groups of relative responders, a nested two-way analysis of variance was used. Graphic plots and Pearson correlation coefficients (r) were used to evaluate the nature and degree of relationship between any two variables.

RESULTS

1. Blood Levels

Butaperazine. All groups of nonresponders had significantly lower blood levels of butaperazine than the comparison groups of relative responders.

Let us first examine the blood levels of patients in the chronic nonresponder groups compared to relative responder groups who were all treated with the same standard dose of butaperazine. The patients first underwent a drug-free washout period and then received one acute dose of 40 mg of butaperazine. Several days later they began a regimen of 40 mg of butaperazine twice a day. After the acute 40-mg dose, chronic nonresponders had significantly (t test for Welch t) lower peak levels of butaperazine in plasma ($p < .001$) and red cells ($p < .05$) than did relative responders (Figure 1). On the 40-mg b.i.d. dosage schedule, chronic nonresponding schizophrenics also showed significantly lower steady-state butaperazine levels in plasma ($p < .01$) and red cells ($p < .05$) than did relative responders (Figure 2). Note the good correspondence of the results after the acute test dose and during the steady-state administration. The differences between the two groups were apparent in both plasma and red cell levels. Not only were butaperazine levels in chronic nonresponders statistically significantly lower on average but, as inspection of the graph shows, many nonresponders had plasma levels substantially lower than those of any patient in the relative responder group.

These low blood levels in nonresponders were not due to any special characteristics of Manteno State Hospital or a chronic psychiatric ward. One of the patients admitted to the Manteno clinical investigation unit (CIU) was more similar to the relative responders we studied at other hospitals; she was a chronic schizophrenic woman who had been functioning in the community but had relapsed after she stopped taking her medication for several months. She was subsequently rehospitalized and was sent to the CIU after a few days' stay on the Manteno admission ward. She had a good clinical response to butaperazine. Her mean steady-state plasma butaperazine level of 191 ng/ml was in the "normal" range of relative responders studied at other hospitals.

From time to time we have also had nonresponding patients referred to us from more acute hospitals for evaluation of their neuroleptic blood levels. Usually these patients had been hospitalized for several months, had been treated with one or more neuroleptic drugs, and had shown little clinical improvement. They were referred to one of us (J.M.D.) for blood level studies. These patients also received the 40-mg dose of butaperazine for an acute pharmacokinetic curve. Peak blood levels of butaperazine in these patients are also shown in Figure 1. Mean peak plasma levels (62 ± 15 ng/ml) and RBC levels (26 ± 18 ng/ml) were both significantly ($p < .01$ and $p < .05$, respectively) lower in this group of acute nonresponders than in the relative responders, and the level of butaperazine in the more acute nonresponders seemed to be quite similar to that of the chronic nonresponders.

Overall, 85 percent of the nonresponders had plasma butaperazine levels below 150 ng/ml after an acute 40-mg dose compared to only 29 percent of the relative responders; and 92 percent had steady-state plasma butaperazine levels below 150 ng/ml compared to 9 percent of the relative responder group.

To enlarge our sample, we performed additional analyses on blood levels of patients who received several other fixed dosages of butaperazine in the normal range (i.e., 10 to 60 mg in a single dose for acute studies, or twice daily during regular treatment) on a random or predetermined

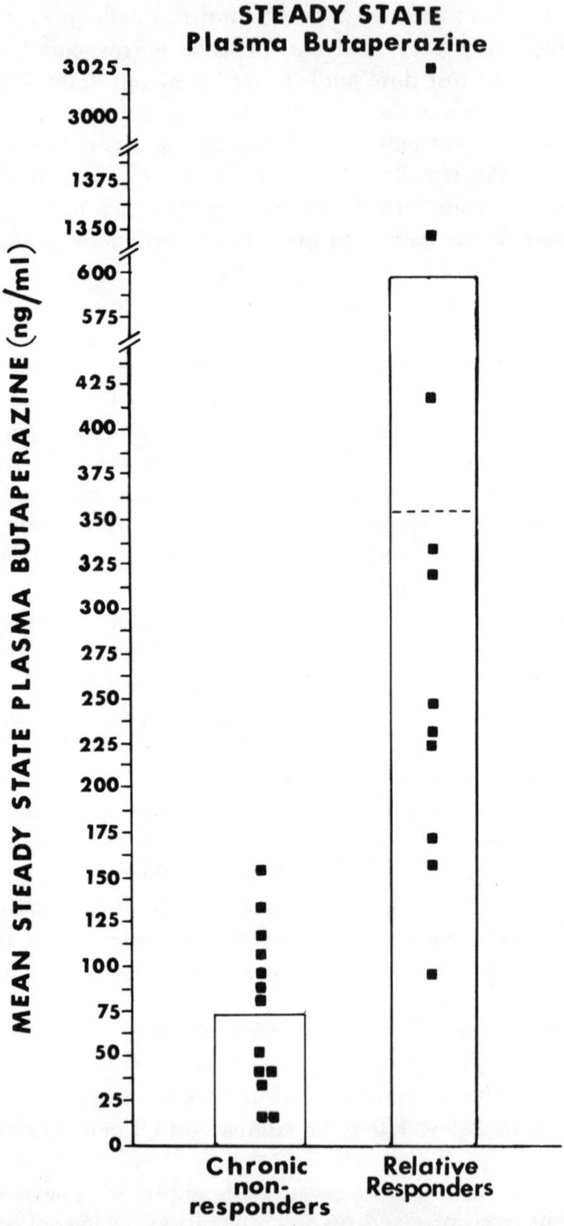

Figure 2. Mean steady-state levels of butaperazine after a daily dosage of 80 mg of butaperazine (40 mg twice a day) for one to three weeks. (a) ■ Plasma, (b) ● RBC—indicates mean of group with the highest patient's value (> 3000 ng/ml) excluded. For explanation of other symbols see Figure 1.

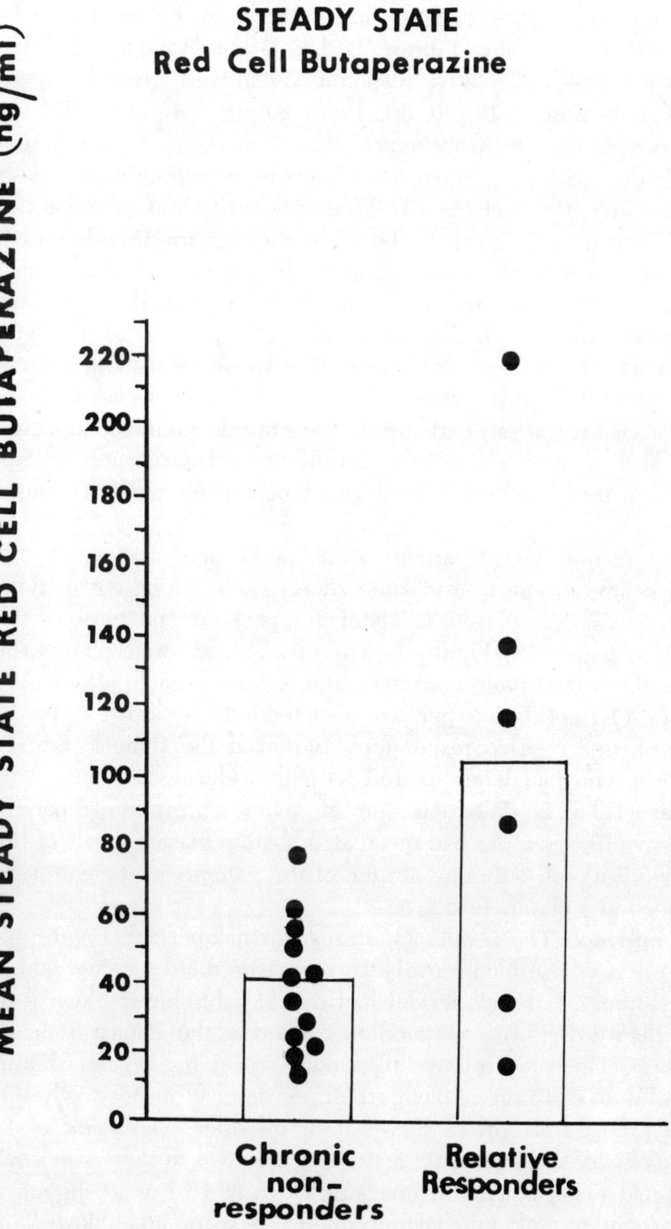

Figure 2 (Continued)

basis (i.e., not by physician's choice which can be influenced by the patient's response). Table 1 presents data for two samples of nonresponders and two samples of relative responders who were given butaperazine in a single acute dose of 10, 20, 30, 40, or 60 mg or received this steady-state fixed dosage on a b.i.d. schedule. Blood level values at different dosages have been equated by expressing results in mg/ml/mg dose since our previous research (Davis et al., 1974) has shown that butaperazine blood levels at different dosages given to the same patients are directly proportional to dose with proportionality constant (k) of about 1. Peak plasma and RBC butaperazine levels after the single dose and also the mean steady-state plasma and RBC levels differed significantly ($p < .05$ to $p < .001$). Levels were lower in the two groups of nonresponders than in the comparison group of relative responders.

Other neuroleptics. Patients in the chronic nonresponding group who were also treated with other neuroleptics, thioridazine, haloperidol or mesoridazine, tended to have lower blood levels of these neuroleptics as well.

Thioridazine. Those patients with low butaperazine levels also tended to have low plasma thioridazine; there was a strong correlation between mean steady-state plasma levels of butaperazine and those of thioridazine ($r = .74$, $p < .025$) (Figure 3). The mean steady-state plasma thioridazine levels of seven chronic nonresponding schizophrenic patients treated with 800 mg of thioridazine per day also tended ($p < .10$) to be lower than those of nine relative responders studied at the Illinois State Psychiatric Institute who had been treated with thioridazine dosages of 400 to 800 mg/day (Table 2). Whereas four of seven schizophrenic patients in the nonresponding sample had mean steady-state plasma levels of thioridazine below 3.5 ng/ml, only one of nine of the patients in the comparison group had such low plasma levels.

Haloperidol. The results are similar for haloperidol (Figure 4). Six nonresponders whose blood levels were measured after a single dose or regular treatment with haloperidol had considerably lower blood levels of this drug than did relative responders studied at the Illinois State Psychiatric Institute. Thirty-six relative responders receiving regular treatment with an oral dose of 15 mg of haloperidol per day had mean steady-state plasma haloperidol levels of 15.3 ± 2.0 ng/ml after one week of treatment. Twenty-six of these patients restudied after two to three weeks of this regimen had mean plasma haloperidol levels of 10.1 ± 1.0 ng/ml. In the six nonresponders, plasma haloperidol levels were much lower (mean 4.0, range 0-9 ng/ml) in spite of the fact that they received much higher dosages (20-60 mg/day). These preliminary data show that haloperidol plasma

Table 1

Butaperazine Levels in Four Groups of Schizophrenic Patients Receiving Various Dosages

	SAMPLE				
Butaperazine Blood Level Type	Nonresponders (NR)		Relative Responders (RR)		Statistical Difference Between Nonresponders and Relative Responders
	CNR	ANR	ISPI-RR	TNI-RR	
(N)	(16)	(24)	(15)	(24)	
Plasma peak, acute dose	2.1 ± 0.4*	1.6 ± 0.4	8.1 ± 0.6	10.3 ± 1.2	$F = 59.75$, $df = 1,75$, $p < .001$
(N)	(16)	(8)	(15)	—	
Red cell peak, acute dose	1.3 ± 0.2	0.7 ± 0.5	3.4 ± 1.1	—	$t' = 2.14$, $df' = 15.1$, $p < .05$
(N)	(18)	—	(8)	(18)	
Plasma, mean steady state	2.4 ± 0.7	—	13.5 ± 8.9	8.5 ± 2.4	$t' = 2.43$, $df' = 27.8$, $p < .025$
(N)	(18)	—	(8)	—	
Red cell, mean steady state	1.2 ± 0.3	—	2.5 ± 0.5	—	$t = 2.45$, $df = 24$, $p < .025$

*Each value represents mean ± s.e.m. of indicated number of patients. Butaperazine levels are expressed in ng/ml/mg dose. Doses ranged from 10-60 mg per dose (i.e. 20-120 mg/day with twice daily administration). See text for detailed description of sample group labels. Statistical significance: F = Nonresponder vs. relative responder effect from 2-way analysis of variance. t = 2-sample t-test values comparing all NR patients vs RR patients. t' = Welch t value calculated for tests when variance between two samples was significantly different. df = degree of freedom. df' = calculated Welch degree of freedom. Probability (p) values are two-tailed from t or Welch t-test or 2-way analysis of variance.

Table 2

Plasma Levels of Thioridazine, Haloperidol, and Mesoridazine In Chronic Nonresponders and Relative Responders

	PLASMA LEVEL OF DRUG	
	Nonresponders	*Relative Responders*
	Thioridazine Levels μg/ml (Steady State)	
(N)	(7)	(9)
Mean ± s.e.m.	3.54 ± .47	4.68 ± .38
	Haloperidol Levels ng/ml (Steady State)	
(N)	(6)	(36)
Mean ± s.e.m.	4.0 ± 1.8	15.3 ± 2.0
	Mesoridazine Levels ng/ml (Single Acute Dose[a])	
(N)	(9)	(10)
Mean ± s.e.m.	317 ± 24	504 ± 79[b]

a = highest value measured after acute dose; b = extrapolated value (see text). Dosages of medication: Thioridazine—nonresponders, 800 mg/day; relative responders, 800 mg/day (seven patients), 600 mg/day (one patient), 400 mg/day (one patient). Responder given 400 mg/day had levels as high as some of patients on 800 mg/day. Haloperidol—nonresponders, 20-60 mg/day; relative responders, 15 mg/day. Mesoridazine—nonresponders, 25 mg i.m.; relative responders, 2 mg/kg i.m. extrapolated back to levels at 25-mg i.m. dosage based on 65-Kg average weight (see text).

levels in chronic nonresponders were several times lower than those in relative responders.

Mesoridazine. Nonresponders also appeared to have lower mesoridazine levels after a single acute dose of this drug (75 mg orally or 25 mg intramuscularly, i.m.). It is more difficult to make a definite statement about this drug because we had no comparison group of relative responders who received the same dose. The only extensive pharmacokinetic data on mesoridazine in the literature come from a study by Gottschalk et al. (1975), who gave considerably higher intramuscular doses of mesoridazine (2 mg/kg i.m., equivalent to 80 to 150 mg total dose) to acute schizophrenics. However, if the relationship between blood levels and dose of mesoridazine is similar to that which Davis et al. (1974) had reported for butaperazine—that is, a directly proportional relationship with a k of about 1—one might legitimately make a rough extrapolation from the peak blood levels obtained by Gottschalk et al. (1976) after the acute 2-mg/kg intramuscular dose of mesoridazine (mean 2.39 μg/ml with the spectrofluorometric method) to the approximate blood levels these patients might have had if they had received only a 25-mg intramuscular

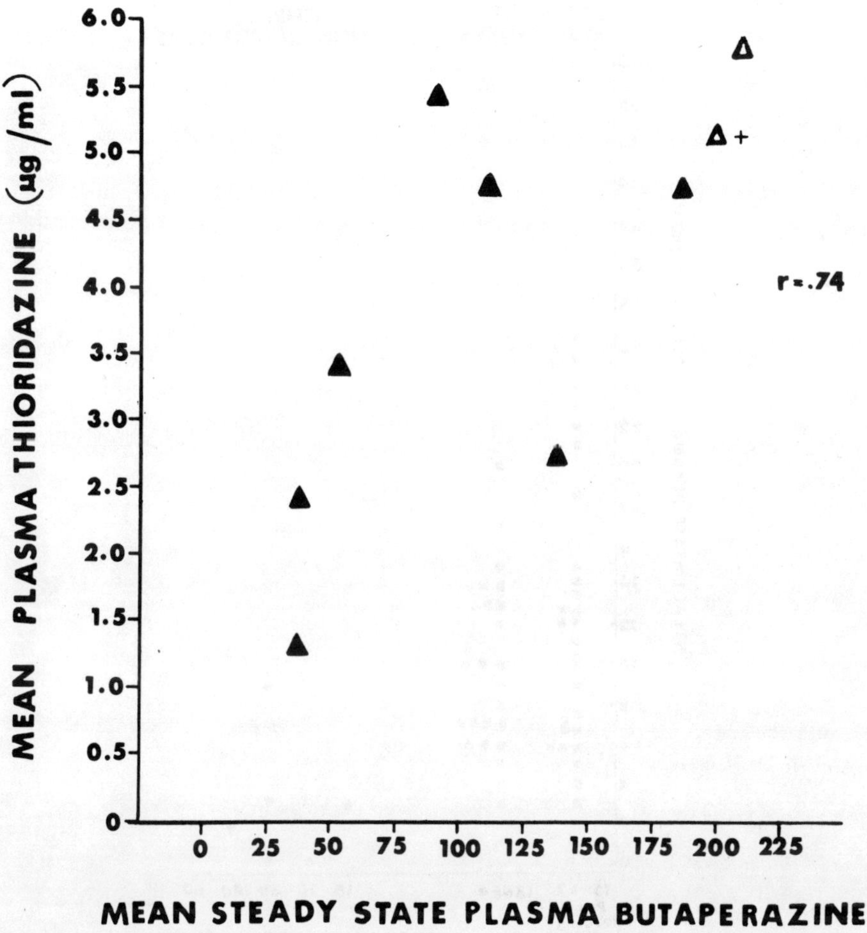

Figure 3. Relationship between steady-state levels of plasma butaperazine (dosage, 40 mg twice a day) and steady-state levels of thioridazine. For explanation of other symbols see Figures 1 and 2. Open symbols (○, Δ) represent patients with RDC diagnosis of major depressive disorder.

dose. Mean values for these extrapolated peak plasma levels range from 390 to 620 ng/ml (depending on weight of subject). These blood levels are considerably higher than the mean peak plasma levels of mesoridazine (317 ng/ml) after the 25-mg intramuscular dose given to nine chronic non-responding schizophrenic patients at Manteno.

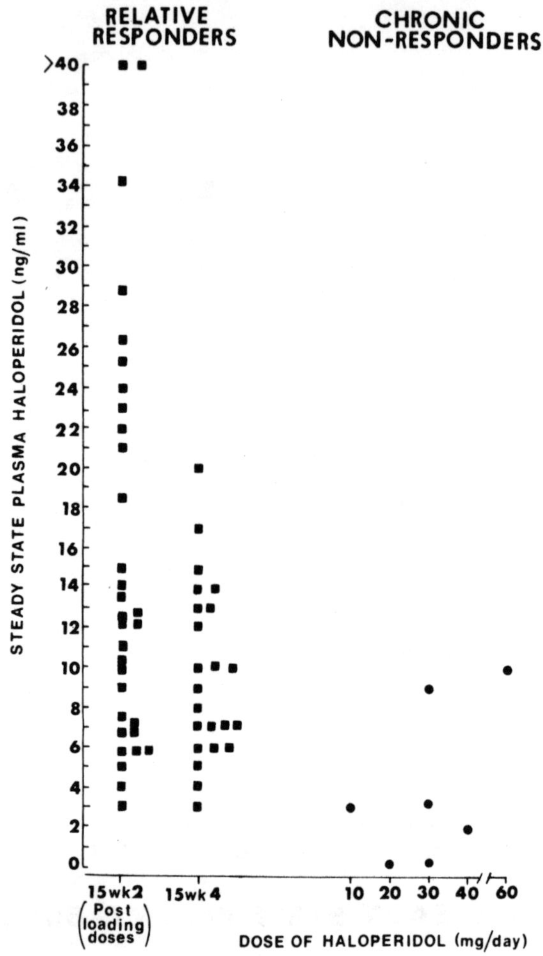

Figure 4. Steady-state haloperidol levels in relative responders and chronic nonresponders. Relative responders were treated with 15 mg of haloperidol/day, and steady-state levels are shown during week 2 and week 3 or 4 of treatment. Nonresponders were treated with 10 to 60 mg of haloperidol/day.

2. *Low Blood Levels of Neuroleptic Drugs: Possible Pharmacokinetic Mechanisms*

Many factors could account for the low blood levels of butaperazine and other neuroleptics we found in chronic nonresponding patients. These include pharmacokinetic factors related to poor absorption of oral drugs, more rapid metabolism or elimination of the drug, as well as differences in the characteristics of the nonresponders vs. relative responders in our samples. Since age and sex characteristics of patients in the relative responder sample and the nonresponder sample at Manteno were the same, differences of this kind could be ruled out, at least in the present study.

More rapid metabolism of the neuroleptic drugs in CNR patients could lead to much lower blood levels. Faster metabolic rates in these patients might be due to hereditary differences in enzyme activity or they might be related to induction of drug-metabolizing enzymes for butaperazine and other neuroleptics during the course of many years of treatment with these drugs. If chronic nonresponders had more rapid *systemic* metabolism of butaperazine, this might be represented by a shorter ß-phase T½ of CNR patients compared to relative responders. However, we found no substantial difference in ß-phase T½ after an acute dose of butaperazine between chronic nonresponders and relative responders in several samples (Table 3). Furthermore, if enzyme induction were an important factor, we would have expected patients who had received more neuroleptic drugs in the past to have lower levels of butaperazine,

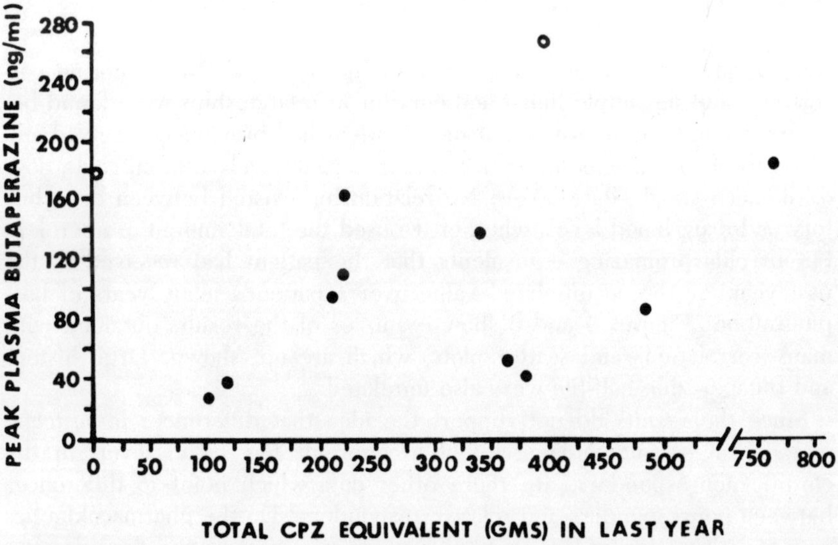

Figure 5. Lack of relationship between drug history and butaperazine levels: peak plasma butaperazine after a single acute 40-mg dose vs. total grams of neuroleptics (converted to chlorpromazine equivalents) during the year prior to the study. For explanation of open symbols see Figure 3.

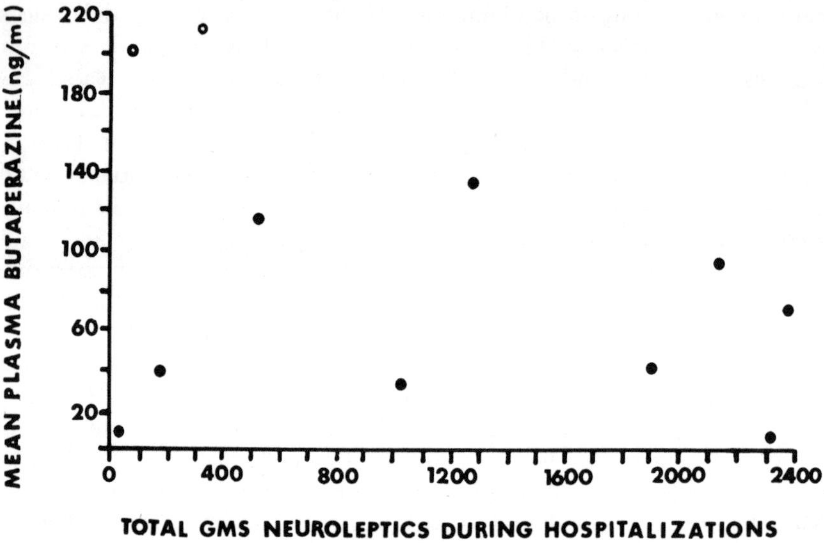

Figure 6. Lack of relationship between drug history and butaperazine levels: mean steady-state plasma butaperazine vs. total grams of neuroleptics during years of hospitalization. For explanation of open symbols see Figure 3.

thioridazine, and mesoridazine. This was not the case. No significant correlations and no simple linear and curvilinear relationships were found between amounts of neuroleptic drugs a patient had previously received and blood levels of these neuroleptics, either at peak levels after an acute dose or at mean steady-state levels. No relationship existed between drug history and drug blood levels whether we used the total amount of neuroleptics or chlorpromazine equivalents that the patient had received in the past year, or the accumulated value over a patient's many years of hospitalization. Figures 5 and 6 show examples of the results obtained with many correlations and scatter plots, which are not shown. Drug history and butaperazine half-life were also unrelated.

Since the results do not support the idea that differences in *systemic* metabolism of butaperazine might account for low blood levels in the chronic nonresponders, are there other data which point to differences between nonresponders and relative responders? Do the pharmacokinetics or metabolism during the absorptive phase (i.e., before the drug reaches the systemic circulation) contribute to much lower blood levels in chronic nonresponders? We have only limited and indirect data to bring to bear on the question of whether processes in the absorptive phase contributed

Table 3

Plasma Butaperazine Half-Life after an Acute Dose in Chronic Nonresponders and Comparison Groups

	β-Phase Half-Life (hr.)		
	Nonresponders (NR)	*Relative Responders (RR)*	
	CNR	*ISPI-RR*	*TNI-RR*
(N)	(10)	(10)	(23)
Mean ± s.e.m.	13.7 ± 1.5	12.2 ± 2.0	11.9 ± 1.5

Nonresponder sample, 40-mg. Relative responder samples, 20 to 60 mg.

to the low blood levels of neuroleptic drugs. If events related to the absorptive phase result in low blood levels of a drug, then one would expect an intramuscular dose of the drug to yield higher blood levels than an equivalent oral dose. One might also expect a low correlation between plasma levels after similar drug doses administered by oral and intramuscular routes. Because of unexpected hypotensive effects of mesoridazine in these patients, we could not give equal oral and i.m. doses of mesoridazine. In the same subjects, however, the correlation between the highest plasma level after 75 mg of orally or 25 mg of intramuscularly administered mesoridazine was very low (r = .03), as was the correlation between the patient's highest plasma level after 25 mg of mesoridazine i.m. and a 40-mg acute dose of butaperazine (r = .05). If events in the absorptive phase were important factors, one would also expect area under the blood level curve (AUC) to be higher after similar intramuscular as compared to oral doses. (Graphic plots of blood levels indicated that ß-phase slopes generally appeared similar after the two routes of mesoridazine administration in the same subject, although our limited sampling points did not permit accurate calculation to T½s). If blood levels of mesoridazine were directly proportional to dosage, we could compare AUC/mg dose for intramuscular vs. oral mesoridazine, and see whether this ratio is greater or less than 1.0. Using this assumption, the AUC_{0-25} hours were calculated and compared for the two routes by the triangulation method; six or eight nonresponders had ratios of intramuscular dose/oral dose of AUC/mg greater than 1.0, and only one nonresponder had a substantially greater AUC/mg after oral mesoridazine. There are important methodological deficiencies that do not permit a definite interpretation of the significance of these data in regard to changes in the absorptive phase. But our preliminary results would be consistent with the suggestion that differences between responders and nonresponders in

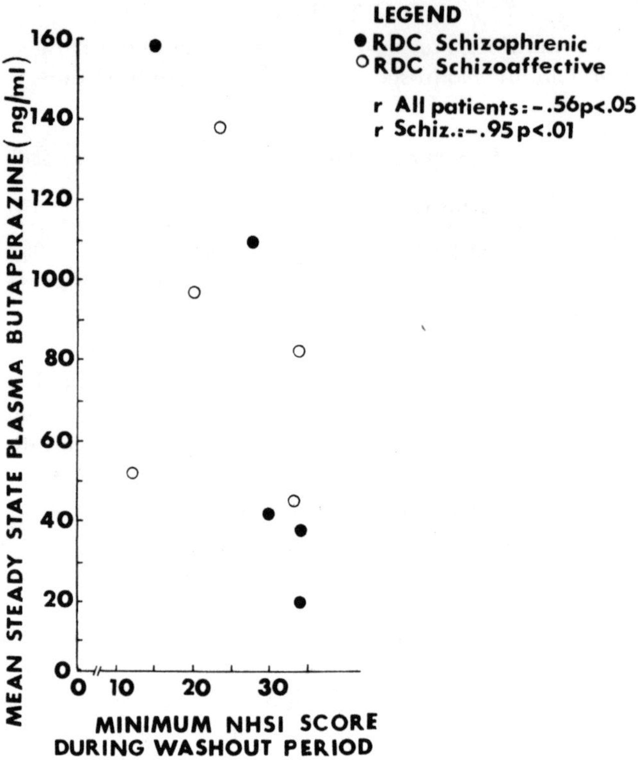

Figure 7. Relationship between psychopathology manifest during drug-free washout (lowest NHSI score) and steady-state plasma butaperazine levels during subsequent treatment with this medication. • Patients with RDC diagnosis of chronic schizophrenia. ○ Patients with RDC diagnosis of chronic schizoaffective disorder.

the pharmacokinetics of the absorptive phase after oral administraton of a neuroleptic may contribute to the low blood levels we have documented in chronic nonresponding schizophrenic patients.

3. *Blood Levels and Clinical Response*

What is the clinical significance of these low drug blood levels in chronic nonresponders? Are these levels directly related to the poor clinical response of the nonresponding schizophrenic patients? If low blood levels were a decisive immediate cause of the patients' failure to benefit from treatment with neuroleptics, one might make the following predictions: (1) Nonresponders with the lowest drug blood levels should have the most severe schizophrenic psychopathology and show the least improvement after neuroleptic medication, compared to those nonresponding patients whose blood levels were only slightly below the "normal" level of relative responders; and (2) if blood levels in these patients could be raised into the "normal" range by increasing the dosage of neuroleptic medication or changing the route of administration, then the psychosis of these intractable nonresponders should improve substantially.

Low plasma levels of butaperazine were related to baseline levels of schizophrenic psychopathology during the drug-free period (Figure 7). Patients with the highest psychopathology scores during the washout period had the lowest steady-state butaperazine levels when they were later put on 80 mg of butaperazine/day, with only one patient deviating from this pattern. Pearson correlation coefficients for the relationship of steady-state blood levels to New Haven Schizophrenia Index (NHSI) Score showed an especially high negative correlation ($r = -.95$) for patients with an RDC diagnosis of chronic schizophrenia.

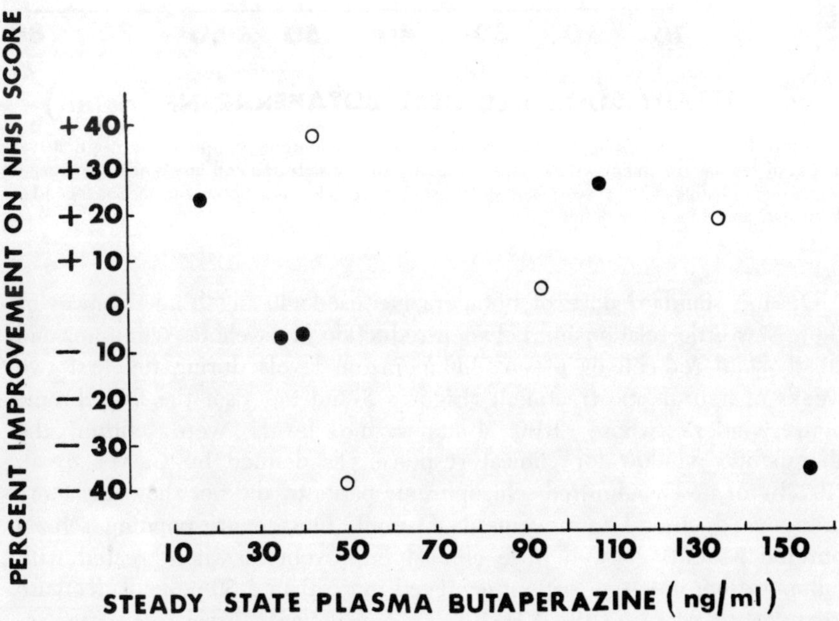

Figure 8. Relationship between improvement in schizophrenic symptoms during first two weeks of regular treatment (percentage change from mean NHSI score during pre-drug washout) and mean steady-state plasma levels of butaperazine (dosage 80 mg/day). For interpretation of other symbols see Figure 7.

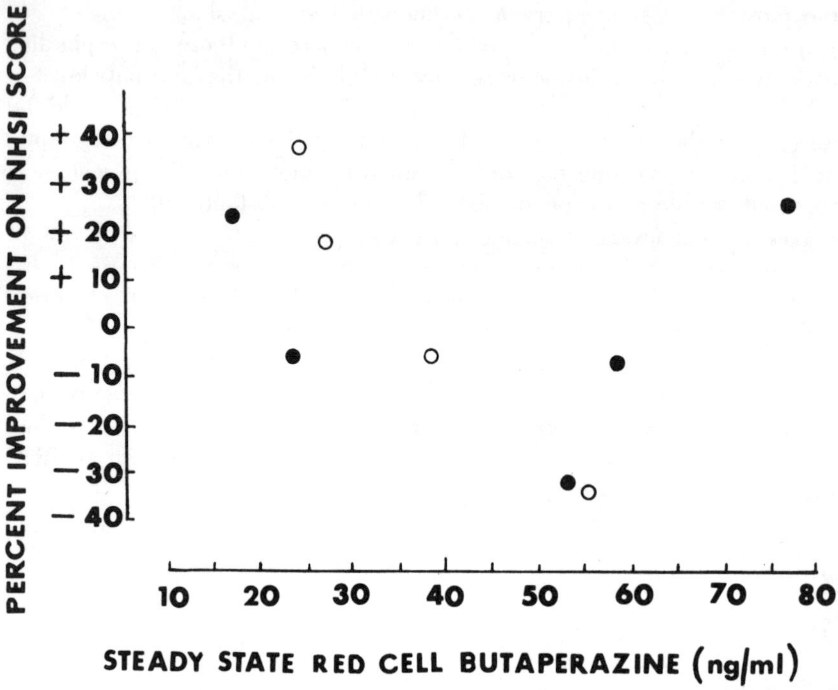

Figure 9. Relationship between improvement in schizophrenic symptoms during first two weeks of regular treatment with butaperazine and steady-state red cell levels of butaperazine (percentage change in NHSI score) and steady-state red cell levels of butaperazine. See legend of Figures 7 and 8 for other details.

On the standard dose of butaperazine used (40 mg b.i.d.), however, there was little relationship between reduction of psychotic symptoms and steady-state red-cell or plasma butaperazine levels during the first two weeks of neuroleptic treatment (Figures 8 and 9). Also, the few chronic nonresponders whose RBC butaperazine levels were within the therapeutic window for clinical response, as defined by Garver et al. (1977b) for newly admitted schizophrenic patients, did not show any more pronounced clinical improvement. Overall, most nonresponding schizophrenic patients showed little clinical improvement when treated with butaperazine; only one patient achieved more than a 30-percent decrease in psychosis score on the NHSI and a few patients' psychoses scores increased during butaperazine treatment.

One could argue that our failure to find any correlation of blood levels with clinical improvement in psychosis, when nonresponders were on the standard dosage of butaperazine, may be due to the fact that most blood levels in CNR patients were very low and that even the few nonresponders with blood levels within the presumed "therapeutic window" for relative responders had blood levels only slightly above these somewhat arbitrary cut-off points. Is it possible to raise neuroleptic blood levels in chronic nonresponders to levels equal to those of relative responders by increasing dosages? Would substantial clinical improvement follow?

Preliminary data from a continuation of the original study do indicate that when these CNR patients are given very high dosages of butaperazine, 160 to 320 mg/day, most of the patients do achieve plasma and red-cell butaperazine levels well within or even above the range of "normal" blood levels achieved by relative responders at lower dosages (40 to 80 mg/day) of the drug (Figure 10). In these later studies, chronic nonresponders began a regular butaperazine regimen on doses of 40 b.i.d., with an increase in dosage every three or four weeks. As Table 4 shows, during one or more of these four-week treatment blocks, most chronic nonresponders appeared to have plasma and red-blood cell butaperazine levels within the "therapeutic window" or levels similar to those at which most relative responders show optimal benefit from therapy with antipsychotic medication. Our quantitative measures of clinical response (reduction of psychosis scores) of the CNR patients on these very high dosages of butaperazine remain to be analyzed. Thus, the second question—whether more "normal" blood levels in chronic nonresponders are associated with substantially greater reduction in psychosis scores—cannot yet be answered. Based on our clinical observations, we can state, however, that no patient improved markedly on the very high doses of butaperazine at which these CNR patients showed more normal blood levels of the drug.

4. *Clinical Response and Prolactin*

Possibly factors other than blood or CNS levels of neuroleptics—perhaps changes in the sensitivity of neuroleptic receptors—are responsible for the relatively poor clinical response to antipsychotic medication of the chronic nonresponding schizophrenic patients. A substantial body of research now demonstrates that there are dopamine and neuroleptic receptors in the tuberoinfundibular system as well as striatum (Seeman et al., 1975; Brown, Seeman, and Lee, 1976) and that dopaminergic influences play a large part in mediating prolactin responses in animals and man (Meites, Lu, and Wuttke, 1972; Smalstig, Sawyer and Clemens, 1974; Frohman and Stachura, 1975). Neuroleptic drugs raise plasma prolac-

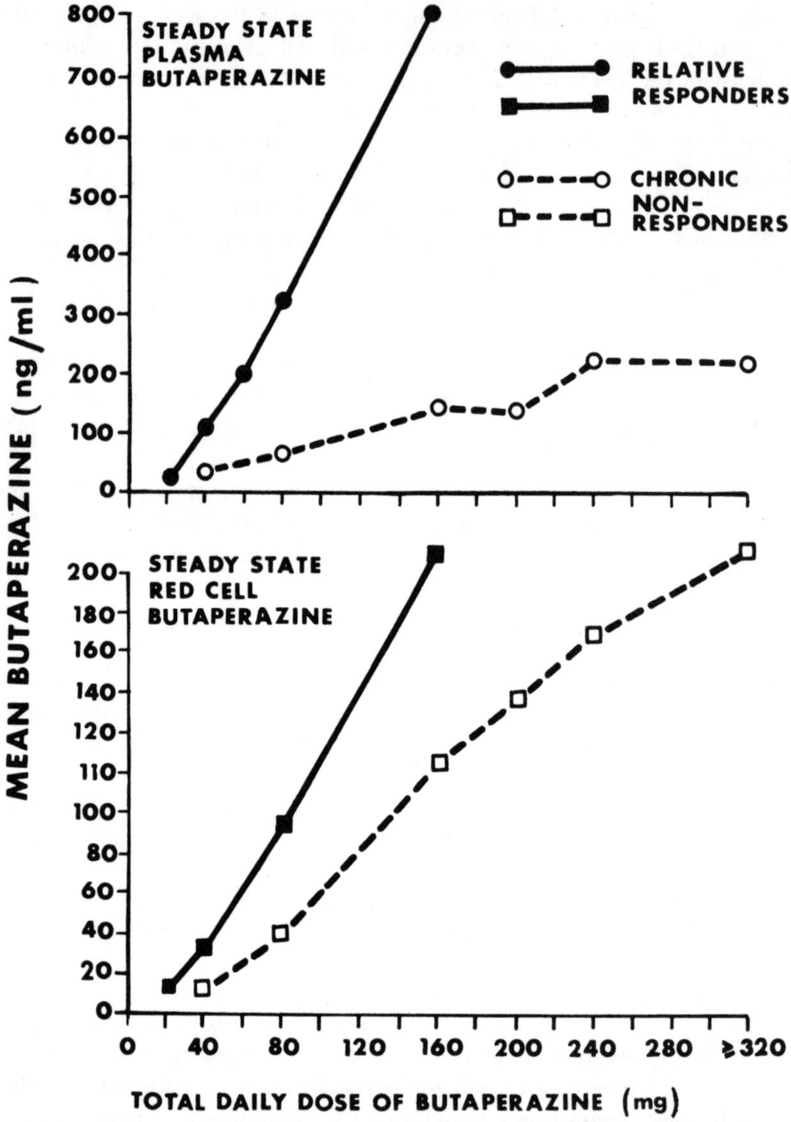

Figure 10. Dose-response curve for plasma and red cell butaperazine levels in relative responders (●—●, ■—■) and chronic nonresponders (○—○, □—□). Each point represents mean butaperazine level. (N varies from 2 to 16 patients for different dosages.)

tin levels through a blockade of brain dopamine receptors and consequent reduction of inhibitory dopaminergic influences on secretions of this hormone (Sachar et al., 1976; Gruen et al., 1978). One study by Meltzer and Fang (1976), done in a short-term hospital, suggests a positive relationship between rise of plasma prolactin and clinical response of schizophrenic patients treated with neuroleptic medication.

These ideas lead to the suggestion that plasma prolactin may reflect the sensitivity of brain dopamine or neuroleptic receptors, at least those in the tuberoinfundibular dopaminergic system. If chronic nonresponders do not benefit from chemotherapy because of decreased sensitivity of brain receptors for antipsychotic drugs (or defects in other "coupling" steps between receptor binding and cellular response), then one might expect chronic nonresponders with the lowest prolactin rise after neuroleptic treatment to experience the least clinical response. Our preliminary results with a small number of patients, however, tend to be in the opposite direction. Patients with the highest levels of prolactin during the first two weeks of regular treatment with the standard dosage (40 mg b.i.d.) of butaperazine showed the poorest clinical response—that is, the lowest percentage of improvement in their psychopathology scores. This was especially true for female patients with an RDC diagnosis of schizophrenia (Figures 11 and 12).

Discussion

Our investigation has gone farther than have most earlier studies to provide evidence that many schizophrenic patients who have consistently shown poor clinical response to treatment with neuroleptic drugs have low blood levels of these drugs. This was shown for several drugs after administration (Curry et al., 1970). Although first-pass metabolism through the liver could be another reason for the lower butaperazine, in several comparisons, relative responders had three to seven times higher plasma levels of butaperazine and two to five times higher red-cell butaperazine levels than nonresponders. Dosage vs. blood level graphs for butaperazine in relative responders, compared to chronic nonresponders, showed a considerable shift to the right in both plasma and red-cell curves of the CNR patients. Plasma levels of other neuroleptics—thioridazine, haloperidol, and mesoridazine—measured in some of the same patients were also lower than in relative responders, although our data for these other neuroleptic drugs are not as extensive.

The very low blood levels of neuroleptics we have documented in chronic nonresponders lead to two important questions: (1) what processes

Table 4
Percentage of Chronic Nonresponders Showing Plasma or Red Cell Butaperazine within Therapeutic Window or Similar to Relative Responders

	Patients Treated with Butaperazine at Dosage of	
Steady-State Plasma Butaperazine	80 mg/day	80 mg/day + Higher Dosages*
100-275 ng/ml	16%	80%
≥ 150 ng/ml	5%	90%
Steady-State Red Cell Butaperazine		
45-90 ng/ml	39%	70%

*Each number in this column represents percentage of patients who had mean blood level in indicated range during one or more three-week periods of treatment with 80 mg/day of butaperazine and/or one of the higher butaperazine dosages.

are responsible for these low levels, and (2) what is their clinical significance? Information about the pharmacokinetics of these drugs in responders and nonresponders, the relationship of blood levels to quantitative measures of clinical response, and the plasma prolactin responses to neuroleptics that we have collected in the current study may begin to answer these questions and point to specific types of additional information needed for more definitive answers.

Mechanisms That Account for Low Blood Levels of Neuroleptic Drugs

There may be many reasons for the low blood levels of neuroleptic drugs in these patients. These can include factors related to: (1) differences in patient characteristics, for example, age and sex, which might affect drug absorption or metabolism of drugs; (2) poor absorption of orally ingested drugs; (3) increased drug metabolism in the gut wall or in the first pass through the liver; (4) faster *systemic* metabolism of the drug (i.e., after the drug reaches the general circulation); (5) changes in drug distribution and storage in body tissues. Our preliminary information bears on a few of these issues. The data presented here support the conclusions that: (a) age and sex differences in the nonresponders and relative responder samples do not account for the differences in blood levels, and (b) differences in *systemic* metabolism of butaperazine are unlikely to be a primary factor explaining the lower blood levels of chronic nonresponders. Our results point to a possible defect in the absorptive phase after oral drug administration, and this needs further investigation.

Cooper et al. (1975) reported a single case of a chronic schizophrenic

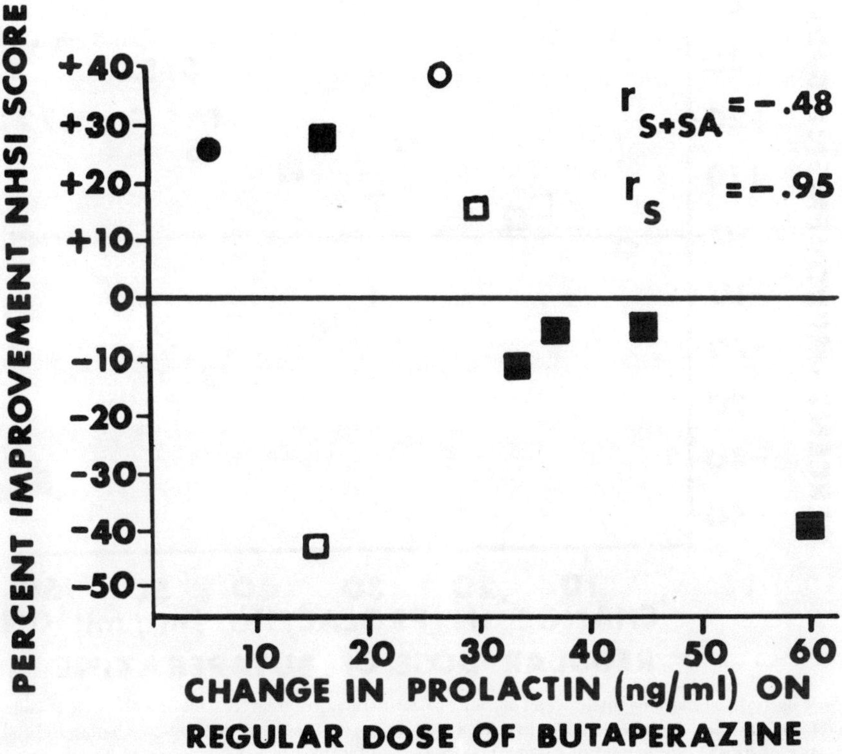

Figure 11. Relationship between plasma prolactin during regular treatment with butaperazine and improvement in schizophrenic symptoms. Blood samples were drawn at 8 a.m. Each plasma prolactin value represents the mean prolactin, based on two to four samples, drawn during the second week of regular butaperazine administration (80 mg/day) minus the mean prolactin in the pre-drug washout period samples. Improvement in schizophrenic symptoms is represented by percentage change in NHSI score during first two weeks of regular treatment. (● ○)Male patients, (□ ■) female patients. (● ■) Patients with RDC diagnosis of chronic schizophrenia. (○ □) Patients with RDC diagnosis of chronic schizoaffective illness. r_{S+SA} = correlation coefficient using all patients; r_S = correlation coefficient using only chronic schizophrenic patients.

patient whose plasma butaperazine levels declined steeply during 28 weeks of treatment with 100 mg/day of butaperazine, which corresponded with a decline in his clinical status; these authors suggested that induction of hepatic drug-metabolizing enzymes for butaperazine was a likely explanation for these blood level changes. If this explanation were also valid for the low blood levels in our sample of chronic nonresponding patients, one would have predicted a shorter β-phase butaperazine T½ in nonresponders compared to relative responders. Our results, however, do *not* support faster *systematic* metabolism as the reason for the low blood levels of

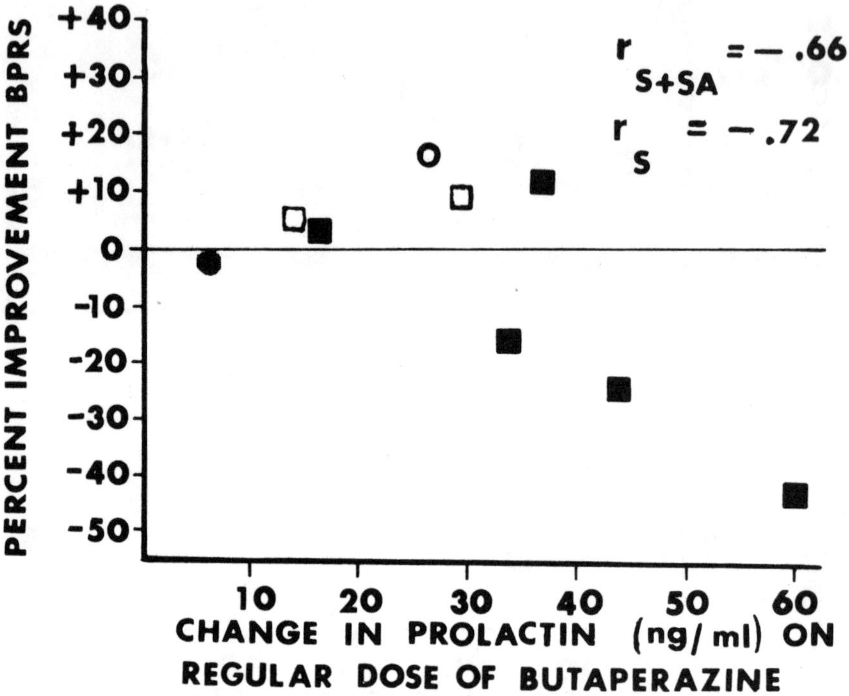

Figure 12. Relationship between plasma prolactin during regular treatment with butaperazine (80 mg/day) and improvement in psychiatric symptoms assessed as percentage change in total score of BPRS. See legend of Figure 11 for other details.

butaperazine in the nonresponders we studied. The ß-phase T½ was not shorter in chronic nonresponders than relative responders, and we also found the quantity of neuroleptics a patient had received unrelated either to the patients' levels of neuroleptics or their butaperazine T½. Although we have no data on ß-phase T½ of thioridazine, two other recent studies do not support the idea that chronic administration of thioridazine results in lower blood levels or more rapid metabolism. Axelsson and Mårtensson (1976) found no systemic differences in thioridazine blood levels or T½ in patients chronically treated with thioridazine for a one- to two-year period, and the Berling group's (1975) data also indicate no systematic trend for increases or decreases in thioridazine levels in chronic schizophrenic patients during continued treatment with the drug. Taken together, our own and others' results suggest that, in most patients, faster *systonic* metabolism of neuroleptics is unlikely to be the primary cause of the very low blood levels found in chronic nonresponders. It may be a factor for a few patients.

These findings shifted our attention to processes in the absorptive phase as a possible explanation of the low drug levels in chronic nonresponders. Mechanisms in the absorptive phase that might be altered in chronic schizophrenics include poorer gastrointestinal absorption of oral medication, extensive drug metabolism in the gut wall, greater first-pass metabolism in the liver, or increased biliary extraction of drugs with subsequent redepositing in the gastrointestinal tract. A substantial body of research with another phenothiazine, chlorpromazine, suggests gut-wall metabolism may be of primary importance. A series of experiments in animals and man reported by Curry and associates has shown that metabolism of chlorpromazine in the gut wall is a major mechanism accounting for the original clinical finding (reported by Curry et al., 1970) that there were much lower levels of chlorpromazine in the patients given the drug by the oral route as compared to the intravenous or intramuscular route. Poor gastrointestinal absorption of oral chlorpromazine, however, was shown not to be an important factor since similar levels of total radioactive (S-35) chlorpromazine were found in animals administered the drug by all routes; in man total urinary levels of chlorpromazine metabolites were similar after intramuscular and oral administration (Curry et al., 1970). Although first-pass metabolism through the liver could be another reason for the lower plasma levels of the parent drug after oral doses, experiments in rats, which showed that plasma levels of chlorpromazine were similar after i.p. administration (in which this step is bypassed), suggested that first-pass metabolism was not the sole explanation. This line of reasoning led to *in vitro* studies in which chlorpromazine was injected into the loop of the rat intestine, with the result that large amounts of the drug were metabolized to biologically inactive metabolites in the gut-wall (Curry, D'Mello, and Mould, 1971). It is quite possible, therefore, that the phenothiazines, butaperazine and thioridazine, may also undergo extensive metabolism in the gut wall, and that increases in gut-wall metabolism could be an important factor contributing to the much lower blood levels of butaperazine and other neuroleptics we report in nonresponders. However, unlike chlorpromazine, butaperazine has also been shown to undergo substantial biliary extraction in animal studies (Bruce et al., 1974), and therefore this process may also be increased in chronic nonresponders. If elements in the absorptive phase were to account, importantly, for low blood levels of butaperazine in chronic nonresponders, one might predict that these patients would have lower peak elevations of butaperazine after a single acute dose, have lower steady-state levels of the drug, but show no appreciable difference in β-phase half-life; this is what our results for butaperazine show. Our suggestions about increases in gut-wall metabolism or other changes in the absorptive phase point to specific types of additional investigations needed to confirm these speculations and identify the most important factor. If we were able, for example, to measure butaperazine sulfoxide and sulfoxone metabolites in blood and urine and found these much higher in chronic nonresponders who also had low levels of the parent drug, this would provide support for the mechanism of gut-wall metabolism. A much higher concentration of butaperazine in feces would suggest poor absorption or increased biliary extraction as the primary mechanism of the low neuroleptic levels.

Clinical Significance of Low Blood Levels

Our attempt to relate neuroleptic blood levels to clinical response and serum prolactin levels suggests that the low levels of neuroleptic drugs in chronic nonresponders are in some way related to their psychoses, but that they may not be the immediate cause of the poor clinical response chronic nonresponding patients show to their current antipsychotic medication. The fact that higher baseline levels of psychopathology during the drug-free washout period correlated strongly with lower steady-state levels of butaperazine during the period of regular drug treatment suggests that some of the factors associated with severe schizophrenic illness may also cause or be related to low blood levels of neuroleptic drugs. The absence of any relationship between blood levels and clinical response at the standard dosage (40 mg b.i.d.), and the preliminary evidence suggesting no greater therapeutic improvement when the blood levels of these chronic nonresponders were brought into the "normal" range with higher dosages of butaperazine, both argue against the idea that low blood levels were the main reason for our patients' continued failure to improve on antipsychotic drugs. This interpretation is based, however, on data from a relatively small sample of nonresponders at the standard dose, and our quantitative data on the relationship between blood levels and clinical response at higher dosages have not been fully analyzed; these conclusions must, therefore, be regarded with the caution appropriate to results that require further validation.

How might this apparent lack of relationship between neuroleptic drug levels and clinical response have come about? We can think of two hypotheses.

First, the absence of relationship between blood levels and clinical response in the CNR patients at this chronic stage of schizophrenic illness may be due to inadequate pharmacotherapy with antipsychotic medication they received at an earlier stage in the evolution of their illness. In a group of more acute nonresponders, studied at several short-term hospitals, we also found very low blood levels of butaperazine, similar to those of the chronic nonresponders at Manteno State Hospital. It is likely, therefore, that many chronic nonresponders also had low blood levels when they were treated with neuroleptic medication at an earlier stage of their illness. Perhaps if these patients had been treated early on with much higher doses of neuroleptics, bringing their blood levels into the therapeutic range, they would have shown a better clinical response in their psychosis; consequently, their illness might not have progressed to a chronic schizophrenia which is more refractory to treatment with neuroleptics. A few clinical studies of high-dose treatment with neuroleptics (Prien, Levine, and Cole, 1969; Clark et al., 1972; Donlon, 1976) for nonresponding schizophrenic patients generally showed that younger ones, or those with fewer years of hospitalization, achieved slightly more benefit from higher doses of neuroleptics than did schizophrenics hospitalized for longer periods of time. These findings are consistent with the idea that less chronic nonresponders may derive greater benefit from high dosages of neuroleptics that raise blood levels into the therapeutic range of relative responders. More systematic studies in acute nonresponders are needed to test this point.

On the other hand, the CNR schizophrenic patients may be physiologically and biochemically different from acute or relapsing schizophrenics. These differences could be intrinsic characteristics of two different types of schizophrenia, or they could be induced by the course of chronic unremitting schizophrenic illness. Several researchers have suggested that acute or relapsing schizophrenia, which is characterized by more prominent affective symptoms, is a disease whose etiology and course are quite different from chronic persistent schizophrenia. Scandinavian investigators distinguish schizophreniform psychosis from schizophrenia, and American investigators refer to *reactive* vs. *process* schizophrenia. Much of the research that supports the dopaminergic-overactivity theory of schizophrenia is based on studies with the more acutely ill schizophrenic patients and may be applicable only to this subcategory of schizophrenia. Research by our own group (Smith et al., 1977; Tamminga et al., 1977; Pandey et al., 1977) and others (Kornetsky, 1976) has demonstrated important biochemical and pharmacological differences between acute and chronic schizophrenics which are relevant to the dopamine hypothesis of schizophrenia. That the release of prolactin and growth hormone (Frohman and Stachura, 1975) is partially under the control of dopaminergic influences in the brain is well documented. Whereas acute schizophrenic patients have increased responses to prolactin and growth hormone, compared to normal controls, in response to a single dose of the dopamine agonists apomorphine and l-dopa, chronic schizophrenics do not show this hyperresponsiveness; their prolactin and growth hormone responses do not differ significantly from those of normal controls (Tamminga et al., 1977; Pandey et al., 1977). Intravenous administration of the stimulant drugs, amphetamine or methylphenidate, which release dopamine from presynaptic neurons in the brain, produce clear increases in the schizophrenic symptomatology of actively ill acute schizophrenics (Janowsky and Davis, 1976). This may not be true in chronic schizophrenia. In several chronic schizophrenic patients studied in connection with tardive dyskinesia, we did not find that intravenously administered amphetamine consistently increased their psychotic symptoms (Smith et al., 1977). Kornetsky (1976) similarly reported no effect of fairly high dosages of oral amphetamine on increasing the psychosis of chronic schizophrenic patients. If our CNR patients, who have low blood levels of neuroleptics, are not suffering from a disease due to a primary biochemical defect in the dopaminergic system, their schizophrenic illness may not be substantially ameliorated by neuroleptic drugs that probably exert their therapeutic effects by blocking brain dopamine receptors (Burt, Creese, and Snyder, 1976). The negative correlation of prolactin response and therapeutic response to neuroleptics in the chronic nonresponding schizophrenic patients in our study is also consistent with the suggestion that the cause of their illness may not be a defect in the brain dopaminergic system.

Before we can definitely conclude, however, that higher blood levels of neuroleptic drugs will not substantially benefit many chronic nonresponding schizophrenic patients, we must extend our studies to such other neuroleptic drugs as haloperidol. We should determine whether high dosages of these other drugs will also raise blood levels to those achieved in relative responders, and then correlate these blood levels with quantitative measures of clinical improvement.

REFERENCES

Axelsson, R., and Mårtensson, E., 1976. Serum concentration and elimination from serum of thioridazine in psychiatric patients. *Curr. Ther. Res.*, 19:242-265.

Berling, R., Mjorndal, T., Oreland, L., Rapp, W., and Wold, S. 1975. Plasma levels and clinical effects of thioridazine and thiothixene. *J. Clin. Pharmacol.*, 15:178-186.

Brown, G. M., Seeman, P., and Lee, T. 1976. Dopamine/neuroleptic receptors in basal hypothalamus and pituitary. *Endocrinology*, 99:1407-1410.

Bruce, R. B., Turnbull, J. H., Newman, J. M., Kinzie, P. H., Morris, P. H., and Pinchbeck, F. M. 1974. Butaperazine dimaleate metabolism. *Xenobiotica*, 4:197-207.

Burt, D. R., Creese, I., and Snyder, S., 1976. Dopamine receptor binding predicts clinical and pharmacological potencies of anti-schizophrenic drugs. *Science*, 192:481-483.

CLARK, M. L., RAMSEY, R., RAHHAL, D. K., SERAFETINIDES, E. A., WOOD, F. D., and COSTILOE, J. P. 1972. Chlorpromazine in chronic schizophrenia. *Arch. Gen. Psychiatry*, 27:479-483.

COOPER, T. B., SIMPSON, G. M., HAHER, E. J., and BERGNER, P. E. 1975. Butaperazine pharmacokinetics. *Arch. Gen. Psychiatry*, 32:903-905.

CURRY, S. H., DAVIS, J. M., JANOWSKY, D. S., and MARSHALL, J. H. L., 1970. Factors affecting chlorpromazine plasma levels in psychiatric patients. *Arch. Gen. Psychiatry*, 22:209-215.

CURRY, S. H., DERR, J. E., and MALING, H. M., 1970. The physiological disposition of chlorpromazine in the rat and dog. *Proc. Soc. Exp. Biol. Med.*, 134:314-318.

CURRY, S. H., MARSHALL, J. H. L., DAVIS, J. M., and JANOWSKY, D. S., 1970. Chlorpromazine plasma levels and effects. *Arch. Gen. Psychiatry*, 22:289-296.

CURRY, S. H., D'MELLO, A., and MOULD, G. P. 1971. Destruction of chlorpromazine during absorption in the rat *in vivo* and *in vitro*. *Br. J. Pharmacol.*, 42:403-411.

DAVIS, J. M. 1974. Dose equivalence of anti-psychotic drugs. *J. Psychiatr. Res.*, 11:65-69.

DAVIS, J. M., JANOWSKY, D. S., SEKERKE, H. J., MANIER, H., and EL-YOUSEF, M. K. 1974. The pharmacokinetics of butaperazine in serum. In I. S. Forest, C. J. Carr, and E. Usdin (eds.), *Phenothiazines and Structurally Related Drugs. Advances in Biochemical Pharmacology*, vol. 9, pp. 433-443. New York: Raven Press.

DONLON, P. T. 1976. High dosage neuroleptic therapy. *Int. Pharmacopsychiatry*, 11:235-245.

FORSMAN, S., MÅRTENSSON, E., NYBERG, G., and ÖHMAN, R., 1974. A gas chromatographic method for determining haloperidol. *Naunyn Schmiedelbergs Arch. Pharmacol.*, 286:113-124.

FROHMAN, L. A. and STACHURA, M. E. 1975. Neuropharmacologic control of neuroendocrine function in man. *Metabolism*, 24:211-234.

GARVER, D. L., DAVIS, J. M., DEKIRMENJIAN, H., JONES, F. D., CASPER, R., and HARASZTI, J. 1976. Pharmacokinetics of red blood cell phenothiazine and clinical effects. *Arch Gen. Psychiatry*, 33:862-866.

GARVER, D. L., DAVIS, J. M., DEKIRMENJIAN, H., and SMITH, R. C. 1977a. Phenothiazine red cell levels and clinical response. Paper presented at 16th Annual Meeting, American College of Neuropsychopharmacology, San Juan, Puerto Rico.

GARVER, D. L., DEKIRMENJIAN, H., DAVIS, J. M., CASPER, R., and ERICKSEN, S., 1977b. Neuroleptic drug levels and therapeutic response: Preliminary observations with red blood cell bound butaperazine. *Am. J. Psychiatry*, 134:304-307.

GOTTSCHALK, L. A., DINOVO, E., BIENER, R., BIRCH, H., SYBEN, M., and NOBLE, E. P. 1976. Plasma levels of mesoridazine and its metabolites and clinical response after a single intra-muscular drug dose. In L. A. Gottschalk and S. Merlis (eds.), *Pharmacokinetics of Psychiatric Drugs*, pp. 171-190. New York: Spectrum.

GRUEN, P. H., SACHAR, E. J., LANGER, G., ALTMAN, N., LEIFER, M., FRANTZ, A., and HALPERN, F. S. 1978. Prolactin responses to neuroleptics in normal and schizophrenic subjects. *Arch. Gen. Psychiatry*, 35:108-116.

JANOWSKY, D. S., and DAVIS, J. M. 1976. Methylphenidate, dextroamphetamine, and levoamphetamine: Effect on schizophrenic symptoms. *Arch. Gen. Psychiatry*, 33:304-308.

JANOWSKY, D. S., DAVIS, J. M., and KORNETSKY, C. 1976. Hyporesponsivity of chronic schizophrenic patients to dextroamphetamine. *Arch. Gen. Psychiatry*, 33:1425-1428.

KORNETSKY, C. 1976. Hyporesponsivity of chronic schizophrenic patients to dextroamphetamine. *Arch. Gen. Psychiatry*, 33: 1425-1428.

MEITES, J., LU, K. H., and WUTTKE, W., 1972. Recent studies of functions and control of prolactin secretion in rats. *Recent Prog. Horm. Res.*, 28:471-526.

MELTZER, H. Y., and FANG, V. S. 1976. The effects of neuroleptics on serum prolactin in schizophrenic patients. *Arch. Gen. Psychiatry*, 33:279-286.

PACHA, W. L. 1969. A method for fluorimetric determination of thioridazine (Mellaril) or mesoridazine (Lidanil) in plasma. *Experientia*, 25:103-104.

PANDEY, G. N., GARVER, D. L., TAMMINGA, C. A., ERICKSEN, S., ALI, S. I., and DAVIS, J. M. 1977. Postsynaptic supersensitivity in schizophrenia. *Am. J. Psychiatry*, 134:518-522.

PRIEN, R. F., LEVINE, J., and COLE, J. O., 1969. High dose trifluoperazine therapy in chronic schizophrenia. *Am. J. Psychiatry*, 126:305-313.

RIVERA-CALIMLIM, L., NASRALLAH, H., STRAUSS, J., and LASAGNA, L. 1976. Clinical response and plasma levels: Effects of dose, dosage schedules, and drug interactions on plasma chlorpromazine levels. *Am. J. Psychiatry*, 133:646-652.

RITSCHEL, W. A. 1976. *Handbook of Basic Pharmacokinetics*, pp. 189-190. Hamilton, Ill.: Drug Intelligence Publications.

SACHAR, E. J., GRUEN, P. H., ALTMAN, N., HALPERN, F. S., and FRANTZ, A. G. 1976. Use of neuroendocrine techniques in psychopharmacological research. In E. J. Sachar (ed.), *Hormones, Behavior, and Psychopathology*, pp. 161-176. New York: Raven Press.

SCHAFFER, M. H., TAMMINGA, C. A., and DAVIS, J. M. 1977. Modified New Haven Schizophrenia Scale. Mimeographed.

SEEMAN, P., CHAU-WONG, M., TEDESIO, J., and WONG, K. 1975. Brain receptors for antipsychotic drugs and dopamine: Direct binding assays. *Proc. Natl. Acad. Sci. USA*, 72:4376-4380.

SMALSTIG, E. B., SAWYER, B. D., and CLEMENS, J. A. 1974. Inhibition of rat prolactin release by apomorphine *in vivo* and *in vitro*. *Endocrinology*, 95:123-129.

SMITH, R. C., TAMMINGA, C. A., HARASZTI, J., PANDEY, G. N., and DAVIS, J. M. 1977. Effects of dopamine agonists in tardive dyskinesia. *Am. J. Psychiatry*, 134:763-768.

SPITZER, R. L., ENDICOTT, J., ROBINS, E., KURIANSKY, J., and GURLAND, B. 1975. Preliminary report on reliability of research diagnostic criteria applied to psychiatric case records. In A. Sudilovsky, S. Gershon, and B. Beer (eds.), *Psychopharmacology: Pre-clinical and Clinical Correlations*, pp. 1-48. New York: Raven Press.

TAMMINGA, C. A., SMITH, R. C., PANDEY, G., FROHMAN, L. A., and DAVIS, J. M. 1977. A neuroendocrine study of supersensitivity in tardive dyskinesia. *Arch. Gen. Psychiatry*, 34:1199-1203.

9

CLINICALLY SIGNIFICANT INTERACTIONS WITH PSYCHOTROPIC DRUGS

HERSHEL JICK, M.D.

Few topics have received more attention in clinical pharmacology in the past ten years than has the topic of drug interactions. Some interactions can be demonstrated from pharmacokinetic studies. Others have merely been suggested on theoretical grounds. Mechanisms by which drug interactions may occur include modifications of gastrointestinal absorption, protein binding, renal excretion, metabolism, and end-organ response. There is, in addition, another mechanism by which multidrug therapy may lead to clinically important events, that is, by exerting a cumulative effect on end organs.

In the area of psychopharmacology there is a voluminous literature concerning drug interactions that appear to lead to serious toxicity. Perhaps most frequently implicated are the monoamine oxidase (MAO) inhibitors (Marley, 1977). It is generally believed that these drugs are contraindicated in patients receiving other psychopharmacologic agents in general, and in patients receiving tricyclic antidepressants in particular (Marley, 1977).

The concern about the toxicity of MAO inhibitors has led to a marked decrease in their use. (In our study of more than 26,000 medical inpatients, fewer than 20 have received MAO inhibitors.) The concern about drug interactions is not, however, limited to MAO inhibitors. Virtually all other psychotropic drugs have been repeatedly implicated in a large variety of drug interactions (Grahame-Smith, 1977).

The complexity and substance of this subject has been thoroughly and admirably reviewed by Grahame-Smith (1977) and others (Marley, 1977).

I shall discuss the findings of our own research program which relates specifically to medical inpatients. Our research group now known as the Boston Collaborative Drug Surveillance Program (BCDSP) has been collecting information on clinical drug effects in hospitalized medical patients for more than ten years (Jick et al., 1970). The details of our methods have been repeatedly reported (Jick et al., 1970). This data base provides an opportunity to explore the clinical significance of proposed drug interactions. With the aid of a computer, it is possible to identify patients who received any combination of drugs and to evaluate their clinical course in relationship to patients who received any of the drugs alone. That the data are well suited to demonstrate clinically significant drug interactions is illustrated by a number of studies we have already published. As an example of a special analysis designed to evaluate the influence of one drug on the effect of another, we have evaluated the possible interaction between chloral hydrate and warfarin (Boston Collaborative Drug Surveillance Program, 1972a). All monitored patients who were warfarinized during hospitalization were identified and divided into three groups—those who received chloral hydrate continuously during hospitalization, those who received it occasionally, and those who never received it. The initial loading dose of warfarin, the dosage during days 2 to 4 of warfarinization, and the maintenance dosage were calculated for patients in each of the three groups. The results showed that the loading doses and maintenance dosages were similar in the three groups. However, during days 2 to 4 of warfarinization patients receiving chloral hydrate continuously required substantially less warfarin compared with those receiving no chloral hydrate. Those taking chloral hydrate occasionally received an intermediate amount of warfarin. These data are consistent with the mechanism of interaction proposed by Sellers and Koch-Weser (1970) that a transient rise in prothrombin time follows the displacement of warfarin from plasma albumin by chloral hydrate metabolites. This rise is caused by an increase in the level of unbound (active) warfarin, which subsequently falls as increased metabolic inactivation leads to a reduction in the half-life of the drug in the plasma. Incidentally, we examined the relationship of barbiturate administration in the same manner and found no significant differences in warfarin dosage between patients who received barbiturates and those who did not.

In an analogous fashion it is possible to perform a variety of analyses with these data to evaluate proposed interactions. We have not yet had time for a substantial number of *detailed* evaluations of certain proposed interactions. However, we have carried out some preliminary analyses in certain areas. It is our impression, for example, that patients who are taking antacids do not respond differently to a wide variety of drugs such as barbiturates, whose absorption from the gastrointestinal tract has been proposed to be influenced by the presence of antacid substances. There is, in addition, little gross evidence for a substantial effect of the large number of inducers or inhibitors of drug-metabolizing enzymes on the usual clinical course of most patients. Indeed, in our experience with more than 32,000 medical inpatients, a well-defined interaction involving drug-metabolizing enzyme systems has been implicated by the attending physician in an adverse event in less than two dozen instances. This does not mean that such interactions do not occur substantially more often, and future thorough evaluations of the data may provide better quantification of the extent of this problem.

Another proposed drug interaction of substantial clinical importance has been evaluated within our data—the interaction between potassium chloride and spironolactone (Greenblatt and Koch-Weser, 1973). An additional factor involved in this interaction is renal function. Among some 13,000 patients who were studied, 5.9 percent received spironolactone. Hyperkalemia developed in 16 percent of patients who received potassium chloride concomitantly compared with 6 percent of those who did not. In addition, hyperkalemia developed in 20 percent of patients with admitting blood urea nitrogen (BUN) values of 50 mg/100 ml or higher. Of patients with such BUN values who also received potassium chloride, 42 percent developed hyperkalemia. These data provide evidence for a profound, clinically important interrelationship between potassium-sparing diuretics, potassium chloride supplements, and renal function. Indeed, of all of the interactions we have evaluated, this one seems to be the most commonly occurring and the most serious.

Other apparent interactions we have studied in detail may be classified as unexpected or newly discovered. Clues regarding the possible existence of these interactions were obtained from routine scans of the BCDSP data base. These scans are designed to provide initial clues on unsuspected drug effects. One of these scans, for example, showed a strong association between allopurinol and allergic skin reactions (Boston Collaborative Drug Surveillance Program, 1972b). A detailed evaluation revealed that the association existed exclusively in allopurinol recipients who were also receiving ampicillin at the same time. Patients taking allopurinol in the absence of ampicillin developed rashes at the same rate as the population at large. This finding led to a detailed evaluation of the possible interaction between the two drugs. The frequencies of rashes among allopurinol recipients and nonrecipients were 22.4 and 7.5 percent, respectively ($p < 0.00005$). Apart from allopurinol, no other drugs were significantly associated with ampicillin rashes. The data thus suggest that the allergenicity of ampicillin is enhanced by allopurinol or, alternatively, by hyperuricemia. The relationship cannot be explained without invoking interaction because the frequency of drug-attributed rashes among recipients of allopurinol who did not receive ampicillin was similar to that observed among ampicillin nonusers in general.

It is important to note that the technique used to identify these proposed interactions—namely, intensive monitoring—is the only one likely to do so in the absence of laboratory findings that suggest that an interaction might be expected.

We have explored to some degree two other areas related to drug interactions. The first relates drug effects to cigarette smoking. We have repeatedly observed, in our routine scans, that cigarette smokers seem to react differently from nonsmokers to certain drugs. We have reported the results of detailed evaluations of smoking in relation to propoxyphene efficacy (Boston Collaborative Drug Surveillance Program, 1973a) and to chlordiazepoxide, diazepam (Boston Collaborative Drug Surveillance Program, 1973b), and chlorpromazine toxicity (Swett, 1974). In each case the results were consistent with a decrease in pharmacological effects among smokers for the drugs studied.

Another area of drug interaction seems to be clinically relevant if one defines drug interaction as it is normally defined—a pharmacological response that cannot be explained by the action of a single drug but is due to two or more drugs acting simultaneously. This definition includes effects that result from the cumulative effects of two or more drugs that have similar pharmacological actions. In our study, more than 90 percent of the reported interactions are of the "cumulative" variety and they account for substantial morbidity. In particular, the administration of multiple central nervous system (CNS) depressant drugs is quite common and leads not infrequently to substantial morbidity and, occasionally, to mortality (Porter, 1977).

To provide a crude estimate of the clinical significance (in medical patients) of drug interaction with psychotropic drugs that involves the mechanism of cumulative effects, I have obtained data on the rate of CNS depression with two of the most commonly used psychotropic drugs—chlorpromazine and amitriptyline—when given with certain other CNS-depressant drugs. Table 1 gives the frequency of exposure to ten important drugs that have an effect on the central nervous system. Tables 2 and 3 provide crude data on the overall incidence of clinically diagnosed CNS depression in patients who received chlorpromazine and amitriptyline according to the number of other CNS-active drugs (listed in Table 1) given to these patients. Although the analysis is crude, it does demonstrate the point that the frequency of this event is directly correlated with the number of drugs received.

Table 1

Number of Patients Exposed to Psychotropic Drugs among 26,294 Hospitalized Medical Patients

Drug	# Exposed	%
1. Diazepam	6,130	23.3
2. Chlordiazepoxide	2,526	9.6
3. Phenobarbital	1,650	6.3
4. Chlorpromazine	828	3.1
5. Amitriptyline	373	1.4
6. Hydroxyzine	302	1.1
7. Meprobamate	196	0.7
8. Thioridazine	168	0.6
9. Promazine	155	0.5
10. Imipramine	146	0.5

Table 2

CNS Depression in Patients Receiving Chlorpromazine

Number of Other CNS-Active Drugs	CNS Depression #	%
0	24/233	10.3
1-2	43/347	12.4
3-4	14/105	13.3
5+	7/36	19.4

Table 3

CNS Depression in Patients Receiving Amitriptyline

Number of Other CNS-Active Drugs	CNS Depression #	%
0	7/86	8.1
1-2	18/164	11.0
3-4	11/71	15.5
5+	2/6	33.3

The clinical circumstances surrounding the use of multidrug therapy are terribly complex and specific guidelines for the use of this or that combination are difficult to define, but it should be obvious that the clinical course of patients receiving combinations of psychotropic drugs must be watched carefully. Should untoward events occur, there should be an immediate evaluation of all drugs being prescribed to explore the possibility that the untoward events are caused by the combined effects of the drugs.

REFERENCES

Boston Collaborative Drug Surveillance Program 1972a. Interaction between chloral hydrate and warfarin. *N. Engl. J. Med.*, 286:53-55.

Boston Collaborative Drug Surveillance Program 1972b. Excess of ampicillin rashes associated with allopurinol or hyperuricemia. *N. Engl. J. Med.*, 286:505-507.

Boston Collaborative Drug Surveillance Program 1973a. Decreased clinical efficacy of propoxyphene in cigarette smokers. *Clin. Pharmacol. Ther.*, 14:259-263.

Boston Collaborative Drug Surveillance Program 1973b. Clinical depression of the central nervous system due to diazepam and chlordiazepoxide in relation to cigarette smoking and age. *N. Engl. J. Med.*, 288:277-280.

GRAHAME-SMITH, D. G. 1977. General aspects of drug interactions in psychopharmacology. In D. G. Grahame-Smith (ed.), *Drug Interactions*, pp. 147-157. London: Macmillan.

GREENBLATT, D. J., and KOCH-WESER, J. 1973. Adverse reactions to spironolactone. A report from the Boston Collaborative Drug Surveillance Program. *JAMA*, 225:40-43.

JICK, H., MIETTINEN, O. S., SHAPIRO, S., LEWIS, G. P., SISKIND, V., and SLONE, D. 1970. Comprehensive drug surveillance. *JAMA*, 213:1455-1460.

MARLEY, E. 1977. Monoamine oxidase inhibitors and drug interactions. In D. G. Grahame-Smith (ed.), *Drug Interactions*, pp. 171-194. London: Macmillan.

PORTER, J., and JICK, H. 1977. Drug-related deaths among medical inpatients. *JAMA*, 237:879-881.

SELLERS, E. M., and KOCH-WESER, J. 1970. Potentiation of warfarin-induced hypoprothrombinemia by chloral hydrate. *N. Engl. J. Med.*, 283:827-831.

SWETT, C. 1974. Drowsiness due to chlorpromazine in relation to cigarette smoking. A report from the Boston Collaborative Drug Surveillance Program. *Arch. Gen. Psychiatry*, 31:211-213.

10

IMPORTANCE OF BLOOD LEVELS OF NEUROLEPTIC DRUGS IN THE TREATMENT OF SCHIZOPHRENIA

EDWARD F. DOMINO, M.D.

It is now generally agreed that roughly two of three schizophrenic patients improve on antipsychotic medication. The antipsychotic drugs used are primarily dopamine antagonists; they block the actions of dopamine in various areas of the brain and can also block dopamine receptors peripherally. From a functional point of view, however, dopamine has a predominantly central role. The blockade of dopamine receptors results in both the good as well as the bad effects of antipsychotic medication. These drugs act on neurons (hence "neuro") to take hold of or bind (hence "leptic") dopamine receptors. The term "neuroleptic" has been used widely, especially in Europe; I prefer it to "antipsychotic" because these drugs work in all kinds of people and animals to block dopamine receptors. The term "major tranquilizer" for these drugs seems to be disappearing, for neuroleptics do not always calm and tranquilize.

Although the quality of life has improved for at least two of three of our schizophrenic patients, we should be reminded that these patients are not always restored to perfectly normal lives. Deficits still remain. The families of these patients—especially their young children—must bear a burden that is unknown to families free of mental disease, particularly schizophrenia.

Grunebaum (1977) expresses the concerns some of us have for the children of schizophrenic patients, whether or not their parents are on medication. Are these children at risk because of genetic as well as environmental factors? Are the community mental health programs throughout our country unnecessarily exposing more families to the burden of schizophrenia? What are we really doing for the one of three patients who is a poor responder to neuroleptic therapy? Process schizophrenia has a steady downhill course. Neuroleptics do help, but mainly by reducing the severity of symptoms. We desperately need long-term follow-up studies to document the impact neuroleptic drugs are having on the schizophrenic patients who have been taking these medications over 10- to 20-year periods.

We have known that one-third of psychotic patients get better, one-third stay the same, and one-third get worse, since the days of the American revolution when King George III of England would periodically go mad (his illness was probably caused by acute intermittent porphyria; he had red-wine-colored urine). I suspect that in the last 200 years we have not advanced greatly as far as process schizophrenia is concerned. Some of these patients probably have a disease that does not respond to dopamine antagonists (Domino, 1978), hence the continuing need for basic research at institutions such as the Texas Research Institute of Mental Sciences (TRIMS).

It is my belief that further knowledge of the clinical pharmacology of central dopamine antagonists will improve our present therapy, especially in some nonresponders. By measuring blood levels, developing better ways of administering drugs, and knowing more about drug metabolism, we can treat our patients better. Dr. Kinard (in this volume) indicated that red-cell levels of butaperazine provide better correlates with clinical response than do plasma levels; he suggested that psychiatrists keep the red cells and give the plasma to the internists. As a pharmacologist, I am not ready to get rid of either the red cells or the plasma, or any other tissue or fluid, until we are certain what correlates best with clinical response. Obviously, what is important is the brain concentration of a drug. Presently there is no easy means for an ethical pursuit of such research. For the time being, then, some of us are looking at total levels of drug in the plasma, some of us are looking at free and bound plasma levels, and some of us are looking at red cells, white cells, and muscle biopsies, hoping to ascertain what is going on in the human brain.

Perhaps the future will give us the methods we really need. "I have a dream," said Martin Luther King; my dream is that some day we will have a chemical test of cerebrospinal fluid, blood, or urine that will pinpoint types of schizophrenia as, for example, schizophrenic dopamine disease, schizophrenic indole disease, or schizophrenic endorphine disease. Some day it may be possible that, with a radiolabeled neuroleptic drug that emits gamma rays, a patient will wear a special "space helmet" geared to external measurement of drug content in the brain by appropriate gamma counters. Perhaps we will be able to obtain a CAT (computerized axial tomography) scan distribution of the drug in the brain.

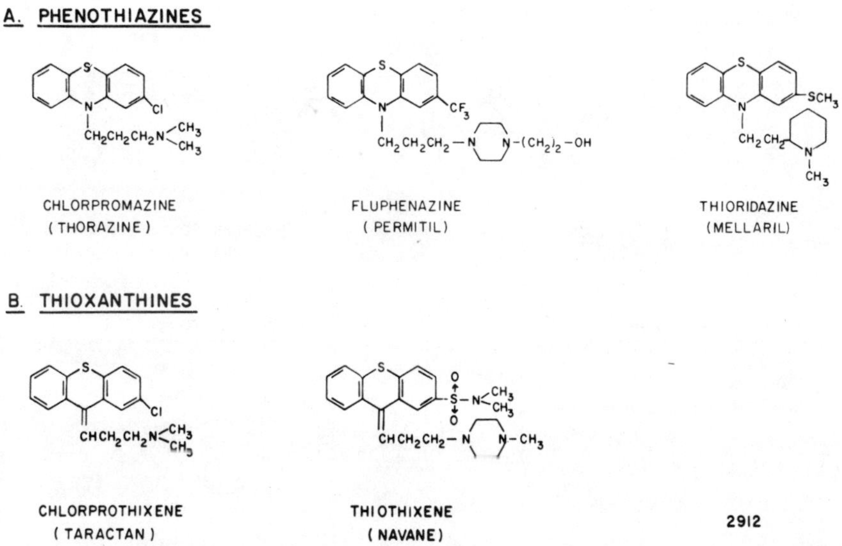

Figure 1. Chemical structures of some substituted phenothiazine and thioxanthine neuroleptics used in treating schizophrenia.

That is all a dream, but a dream that could be converted to reality with some of the methodology we currently have.

For the present, we must be satisfied with measuring the blood levels of neuroleptic drugs. Most of the work has been done on total plasma levels. Admittedly, total plasma levels have limited value, but they at least provide the means for monitoring dosage levels and they can indicate whether the patient is indeed taking the medication.

This paper is directed to the clinicians who are privileged to be on the front lines of daily patient care. Perhaps we can help them in the care of the patient who is not responding well to currently available neuroleptic medication. A recent review by Davis, Erickson, and Dekirmenjian (1978) of the relationship of drug plasma levels to clinical response should be consulted for detailed references.

As illustrated in Figures 1 and 2, there are five major classes of neuroleptic drugs available in the United States for prescription. They include substituted phenothiazines, thioxanthines, butyrophenones, one dihydroindolone, and one dibenzoxazepine. Of the substituted phenothiazines, chlorpromazine, fluphenazine, and thioridazine represent the major prototypes. There are two prototype thioxanthines, chlorprothixene and thiothixene. Of the two butyrophenone neuroleptics available, haloperidol is used primarily by psychiatrists. Anesthesiologists,

C. BUTYROPHENONES

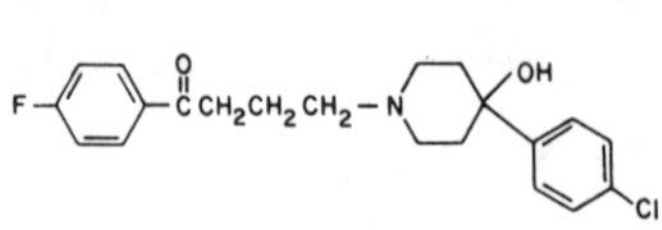

HALOPERIDOL
(HALDOL)

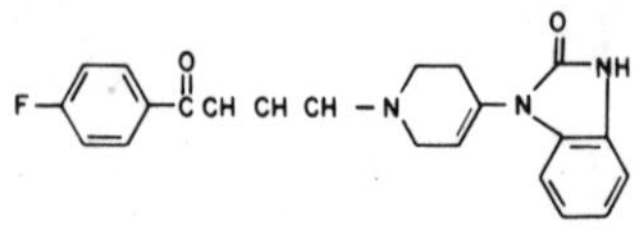

DROPERIDOL
(INAPSINE)

D. DIHYDROINDOLONE

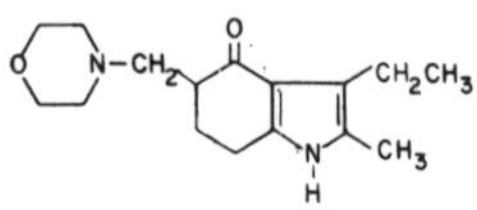

MOLINDONE
(MOBAN)

E. DIBENZOXAZEPINE

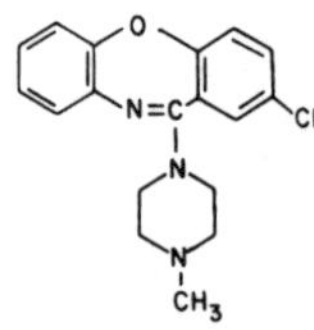

LOXAPINE
(LOXITANE)

Figure 2. Chemical structures of some substituted butyrophenone, dihydroindolone, and dibenzoxazepine neuroleptics used in treating schizophrenia.

however, have long been familiar with the butyrophenone droperidol; because of its shorter duration of action, droperidol is finding increased use, particularly among emergency room physicians. Recently, molindone and loxapine have become available for prescription use.

It is a fact that all neuroleptic drugs are equally effective in benefiting two of three schizophrenic patients; it is also a fact, however, that sometimes patients who do poorly on phenothiazines do well with other classes of neuroleptics. This phenomenon is, in part, the reason we have so many different kinds of neuroleptics. Of course, economic considerations, including fierce competition among pharmaceutical companies, are the chief reason for the large number of dopamine-blocking neuroleptic drugs.

There is a marked individual variability in the blood levels of different patients given the same dose of a neuroleptic. Figure 3 illustrates data on the steady-state plasma levels of chlorpromazine given to 26 patients in a dosage of 400 mg per day (Cooper and Simpson, 1976). The steady-state levels of chlorpromazine varied from 0 to about 235 ng/ml! Obviously, the patients with no chlorpromazine in their plasma were getting inadequate doses, while at the other extreme some patients were getting too much.

Another important concept involves the ratio of active to inactive drug metabolites. Chlorpromazine is an especially complicated drug from this

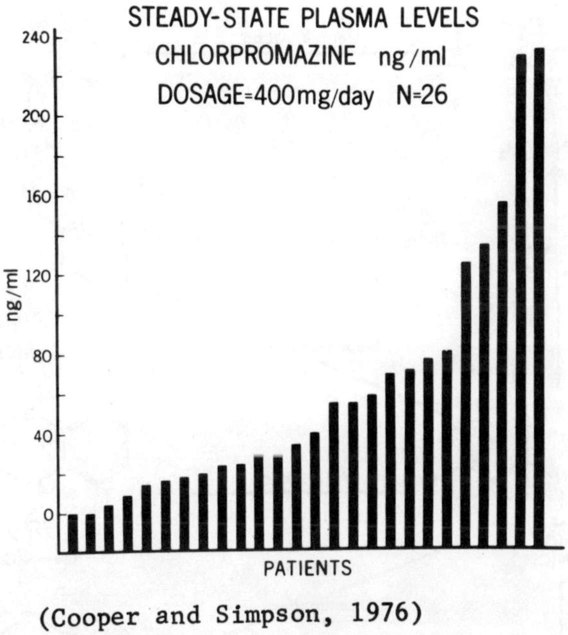

Figure 3. Steady-state plasma levels of chlorpromazine. Height of each vertical bar represents the plasma levels of 26 different patients each given 200 mg of chlorpromazine twice a day. Note marked variability. From Cooper and Simpson (1976).

point of view. Figure 4 presents some of the major pathways of chlorpromazine biotransformation; these include demethylation, hydroxylation, sulphoxidation, deamination, and conjugation. Many different metabolites are formed. The sulfoxides are considerably less active pharmacologically than the hydroxides (Manian, Efron, and Goldbert, 1965; Manian, Efron, and Harris, 1971). Sakalis et al. (1973) and Mackay, Healey, and Baker (1974) have suggested that the plasma ratio of active (chlorpromazine and 7-hydroxychlorpromazine) to less active (chlorpromazine sulfoxide) compounds may predict therapeutic response. There are, however, a number of problems. Other investigators have found only trace amounts of hydroxylated chlorpromazine in the plasma; it is evident much more research is needed in this area.

Kaul and Clark (1976) reported on the absorption and disappearance of chlorpromazine and its sulfoxide in sonicated whole blood of schizophrenic patients given 120 mg of chlorpromazine per square meter of body surface. Blood chlorpromazine levels peaked at two hours at approximately

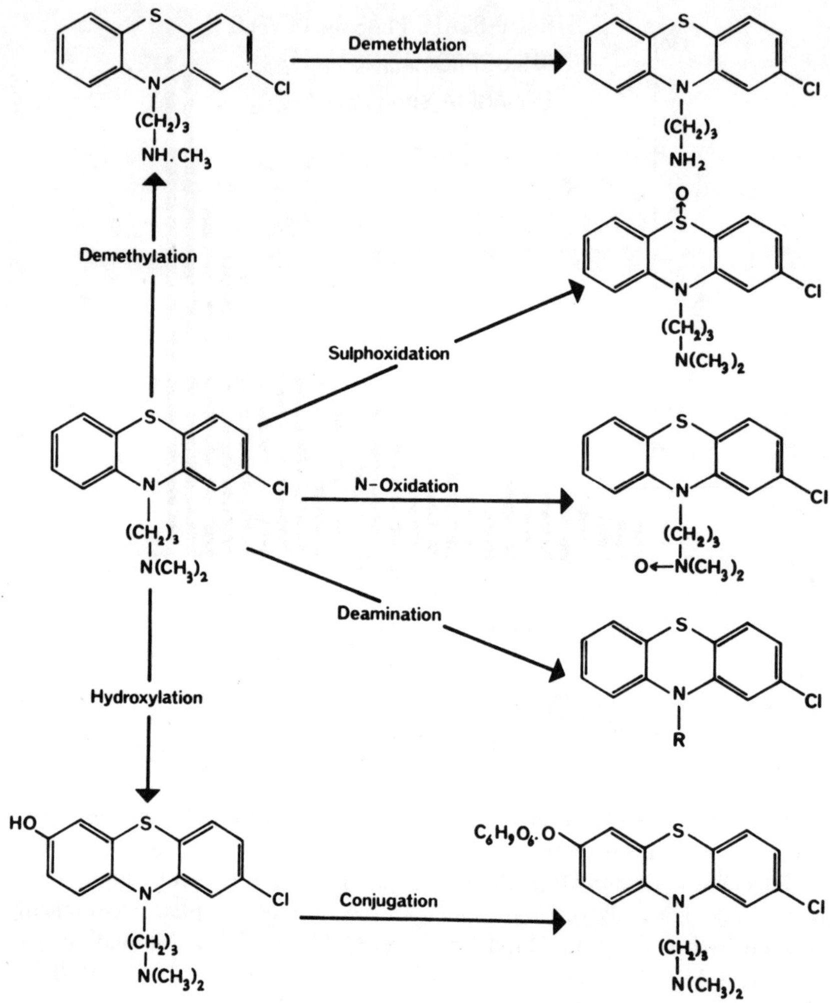

Figure 4. Major pathways of biotransformation of chlorpromazine. From Curry (1976).

155 ng/ml, and reached a plateau of about 40 ng/ml eight hours later. Chlorpromazine sulfoxide levels follow a similar time course and peak at about 45 ng/ml at two hours. Schooler et al. (1976) reported a multidisciplinary collaborative study involving the correlation of the levels of chlorpromazine and 18 metabolites in the plasma of acute schizophrenics over a 28-day period. The effort of measuring all these metabolites is remarkable. In this study the chlorpromazine-treated patients improved signifi-

cantly in contrast to those subjects receiving a placebo. Generally, the plasma levels of most of the metabolites were low early in the course of treatment, but the pattern of change was not uniform for all the compounds. The glucuronides tended to reach their highest levels later in the course of treatment than the other metabolites measured. These investigators found no simple relationship between plasma levels and clinical response. In general, patients improved over time as the plasma levels of most of the metabolites, especially the hydroxyglucuronides, increased.

It is important to know that chlorpromazine is biotransformed in both the intestine and the liver and that the degree of biotransformation varies with each patient. In general, oral administration of chlorpromazine produces much lower plasma levels than intravenous (i.v.) or intramuscular (i.m.) administration (Curry, 1976). A dose of 100 mg of chlorpromazine i.m. in the human leads to plasma levels about three times greater than 100 mg given orally. This phenomenon has been explained in part by a "first-pass" effect in which chlorpromazine is biotransformed in both the gut and liver. It is well known clinically that the degrees of sedation and hypotension are greater with parenteral than with oral chlorpromazine. The plasma findings, then, reinforce a well-known clinical observation: patients with very active chlorpromazine-biotransforming mechanisms in the gut and liver tend to show very low plasma, and hence brain, levels of chlorpromazine. If patients form a greater number of inactive metabolites, they tend to be nonresponders. It follows that plasma levels of both chlorpromazine and its active metabolites would be low in some nonresponders to neuroleptic drugs.

Since chlorpromazine and other phenothiazines induce their own metabolism, some patients will show lower plasma levels after many weeks of constant drug therapy, rather than early in therapy. Cooper and Simpson (1976) described such a pattern in a patient given butaperazine. An initial blood pharmacokinetic study was carried out with a loading dose of 40 mg of butaperazine; blood was collected over a 24-hour period. Adequate blood levels (peaking at 400 ng/ml at two hours) were obtained. One patient had a good clinical response during the first two months of daily butaperazine, but later his clinical state deteriorated. When this happened, his plasma levels of butaperazine were not measurable in spite of oral doses as large as 100 mg per day. After the patient had completed 16 weeks on medication, another 40-mg butaperazine pharmacokinetic study was done; the resultant blood levels were markedly reduced, suggesting an enzyme-inductive effect. Curry (1976) has corroborated the findings that suggest enzyme induction. Ten subjects treated with 100 mg of chlorpromazine twice a day for 36 days tended to have reduced plasma chlorpromazine levels. Obviously, more research of this type needs to be carried out in drug nonresponders with a history of a good drug response.

Davis, Erickson, and Dekirmenjian (1978) have reviewed the concept of a therapeutic window, the therapeutic drug plasma concentration range. It is apparent that very low plasma levels of a drug will be ineffective and very high levels toxic. If one were to plot clinical benefit on the y axis and plasma concentration on the x axis, an inverted U-shaped curve would describe the therapeutic window in which a plasma level too low or too high would be unsatisfactory. The plasma or serum concentration of the lithium ion is an excellent example of the therapeutic-window concept. Concentrations of 0.8 to 1.8 mEq/l are generally therapeutic, while lower levels are ineffective and higher levels toxic; the therapeutic window for most neuroleptic drugs has not been determined. In the case of chlorpromazine, plasma levels of about 30 to 150 ng/ml are generally in the therapeutic range. It should be noted, however, that clinical response does not correlate directly with plasma chlorpromazine levels, perhaps because of such factors as the ratio of active to inactive metabolites. The fact some patients have a desirable effect at 30 ng/ml and others require 150 ng/ml of chlorpromazine should not detract from the importance of measuring plasma levels. The crucial point is that patients with plasma levels outside the therapeutic window are getting either an inadequate or a toxic dosage of chlorpromazine. Furthermore, nonresponders with plasma levels at the high end of the therapeutic window should be taken off medication, because the danger of developing tardive dyskinesia does not warrant continued medication.

The drug package insert, which is reproduced for all prescription drugs in the *Physicians' Desk Reference* (PDR), is essentially a contract between the drug manufacturer and the Food and Drug Administration; neither patient nor physician participate. Both the drug company and FDA are interested in recommending dosage ranges that benefit the largest number of people with the least number of side effects. The dose limits placed on each drug do not take into account the nonresponder who may have negligible blood levels (and no side effects) with a maximum dose. I have seen a patient who easily tolerated 100 mg of fluphenazine per day and did well, yet his physician was under great pressure from various health professionals to reduce the dose to a therapeutically ineffective level not to exceed 20 mg per day because of PDR recommendations. This ridiculous situation exists with most psychotropic drugs simply because we do not measure blood levels.

One of the problems the clinician faces is that relatively simple chemical assays may not be specific enough. The analytic chemist performing an assay must know what he is measuring—is it the parent drug or its metabolites, both active and inactive? Gottschalk et al. (1976) measured the plasma levels of mesoridazine following a single 2 mg/kg i.m. dose given to ten acute schizophrenic patients. Plasma mesoridazine levels were measured fluorometrically and gas chromatographically. With both methods peak plasma levels were obtained four hours after i.m. injection (Figure 5). The fluorometric method, however, measured both mesoridazine and its metabolite, sulforidazine, and gave levels about twice as high as the more specific gas chromatographic method which measured both compounds separately.

Another point that must be made is that the blood concentrations of psychoactive drugs in general are very low. Only in the last ten years have we been able to develop chemical assay techniques that are sensitive and specific. Drugs like haloperidol or fluphenazine that are usually given in doses of less than 25 mg per day represent special problems from the perspective of assay sensitivity; there are now, however, very sensitive gas chromatographic-mass spectrometric assays that can easily measure such levels. If we can manage to send an automatic gas chromatographic mass spectrometer to Mars to assay the planet's atmosphere, we can

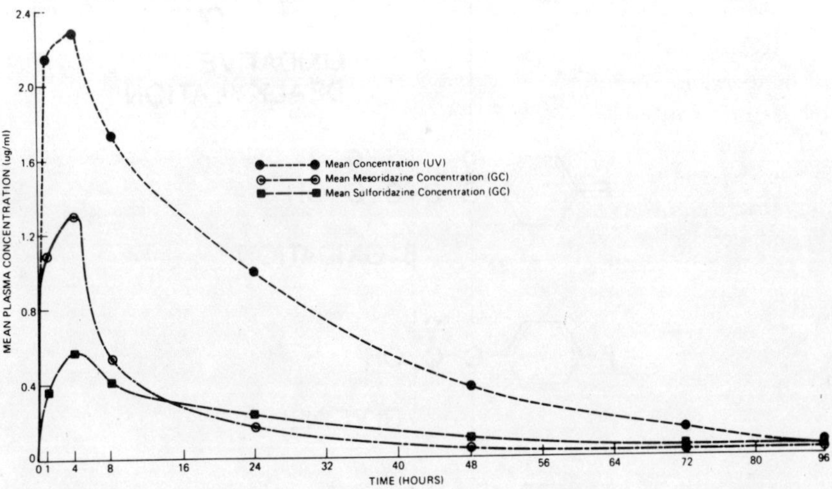

Figure 5. Mean plasma concentrations of mesoridazine and its metabolite sulforidazine in ten acute schizophrenic patients. A single dose of 2 mg/kg of mesoridazine was given intramuscularly. Plasma levels were measured via two different methods of which the fluorometric method was obviously measuring more than mesoridazine. From Gottschalk et al. (1976).

surely manage in the near future to extend such facilities to the physician and patient.

One of the advantages of haloperidol is that all of its metabolites are inactive. Hence one need only be concerned with levels of haloperidol. Forsman and Öhman (1976) have suggested that haloperidol is biotransformed by oxidative dealkylation and subsequent ß-oxidation (Figure 6). These investigators determined the serum profiles of haloperidol concentrations after a total of 10 mg administered intravenously, then orally six weeks later (Figure 7). Note that in this subject serum levels peaked at 5 ng/ml in about five hours and lasted for several days. Much higher serum levels were obtained with the same 10-mg dose of haloperidol given intravenously. The investigators also measured the steady-state concentrations of haloperidol in 11 different patients given 6 mg of haloperidol daily. As Figure 8 shows, a tenfold range in serum concentra-

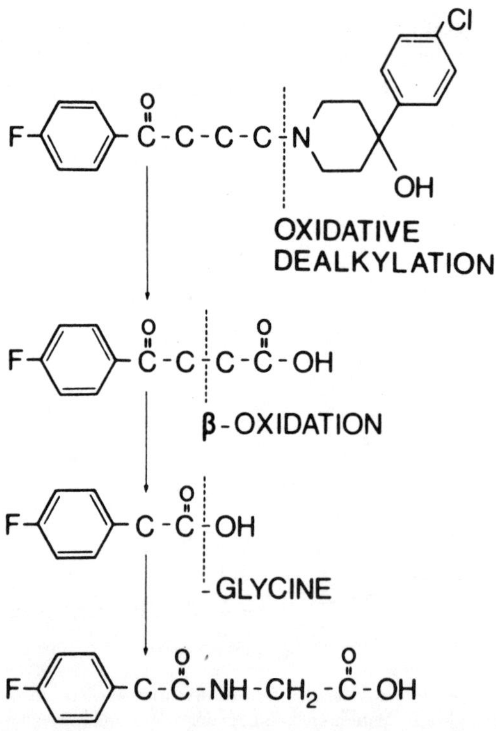

Figure 6. Suggested metabolic pathway of haloperidol biotransformation in man. From Forsman and Öhman (1976).

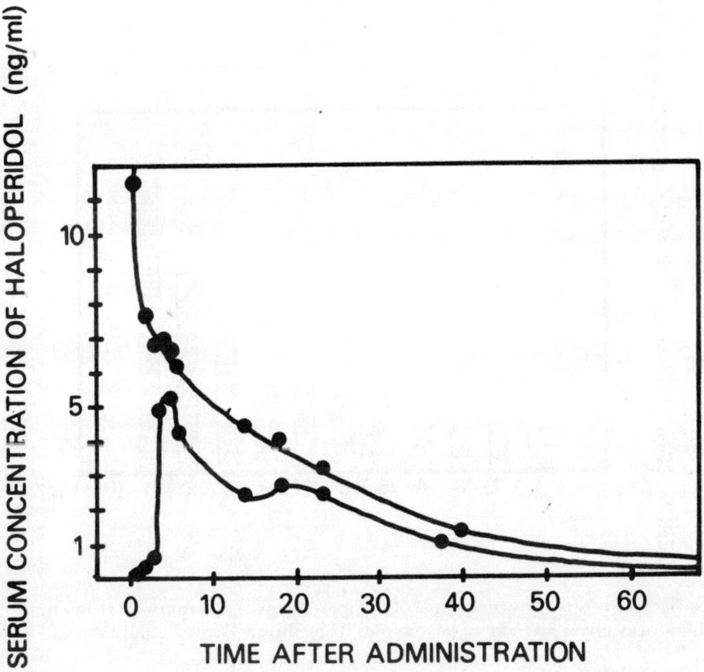

Figure 7. Serum concentrations of haloperidol after intravenous and oral administration. Haloperidol was given to a normal volunteer in a dose of 10 mg i.v. Six weeks later the same dose was given orally. Time is in hours. From Forsman and Öhman (1976).

tions was obtained. Little wonder we need to individualize dosage and observe our patients carefully. Presently most clinicians will not be able to obtain blood levels of neuroleptic drugs in patients because the assays used are fairly complicated for a hospital clinical laboratory.

We need to devote much more effort to a rational use of these drugs based upon their clinical pharmacology. This can only come about if support is available for applied research by each state department of mental health; it will not come from the federal level where other "higher" priorities exist. We can do a great deal to spread the message for extended research at our own local hospitals and at mental health research centers like TRIMS.

There is an interesting correlation between plasma chlorpromazine levels and pupil size which might be useful; whether it applies to other neuroleptic drugs is not known. I frequently ask psychiatrists whether chlorpromazine constricts or dilates the pupils; they usually reply that it

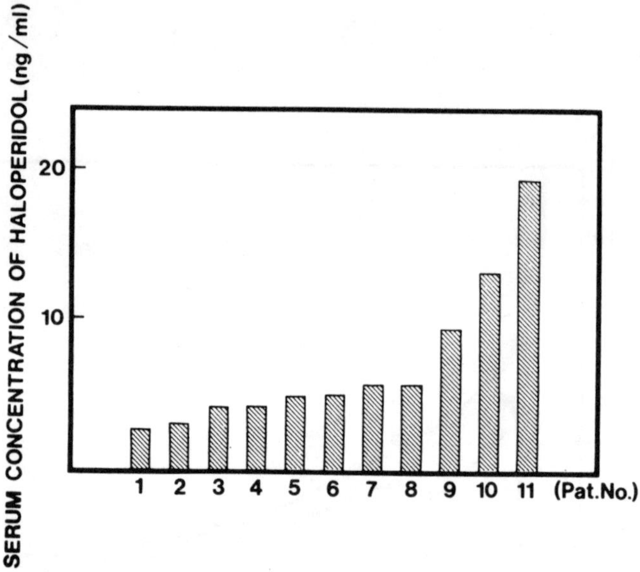

Figure 8. Steady-state concentration of haloperidol in the serum of 11 different patients. Each patient was given 6 mg/kg of haloperidol daily. From Forsman and Öhman (1976).

has a dilating effect. It does not. Chlorpromazine, like morphine, constricts the pupils, but the mechanism for this action has yet to be worked out; we do not even know whether it is a local or central action. Sakalis et al. (1972) studied the physiological (including pupil diameter) and clinical effects of chlorpromazine and their relationship to plasma levels in ten psychotic patients. After obtaining baseline control measures, each patient received 100 mg of chlorpromazine orally every eight hours for five to six weeks. Blood samples and various physiologic measures were taken at 0, 2, 4, and 6 hours after the morning dose. Pupil diameter was measured using the disc comparison method under both dim and bright light with each patient fixating on a reference point.

Under dim illumination, the mean pupil diameter pretreatment was about 5 mm, and under bright illumination about 3.3 mm. After chlorpromazine administration at 8 a.m. or 0 time (steady-state level), the mean pupil size over 36 days of treatment tended to be slightly smaller than before drug administration. This slight change, however, would not be picked up by casual clinical examination. Two hours after chlorpromazine ingestion, mean pupil diameter decreased about 0.6 mm under dim and 0.3 mm under bright illumination. There was no evidence of tolerance to this miotic effect after 36 days of continuous eight-hour 100-mg chlorpromazine treatments. The within-patient correlations between plasma chlorpromazine levels and pupil diameter were $r = -0.5$ ($p < 0.001$) for dim, and $r = -0.35$ ($p < 0.05$) for bright illumination.

Smolen et al. (1975) reported on the use of the miotic response of the pupil as a measure of bioavailability of various forms of chlorpromazine given to normal human volunteers. Very low oral doses of chlorpromazine (about 10 mg total/70 kg) could be detected on the basis of pupilometry. The effects of both intravenous and oral routes of chlorpromazine administration on pupil size were studied. An i.v. dose of 10 mg/70 kg over a 30-minute period produced at least 11 times greater miotic response than a 10 mg/70 kg oral dose of chlorpromazine syrup. Oral doses of 5 to 100 mg produced progressively greater miotic responses. The time course for intensity of pupil response to 100 mg of chlorpromazine syrup and tablets compared favorably with the average temporal blood chlorpromazine levels reported by Hollister et al. (1970) for 150 mg of chlorpromazine syrup. This result confirms the finding of Sakalis et al. (1972) that plasma levels of chlorpromazine correlate with pupil constriction. The oral dose of chlorpromazine to produce maximal miosis has not been established. Whether schizophrenic patients given very large doses of chlorpromazine show dose-related pupillary constriction or evidence of tolerance development beyond 36 days is not known. It might be of value, however, to check the pupil size of patients under standard lighting conditions as a clinical test of chlorpromazine bioavailability. It is noteworthy that Sakalis et al. (1972) commented that the physiologic measure that correlated most consistently with plasma chlorpromazine was pupil diameter. They suggested its use as a routine clinical indicator of chlorpromazine effects; I also recommend it, especially when measured under dim illumination.

In conclusion, the measurement of blood levels of neuroleptic drugs has a place in the treatment of schizophrenia, particularly in nonresponders, or in patients showing severe pharmacological side effects to reasonable dosages. In the future, psychiatrists will probably use the blood level data of neuroleptics just as they now use lithium ion levels to monitor therapy. One of the key issues for the future is to determine what to measure; do we look to the parent drug or a ratio of its active and inactive metabolites? And by what means do we accomplish these measures? These are important questions in clinical psychopharmacology that can only be answered by more research.

REFERENCES

Cooper, T. B., and Simpson, G. M. 1976. Plasma/blood level monitoring techniques in psychiatry. In L. A. Gottschalk and S. Merlis (eds.), *Pharmacokinetics of Psychoactive Drugs: Blood Levels and Clinical Response*, pp. 23-31. New York: Spectrum Publications.

CURRY, S. H. 1976. Metabolism and kinetics of chlorpromazine in relation to effect. In G. Sedvall, B. Uvnas, and Y. Zotterman (eds.), *Antipsychotic Drugs: Pharmacodynamics and Pharmacokinetics*, pp. 343-352. Oxford: Pergamon Press.

DAVIS, J. M., ERICKSON, S., and DEKIRMENJIAN, H. 1978. Plasma levels of antipsychotic drugs and clinical response. In M. A. Lipton, A. DiMascio, and K. F. Killam (eds.), *Psychopharmacology: A Generation of Progress*, pp. 905-915. New York: Raven Press.

DOMINO, E. F. 1978. Acute pharmacological effects of chlorpromazine in neuroleptic therapy resistant chronic schizophrenic patients. In P. Deniker, C. Radouco-Thomas, and A. Villeneuve (eds.), *Proceedings of the 10th Congress of the Collegium Internationale Neuro-Psychopharmacologicum*, pp. 321-330. Oxford: Pergamon Press, 1978.

FORSMAN, A., and Öhman, R. 1976. Some aspects of the distribution and metabolism of haloperidol in man. In G. Sedvall, B. Uvnas and Y. Zotterman (eds.), *Antipsychotic Drugs: Pharmacodynamics and Pharmacokinetics*, pp. 359-365. Oxford: Pergamon Press.

GOTTSCHALK, L. A., DINOVO, E., BIENER, R., BIRCH, H., SYBEN, M., and NOBLE, E. P. 1976. Plasma levels of mesoridazine and its metabolites and clinical response in acute schizophrenia after a single intramuscular drug dose. In L. A. Gottschalk and S. Merlis (eds.), *Pharmacokinetics of Psychoactive Drugs: Blood Levels and Clinical Response*, pp. 171-189. New York: Spectrum Publications.

GRUNEBAUM, H. 1977. Children at risk for psychosis and their families: Approaches to prevention. In M. F. McMillan and S. Henao (eds.), *Child Psychiatry—Treatment and Research*, pp. 172-189. New York: Brunner/Mazel.

HOLLISTER, L. E., CURRY, S. H., DERR, J. E., and KANTER, S. L. 1970. Studies of delayed action medication. V. Plasma levels and urinary excretion of four different dosage forms of chlorpromazine, *Clin. Pharmacol. Ther.*, 11:49-59.

KAUL, P. N., and CLARK, M. L. 1976. A novel approach to quantitative determination of subnanomoles of psychoactive drugs in blood. In L. A. Gottschalk and S. Merlis (eds.), *Pharmacokinetics of Psychoactive Drugs: Blood Levels and Clinical Response*, pp. 3-14. New York: Spectrum Publications.

MACKAY, A. V. P., HEALEY, A. F., and BAKER, J. 1974. The relationship of plasma chlorpromazine and its 7-hydroxy and sulphoxide metabolites in a large population of chronic schizophrenics. *Br. J. Clin. Pharmacol.*, 1:425-430.

MANIAN, A. A., EFRON, D. H., and GOLDBERT, M. E. 1965. A comparative pharmacological study of a series of monohydroxylated and methoxylated chlorpromazine derivatives. *Life Sci.*, 4:2425-2438.

MANIAN, A. A., EFRON, D. H., and HARRIS, S. R. 1971. Appearance of monohydroxylated chlorpromazine metabolites in the central nervous system. *Life Sci.*, 10:679-684.

SAKALIS, M. B., CURRY, S. H., MOULD, G. P., and LADER, M. H. 1972. Physiologic and clinical effects of chlorpromazine and their relationship to plasma level. *Clin. Pharmacol. Ther.*, 13:931-946.

SAKALIS, G., CHAN, T. L., GERSHON, S., and PARK, S. 1973. The possible role of metabolites in therapeutic response to chlorpromazine treatment. *Psychopharmacologia*, 32:279-284.

SCHOOLER, N. R., SAKALIS, G., CHAN, T. L., GERSHON, S., GOLDBERG, S. C., and COLLINS, P. 1976. Chlorpromazine metabolism and clinical response in acute schizophrenia: A preliminary report. In L. A. Gottschalk and S. Merlis (eds.), *Pharmacokinetics of Psychoactive Drugs: Blood Levels and Clinical Response*, pp. 199-219. New York: Spectrum Publications.

SMOLEN, V. F., MURDOCK, H. R., JR., and WILLIAMS, E. J. 1975. Bioavailability analysis of chlorpromazine in humans from pupilometric data. *J. Pharmacol. Exp. Ther.*, 195:404-415.

11

MINOR TRANQUILIZER PHARMACOKINETICS

STANLEY A. KAPLAN, PH.D., and MARGARET L. JACK, M.S.

The minor tranquilizers commonly prescribed in the United States include the benzodiazepine and the propanediol classes of compounds (Table 1). All are anxiolytic agents which are available in oral dosage forms; chlordiazepoxide and diazepam are also available as injectable dosage forms.

The benzodiazepine structures are shown in Figure 1. The marketed benzodiazepines differ structurally only in the R_1, R_2, R_3, and R_4 substituents; the remainder of the molecule is identical for all four agents. Diazepam has the methyl group in the R_1 position, chlordiazepoxide has the methylamine and the N-oxide substituents in the R_2 and R_4 positions respectively; both oxazepam and clorazepate have ketone groups in the R_2 position. In addition, oxazepam contains a hydroxyl group at R_3, while clorazepate has the potassium salt of a carboxylic acid at this position. These various substituents impart differences in the physicochemical, pharmacological, and pharmacokinetic properties of the benzodiazepines.

Pharmacological parameters (ED_{50} values) following various testing procedures with the benzodiazepines, meprobamate, and phenobarbital are

Table 1

Minor Tranquilizers Marketed in the U.S.

Drug Class	Generic Name	Trade Name(s)
Benzodiazepines	chlordiazepoxide	Librium, etc.
	diazepam	Valium
	clorazepate	Tranxene
	oxazepam	Serax
Propanediols	meprobamate	Milltown, Equanil, etc.

Table 2

ED_{50} Values (mg/kg) of Various Anxiolytic Agents

Compound	Inclined Screen	Foot Shock	Unanesthetized Cat	Anti-Metrazole
Chlordiazepoxide	100	40	2	8
Diazepam	30	10	0.2	1.4
Clorazepate	75	20	1	1.7
Oxazepam	225	40	1	0.7
Meprobamate	250	250	100	150
Phenobarbital	120	80	10	75

Adapted from Randall and Kappell, 1973.

Table 3
Daily Clinical Doses Recommended for Anxiolytic Response

Drug	Dosage (mg)
Chlordiazepoxide	15-75
Diazepam	4-40
Clorazepate	15-60
Oxazepam	15-45
Meprobamate	800-1250

reported in Table 2 (Randall and Kappell, 1973). One should anticipate lower dose requirements for the more potent compounds, that is, drugs with smaller ED_{50} values. The clinical daily dose requirements for the treatment of anxiety listed in Table 3 reflect pharmacological profiles.

Pharmacokinetics is a tool which traces the fate of drugs, as a function of time, from the moment of administration until the agent has completely cleared the body. The field involves studies of drug absorption, distribution, biotransformation, and elimination. Drug level and/or biotransformation product data generated from blood, tissue, and excreta specimens are used to construct mathematical models suitable to interpreting such data. For an absolute evaluation, data must be obtained after intravenous drug administration. The pharmacokineticist visualizes drug disposition in terms of mathematical models which may not have anatomical or physiological parallels. Ideally this mathematical model, constructed from biological data, will permit quantitation of the kinetic processes involved in absorption, distribution, metabolism, and excretion.

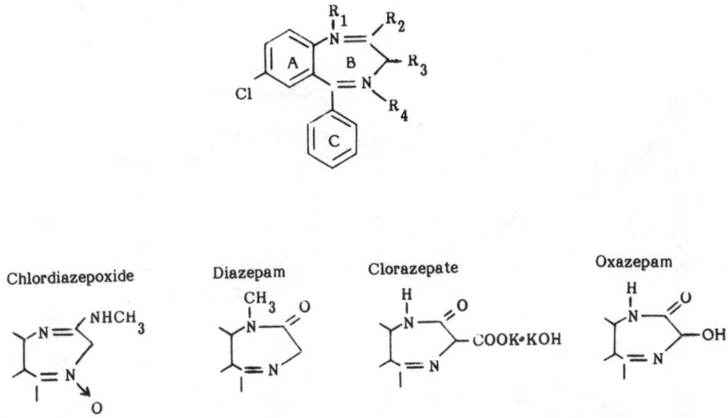

Figure 1. 1,4-Benzodiazepine nucleus and structural skeletons of chlordiazepoxide, diazepam, clorazepate, and oxazepam.

Since the majority of drugs are administered via the oral route, the rate and extent of absorption, that is, the bioavailability after oral administration, is of primary concern. Bioavailability is influenced by the processes of solubility, dissolution rate, and permeability. The plasma peak times and heights may be used as an index of the rate of absorption, whereas the area under the plasma level curves is a measure of the extent of absorption.

The blood level curves of diazepam and desmethyldiazepam following 10-mg single-dose intravenous and oral administrations are presented in Figure 2 (Kaplan et al., 1973). The comparable areas under the intravenous and oral blood level curves for diazepam indicate complete absorption, while the early and sharp blood level peak following oral administration indicates rapid absorption. The desmethyldiazepam blood level curves following intravenous and oral administrations of diazepam are virtually the same, reflecting the completeness of diazepam absorption. The formation rate constants for desmethyldiazepam are shown in Table 4. It should be noted that the initial formation rate constant of desmethyldiazepam is 10 to 20 times more rapid than the slower formation rate constant calculated after the twelfth hour postadministration. The slower formation rate constant of desmethyldiazepam is equal to the overall elimination rate constant of diazepam; such equivalency of rate constants suggests that diazepam is virtually completely converted to the desmethyldiazepam metabolite in man.

Based on data obtained following intravenous administration of diazepam, an open three-compartment pharmacokinetic model system was developed and is presented in Figure 3 with the mean calculated rate

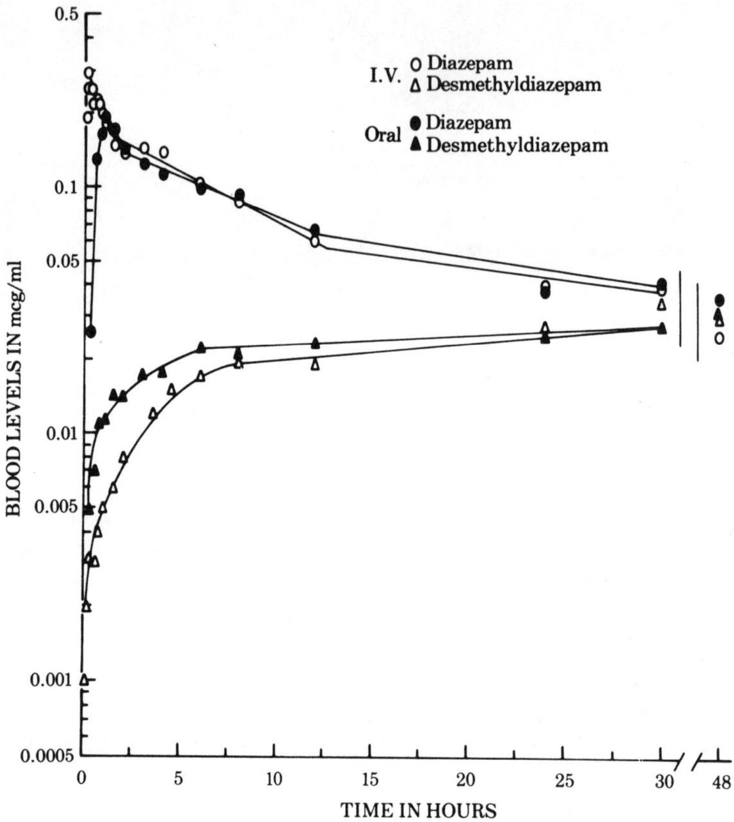

Figure 2. Blood-level curve after single 10-mg intravenous and oral doses of diazepam. From Kaplan et al., 1973.

constants (Kaplan et al., 1973). Compartment 1 is the "central compartment" into which drug is administered and from which elimination occurs. Compartments 2 and 3 are peripheral compartments for which no anatomical designations are given, since they reflect two distinguishable partition phenomena between the blood and distribution and/or binding sites. Overall, the characteristics of the deep peripheral compartment, compartment 3, may be important to the understanding of diazepam's physiological disposition in man. The rate of drug return from compartment 3 to the central compartment may be the rate-limiting step in terms of the elimination of diazepam and the formation of desmethyldiazepam. Therefore, alterations in the binding characteristics of drug to the tissues

Table 4

Formation Rate Constant for Desmethyldiazepam Following Single-Dose Administration of Diazepam

	Subject			
	1	2	3	4
Overall elimination rate constant of diazepam, hour, $^{-1}$	0.019	0.026	0.024	0.021
Formation rate constant of desmethyldiazepam after 12 hr., hour^{-1}	0.020	0.028	0.030	0.016
Initial formation rate constant of desmethyldiazepam, hour^{-1}	0.546	0.427	0.329	0.351

From Kaplan et al., 1973.

or proteins associated with compartment 3 may yield alterations in the pharmacokinetic profile of the drug.

Clorazepate is essentially a prodrug which hydrolyzes to desmethyldiazepam (a metabolite of diazepam and chlordiazepoxide) in the acidic environment of the gastrointestinal tract (Figure 4) (Abruzzo et al., 1977). The pharmacological activity of chlorazepate is ascribed to the hydrolysis product desmethyldiazepam, which is absorbed from the gastrointestinal tract. Therefore, if the drug fails to dissolve in the stomach as a result of pharmaceutical, physiological, or pathological factors, or if it dissolves in a nonacidic environment, a lesser degree of conversion of clorazepate to N-desmethyldiazepam is anticipated. A nonrandomized crossover experimental design was employed with four subjects to evaluate the effects of gastric pH below 3.0 and greater than 6.0 (maintained with sodium bicarbonate) on the absorption characteristics of orally administered dipotassium clorazepate (Abruzzo et al., 1977). Figure 5 represents blood levels of N-desmethyldiazepam in one subject following oral administration of 15 mg of dipotassium clorazepate under controlled gastric pH conditions. As anticipated from theoretical considerations, when the gastric pH was maintained over pH 6, the hydrolysis of clorazepate to N-desmethyldiazepam was slow and incomplete, resulting in incomplete absorption of N-desmethyldiazepam. These blood level maxima of N-desmethyldiazepam were only 14 to 46 percent of the levels achieved from the normally acidic stomach in the same subjects (Abruzzo et al., 1977).

The pharmacokinetic parameters for the anxiolytic benzodiazepines commonly used in the United States are presented in Table 5; these com-

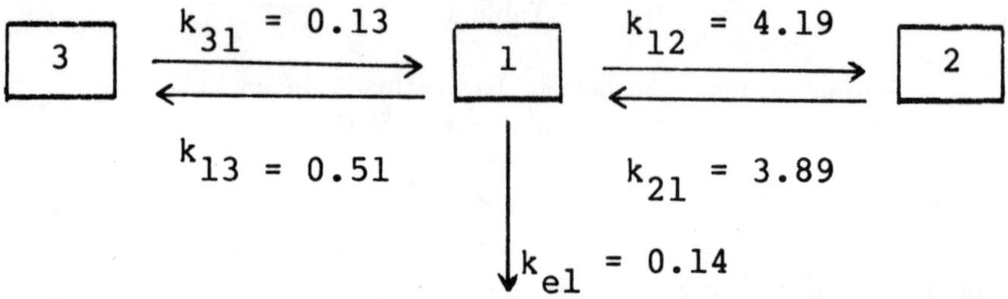

Figure 3. Three-compartment open-model system with mean values of rate constants. Adapted from Kaplan et al., 1973.

pounds are rapidly and completely absorbed, and all are highly protein-bound (> 95 percent). Differences are noted in the volumes of distribution: the more lipophilic the compound, the greater the volume of distribution. Structurally, the $-NHCH_3$ and N → 0 substituents of chlordiazepoxide and the $-OH$ substituents of oxazepam on the benzodiazepine nucleus of these two compounds diminish lipophilicity; diazepam and desmethyldiazepam lack such substituents. The reported half-lives for elimination of oxazepam and chlordiazepoxide are more rapid than those of diazepam and desmethyldiazepam. These differences reflect the influence of the physicochemical properties of the class of compounds on their respective drug disposition profiles.

The structure and mean half-life of meprobamate are presented in Figure 6 (Hollister and Levy, 1964). The published pharmacokinetic data available for this compound are somewhat limited. Meprobamate is reportedly metabolized to hydroxymeprobamate in animals and man (Douglas, Lud-

Table 5

Pharmacokinetic Parameters of Benzodiazepines

Absorption—Rapid and virtually complete (clorazepate is pH-dependent)

	Diazepam	*Desmethyldiazepam*	*Oxazepam*	*Chlordiazepoxide*
Volume of distribution (% body weight)	186	113	64	30
% Protein bound	98.3	96.9	95.7	96.3
Elimination half-life (hours)	21-46	40-61	3-13	6-15
Reference	Kaplan et al., 1973	Abruzzo et al., 1977	Alvan et al., 1977	Boxenbaum, 1977

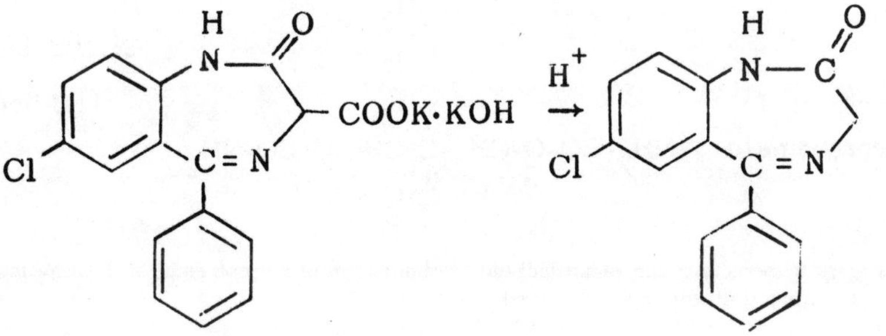

Figure 4. Clorazepate hydrolysis to desmethyldiazepam in an acidic environment. Adapted from Abruzzo et al., 1977.

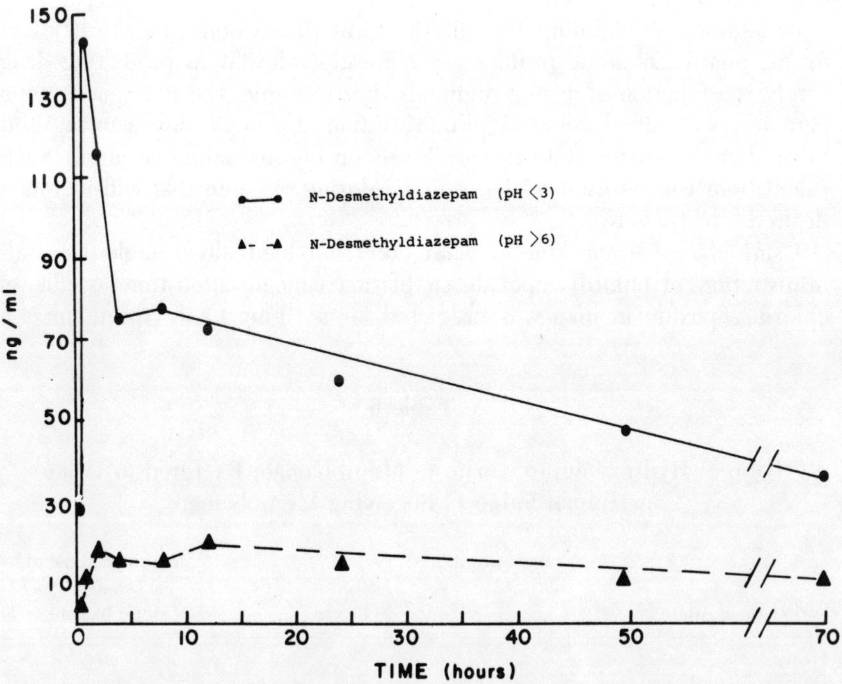

Figure 5. Blood levels of N-desmethyldiazepam in one subject following oral administration of 15 mg of dipotassium clorazepate under controlled gastric pH conditions. From Abruzzo et al., 1977.

Mean half-life of elimination

Meprobamate 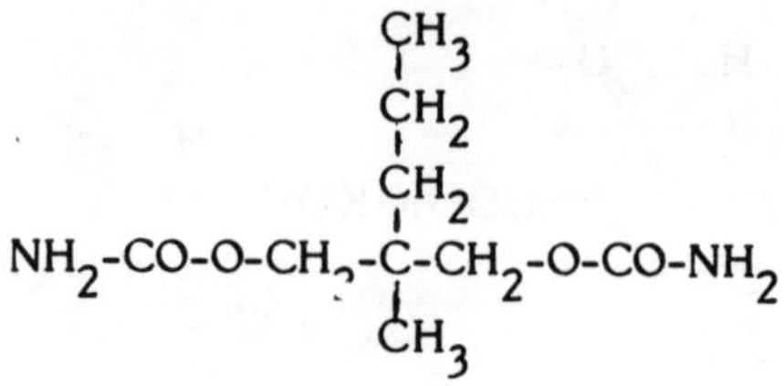 11.3 hour

Figure 6. Structure and mean half-life of elimination of meprobamate in healthy humans. Adapted from Hollister and Levy, 1964.

wig, and Smith, 1963). The ratio of metabolite to parent compound excreted in the urine following single and multiple dose administrations of meprobamate to man are reported in Table 6 (Douglas, Ludwig, and Smith, 1963). The ratio of metabolite (hydroxymeprobamate) to parent compound excreted in the urine is greater on chronic administration than after single-dose administration, which suggests that meprobamate induces its own metabolism.

In addition to defining the physiological disposition characteristics of drugs, pharmacokinetic profiles are clinically relevant in predicting drug levels as a function of dosing regimens. For example, the pharmacokinetic parameters obtained following administration of a single dose can be used to predict the steady-state plasma levels on chronic administration. Such calculations can be used to determine a dosing regimen that will maintain desired blood levels.

Using the pharmacokinetic parameters obtained after single-dose administration of chlordiazepoxide, a plasma concentration-time profile of chlordiazepoxide in man was predicted for a 10-mg t.i.d. (three times a

Table 6

Ratio of Hydroxymeprobamate to Meprobamate Excreted in Urine in Human Subjects Receiving Meprobamate

Period Drug Administered	No. of Subjects	Average Ratio of Excreted Product (Meprobamate = 1)
1 Day	5	.9
Daily for over 30 days	5	1.8

From Douglas et al., 1963.

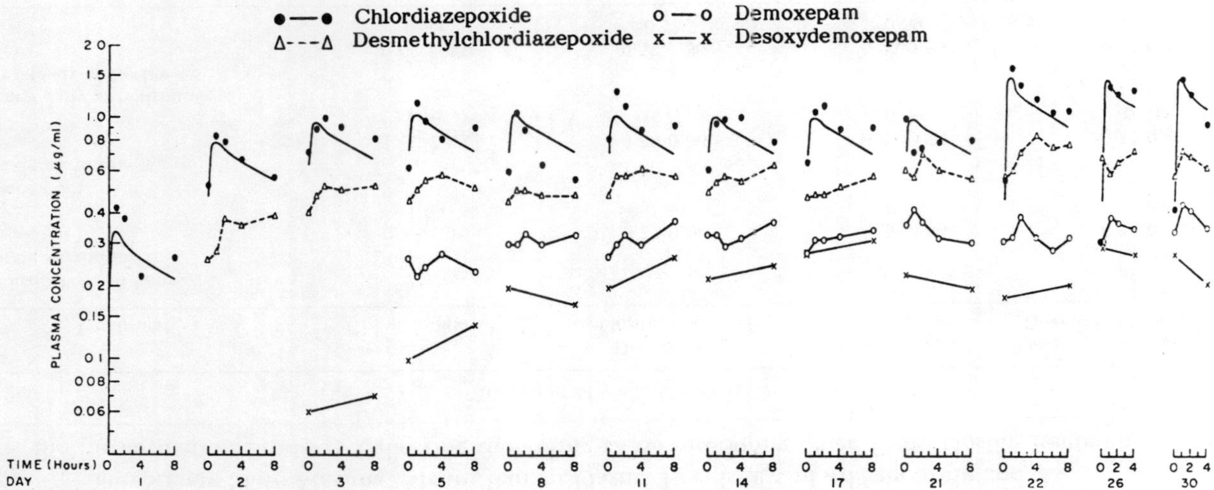

Figure 7. Plasma concentration-time profiles of chlcrdiazepoxide, desmethylchlordiazepoxide, demoxepam, and desoxydemoxepam following oral administration of chlordiazepoxide HCl to one subject. On days 1 through 21, the dosage was 10 mg every eight hours; on days 22 through 36, the dosage was 30 mg every 24 hours (solid line represents calculated chlordiazepoxide plasma level curve). From Boxenbaum et al., 1977a.

Table 7

The Steady-State Maxima, Mean (Range) Plasma Levels of Chlordiazepoxide and Its Biotransformation Products Following the 10 mg-t.i.d. and 30-mg Once Daily Dosing Regimen

Treatment	Compound Measured (μg/ml)			
	Chlordiazepoxide	Desmethyl-chlordiazepoxide	Demoxepam (Lactam)	Desoxydemoxepam (Desmethyldiazepam)
10 mg t.i.d., 0, 8, 16 hours steady-state maximum				
range	0.86-1.48	0.53-0.90	0.20-0.46	0.14-0.38
mean	1.09	0.69	0.35	0.26
30 mg once daily steady-state maximum				
range	1.38-2.89	0.55-0.86	0.23-0.55	0.17-0.43
mean	1.81	0.71	0.39	0.31
30 mg once daily at bedtime 8th hour (steady-state) level				
range	0.62-1.43	0.55-0.86	0.23-0.55	0.17-0.43
mean	0.93	0.71	0.39	0.31

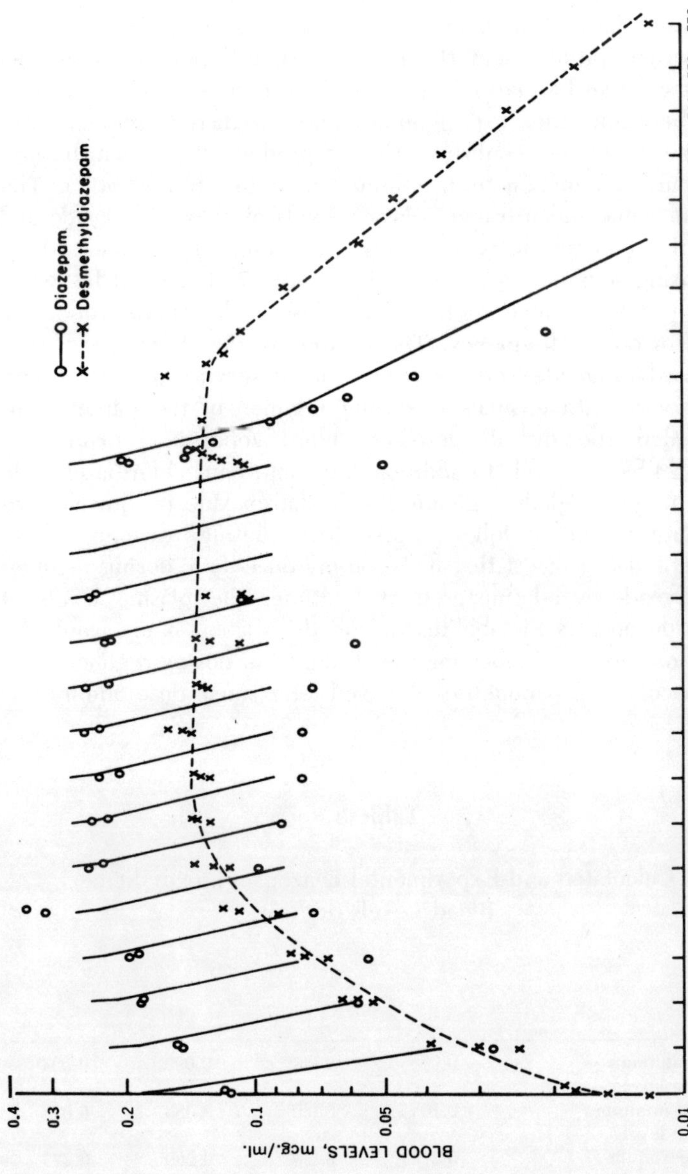

Figure 8. Oral blood-level data of diazepam and desmethyldiazepam in one subject receiving 10 mg of diazepam every 24 hours for 15 days (solid line represents calculated diazepam blood-level curve). From Kaplan et al., 1973.

day) dosing regimen for 21 days followed by 30-mg single daily doses for 11 additional days (Boxenbaum et al., 1977a). The predicted plasma concentration-time profiles and the corresponding experimental plasma levels for intact chlordiazepoxide are shown in Figure 7. The excellent correlation between the experimental and predicted plasma concentration-time profiles confirms the reproducibility, distribution, metabolism, and elimination from administration to administration. The steady-state maxima, mean (range) plasma levels of chlordiazepoxide and its biotransformation products following the 10-mg t.i.d. and 30-mg once-daily dosing regimens are reported in Table 7. It should be noted that the steady-state maxima of a fixed daily dose of chlordiazepoxide vary as a function of dosing frequency. The maxima of the three metabolites desmethylchlordiazepoxide, demoxepam, and desoxydemoxepam, however, do not vary with changes in dosing regimen of the parent compound, provided the overall dose of chlordiazepoxide remains unchanged in a 24-hour period. In addition, the eight-hour chlordiazepoxide plasma level on a once-daily regimen of chlordiazepoxide is equivalent to the steady-state maximum following the t.i.d. dosing regimen. These pharmacokinetic data suggest that if the 30-mg once-daily dosing regimen of chlordiazepoxide is administered at bedtime, the plasma levels of chlordiazepoxide and its metabolites during the waking hours would be identical to those observed following the 10-mg t.i.d. dosing regimen.

The pharmacokinetic parameters observed after single-dose administra-

Table 8

Calculated and Experimental Diazepam Steady-State Blood Levels (μg/ml)

	Subjects			
	1	2	3	4
Calculated minimum steady-state level	0.088	0.066	0.099	0.094
Experimental minimum steady-state level	0.104	0.068	0.085	0.078
Calculated maximum steady-state level	0.212	0.204	0.289	0.277
Experimental maximum steady-state level	0.235	0.210	0.224	0.238

From Kaplan et al., 1973.

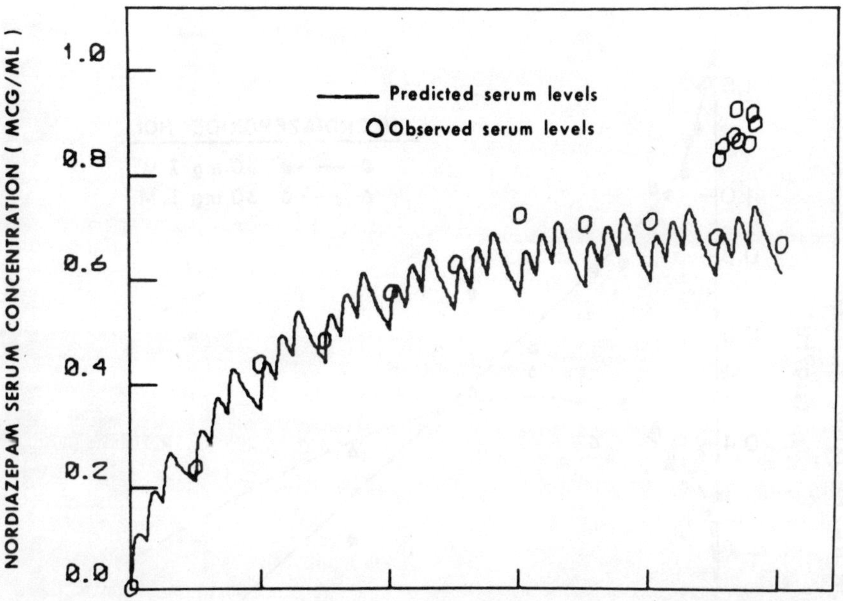

Figure 9. Mean plasma level of N-desmethyldiazepam after administration of 7.5 mg of clorazepate twice a day for ten days. From Carrigan et al., 1977.

tion were used to predict the multiple-dose profile of diazepam. The experimental and predicted blood levels of diazepam are shown in Figure 8 (Kaplan et al., 1973). Comparison of the calculated and experimental minimum and maximum diazepam steady-state levels in four subjects are presented in Table 8. The calculated maximum and minimum steady-state levels are in agreement with the experimental values, again confirming reproducibility of pharmacokinetic parameters from administration to administration.

The predicted and observed steady-state plasma levels of N-desmethyldiazepam resulting from administration of dipotassium chlorazepate (Carrigan et al., 1977) and oxazepam (Alvan, Siwers, and Vessman, 1977) are presented in Figure 9 and Table 9, respectively. The ability to predict steady-state profiles for chlordiazepoxide, diazepam, N-desmethyldiazepam, and oxazepam based on single-dose administration data confirms that unanticipated drug accumulation will not occur after chronic administration of these drugs and that these drugs do not inhibit or induce their own metabolism.

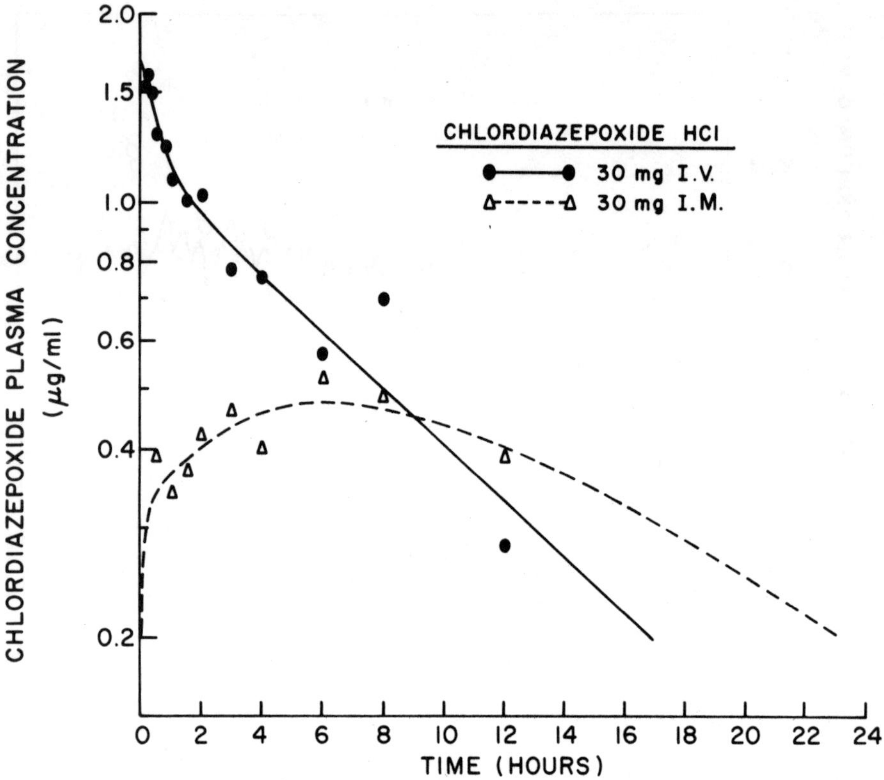

Figure 10. Chlordiazepoxide plasma concentration-time profiles following intramuscular and intravenous administration to one subject. From Boxenbaum et al., 1977b.

Chlordiazepoxide and diazepam may also be administered parenterally. Following intramuscular administration the benzodiazepines are completely absorbed but tend to be absorbed at a slower rate than after oral administration. The plasma levels of chlordiazepoxide after intravenous and intramuscular administrations are shown in Figure 10 (Boxenbaum et al., 1977b). The maximum plasma levels of chlordiazepoxide following intramuscular administration occur over a 4- to 12-hour interval postadministration, reflecting the slow absorption of drug from the site of injection.

Intramuscular diazepam also results in lower maximum plasma levels when compared to the orally administered drug. Assaf (1974) suggests that

Table 9

Comparison of Steady-State Concentrations Observed Following 5 mg Oxazepam Administered Orally t.i.d. and Steady-State Concentrations Predicted from Parameters Obtained Following Single-Dose Administrations

Subject	C_{ss} predicted	C_{ss} observed
	μg/ml	μg/ml
1	67	51.7
2	95	89.5
3	91	42.2
4	189	277.5
5	196	133.0
6	71.5	57.3
7	98.5	36.8
8	119.5	72.0

From Alvan et al., 1977.

Table 10

Mean Diazepam Plasma Levels (ng/ml) Following Single Oral and Intramuscular Administrations

		Mean Plasma Levels of Diazepam (ng/ml) at Time (min) after Administration			
Number of Patients	*Administration*	*15*	*30*	*60*	*90*
40	Orally	75	100	208	177
10	i.m. buttock	96	105	110	100
33	i.m. thigh	80	110	152	149
10	i.m. thigh (exercise)	214	284	272	243

From Assaf et al., 1974.

low plasma levels following intramuscular administration are caused by low blood supply to the resting muscle. Plasma levels of diazepam after oral dosing and intramuscular administration to resting and exercised muscles are shown in Table 10. The resting-muscle diazepam levels are lower than the drug levels observed following oral administration. When the drug was injected into the exercised muscle, however, the plasma levels of diazepam were higher than those observed following oral administration. Dundee, Gamble, and Assaf (1974) suggest that plasma levels of diazepam following intramuscular administration may vary, depending on who injects the drug. Table 11 compares plasma levels of diazepam following intramuscular injection by nurses and doctors.

As a drug class the benzodiazepines are extensively metabolized and their metabolic pathways are similar in that:

1. Substituents are removed from the B ring of the 1,4-benzodiazepine nucleus.

Table 11

Diazepam Plasma Levels (ng/ml) after Intramuscular Injection by Nurses and Physicians

	Minutes after Injection			
Administrator	*15*	*30*	*60*	*90*
Nurse	28 ± 14.1	45 ± 20.3	47 ± 19.5	45 ± 15.4
Physician	90 ± 7.8	121 ± 8.7	124 ± 8.9	100 ± 5.1

From Dundee et al., 1974.

Table 12

Metabolic Pathways of Marketed Benzodiazepines

1. Chlordiazepoxide → desmethyl-chlordiazepoxide → lactam → desmethyl-diazepam → oxazepam → conj.
2. Diazepam → desmethyl-diazepam → oxazepam → conj.
3. Oxazepam → oxazepam → conj.
4. Clorazepate → desmethyl-diazepam → oxazepam → conj.

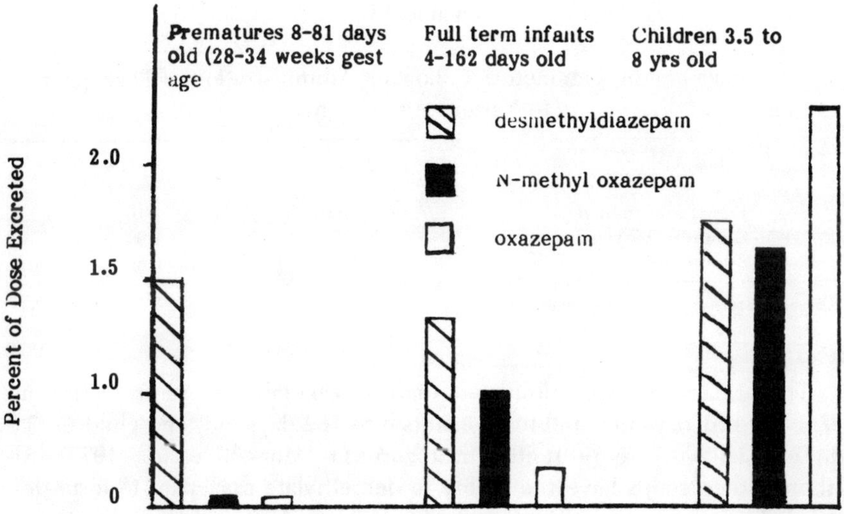

Figure 11. Twenty-four hour urinary excretion profile of diazepam metabolites following a single 0.3-mg/kg intramuscular injection of diazepam. Adapted from Morselli et al., 1973.

2. Position 3 is hydroxylated.
3. The hydroxylated metabolite undergoes glucuronidation and subsequent elimination in the urine.

The metabolic pathways for chlordiazepoxide, diazepam, oxazepam, and clorazepate are described in Table 12. The similarities in pathways are immediately apparent.

The pharmacokinetic profiles discussed here have been obtained from healthy volunteers. In a clinical setting, however, patients of differing age groups may possess a variety of pathological, genetic, and environmental characteristics. Age, disease state, and drug interactions may also affect the physiological disposition profile of a drug. Such variations may be reflected in specific pharmacokinetic parameters which, in turn, may influence the clinical profile of the drug. For example, such metabolic reactions as oxidations, reductions, hydrolyses, and conjugations which readily occur within the livers of children and adults, are negligible in newborns (Vest and Rossier, 1963). Hydroxylation and glucuronidation capabilities, which are major metabolic pathways for the benzodiazepines, seem to be related to the degree of maturation; such alterations in metabolism are reflected in the pharmacokinetic parameters of these drugs.

Table 13

Pharmacokinetic Parameters Following Administration of Diazepam to Various Age Groups.

Subjects	$T_{\frac{1}{2}}$, hr	V_d (l/kg)
Prematures (8-81 days)	40-100	1.10
Children (3-7 yr)	20-45	1.99
Adult (25-43 yr)	21-46	1.86

Adapted from Kaplan et al., 1973; Morselli et al., 1973.

The urinary excretion profiles of diazepam metabolites in premature infants 8 to 81 days old, full-term infants 4 to 162 days old, and children 3.5 to 8 years old, are presented in Figure 11 (Morselli et al., 1973). Although the groups have the ability to demethylate diazepam to form desmethyldiazepam, the ability to hydroxylate and conjugate is limited in both infant groups but not in the older children.

The pharmacokinetic parameters of diazepam in premature infants, children, and adults are presented in Table 13. The long half-life of

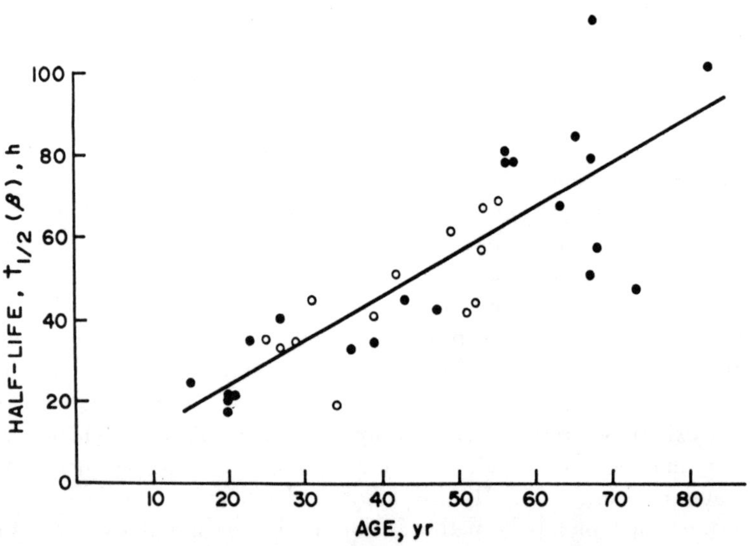

Figure 12. Correlation of diazepam half-life (β) and age. Each symbol represents study of 33 normal individuals. From Klotz et al., 1975.

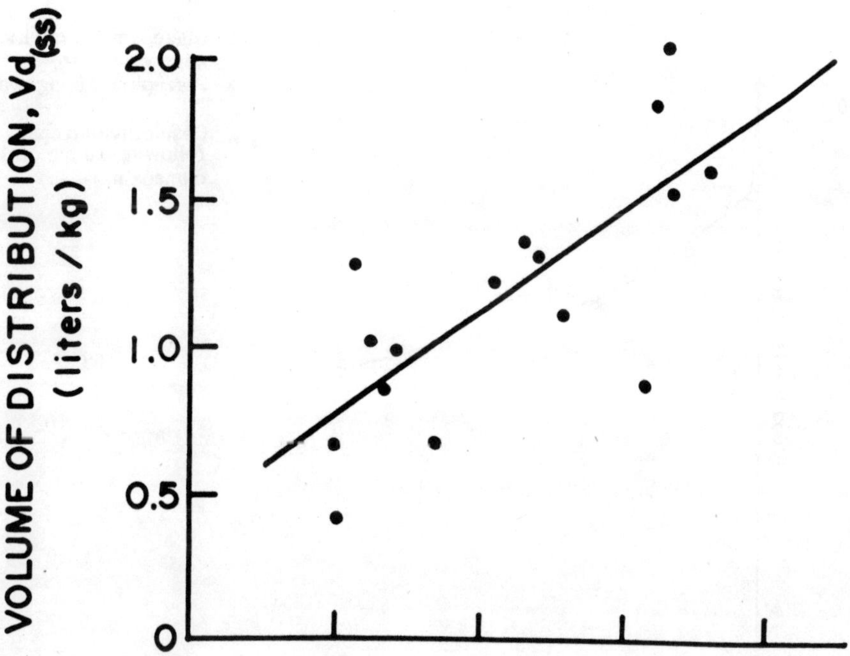

Figure 13. Correlation of volumes of distribution of diazepam and age in normal individuals. From Klotz et al., 1975.

Table 14

Calculated Dosing Regimen to Maintain Steady-State Plasma Levels (γ/ml) Equal to Normal Subjects in Cirrhotic Patients Exhibiting Potential Twofold or Fivefold Increase in Half-Life

	Normal	Cirrhotic		Cirrhotic (corrected)	
		2 x	5 x	2 x	5 x
Dosing interval	24 hr	24 hr	24 hr	31	78
C_{min}	.144	.225	.607	.166	.163
C_{max}	.256	.300	.682	.241	.237

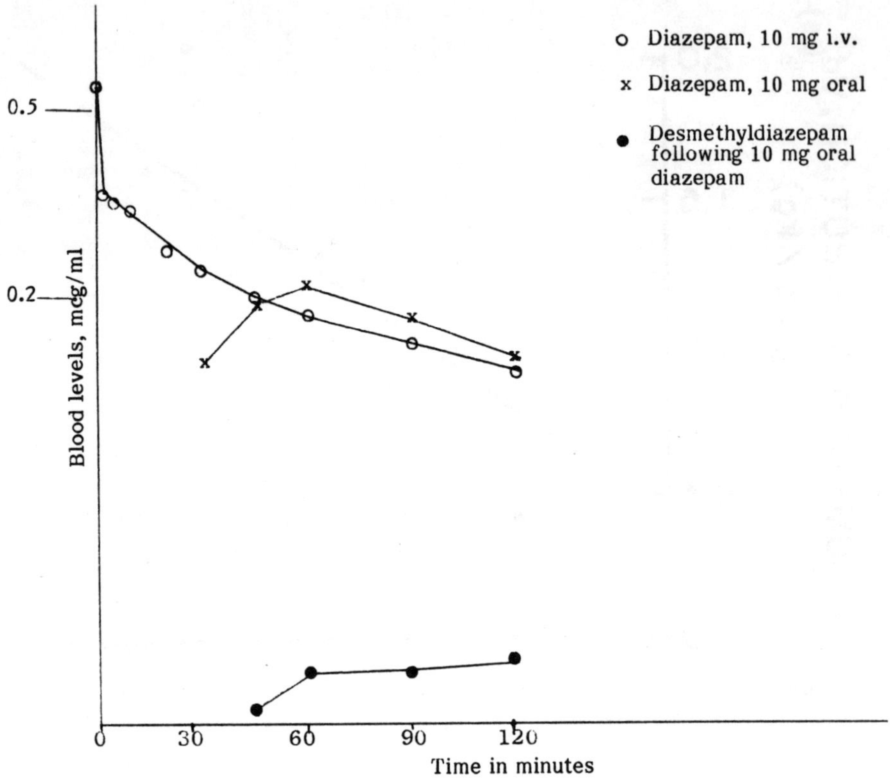

Figure 14. Blood concentration-time profiles of diazepam and N-desmethyldiazepam after intravenous and oral administration to human subjects from 0 to 120 minutes postadministration.

diazepam in premature babies reflects hepatic immaturity. The volume of distribution (Vd) is less for newborns than for adults. Differences in Vd may reflect the lesser amount of plasma proteins and protein-binding capacity in newborns and/or such differences in body composition as greater body water and lower fat content.

The pharmacokinetic parameters of half-life and volume of distribution that differ in the infant also differ in geriatric patients when both groups are compared to young adults. The correlation between the half-life of diazepam and age is shown in Figure 12 (Klotz et al., 1975). There is a marked increase in diazepam half-life with age and, as Figure 13 (Klotz et al., 1975) demonstrates, there is also an increase in volume of distribution. Although these are the same pharmacokinetic parameters that were altered when diazepam was administered to newborns, these parameters are probably changing in the geriatric subject for different reasons. The prolonged half-lives of the benzodiazepines in aging normal subjects reflect alterations in distribution characteristics (Vd) rather than hepatic dysfunction or alterations in protein-binding. Such pharmacokinetic observations may reflect the normal physiological changes of aging such as diminishing lean body mass.

The pharmacokinetics of drugs may be altered in the presence of hepatic disease, and adjustment in dosing schedules may be required. The pharmacokinetic parameters affected by liver disease include protein-binding, extraction ratio, hepatic clearance, and half-life of the administered drug. Renal dysfunction also results in a reduction of plasma proteins. Once the influence of disease state on the pharmacokinetic parameters is established, a new dosing regimen may be calculated to yield desired plasma levels. The steady-state maximum and minimum plasma levels of diazepam following a once-daily dosing regimen for normal and cirrhotic patients with a potential for two- and fivefold increases in half-life, are reported in the first three columns of Table 14. As calculated, the steady-state maximum and minimum plasma levels for the cirrhotic patient would be high when compared to those of the normal. To achieve comparable steady-state levels in the cirrhotic patient, the dosing regimen may be adjusted by considering changes in half-life. The resulting dosing regimen for a two- and fivefold increase in half-life would be a change from once every 24 hours to once every 31 and 78 hours, respectively (Table 14, columns 4 and 5). Corrected, the steady-state maximum and minimum for the cirrhotic patient would then be equivalent to the steady-state levels in normals, and unanticipated drug accumulation would not occur unless there were further changes in the pathological state. Therefore, in spite of changes in the pharmacokinetic parameters of the benzodiazepines with age, hepatic and renal dysfunction, or other pathological states, new dosing regimens may be readily calculated to assure plasma levels associated with clinical efficacy and safety of the drugs.

An intravenous sedative drug for simple surgical procedures should possess the following properties:

1. It must be therapeutically safe in the dosage schedules used and not depress the cardiovascular and respiratory systems.
2. It should be capable of maintaining its full pharmacological effect during the course of the surgical procedure with a single dose.
3. It should blunt consciousness to the point at which amnesia may be

Table 15

Diazepam Profile During First Two Hours After Intravenous and Oral Administration.

I.V. Administration	*Oral Administration*
During 0 to 2 hours postadministration	*During 0 to 2 hours postadministration*
Drug is *distributing* rapidly to body tissues.	Drug is being *absorbed* and is distributing to body tissues.
Blood levels *decline* to about ½ maximum values.	Blood levels are *increasing* due to absorption.
Little or no metabolite present.	Little or no metabolite present.
Patient experiences sedation and amnesia during the 0- to 30-minute interval.	There is no comparable physiological response.

produced and controlled, yet not suppress reflexes to the point at which cooperation of the patient is lost.

4. The sedation should be relatively short-acting so that recovery times are not unduly delayed or prolonged.
5. It should be capable of producing and maintaining adequate sedation and control in all age groups, particularly in the young patient.

Sedative doses of intravenous diazepam have all these properties. Intravenous diazepam is widely used for oral surgery and other minor procedures performed on an outpatient basis. Blood level and clinical effects immediately following intravenous administration differ somewhat from the levels and effects attained after oral administration at the same dose levels; two hours postadministration, however, the blood level and clinical profiles of intravenous and orally administered drug are virtually the same. Comparison of the zero- to two-hour physiological disposition profile of diazepam after intravenous and oral administration is presented in Table 15; the zero- to two-hour blood levels of diazepam following intravenous and oral administrations are highlighted in Figure 14. As noted, the blood levels following intravenous injection are much higher than those following oral administration during the zero- to 30-minute interval. During this time patients receiving intravenous diazepam experience sedation and amnesia; comparable effects are not observed for the same time interval after oral administration. Since metabolite levels are very low or nonexistent during the zero- to two-hour period, the clinical observations of amnesia and sedation must be attributed to high levels of diazepam.

In conclusion, pharmacokinetics has greatly enhanced our knowledge and understanding of drugs and their administration. Pharmacokinetics is a tool that can provide the clinician with a degree of quantitative precision in dosing patients of various ages, disease states, genetic makeup, and environmental histories.

REFERENCES

ABRUZZO, C. W., MACASIEB, T., WEINFELD, R., RIDER, J. A., and KAPLAN, S. A. 1977. Changes in the oral absorption characteristics in man of dipotassium clorazepate at normal and elevated gastric pH. *J. Pharmacokinet. Biopharm.*, 5:377-390.

ALVAN, G., SIWERS, B., and VESSMAN, J. 1977. Pharmacokinetics of oxazepam in healthy volunteers. *Acta Pharmacol. Toxicol.*, 40(1):40-51.

ASSAF, R. A. E., DUNDEE, J. W., and GAMBLE, J. A. S. 1974. Factors influencing plasma diazepam levels following a single administration. *Brit. J. Clin. Pharmacol.*, 343-349.

BOXENBAUM, H. G., GEITNER, K. A., JACK, M. L., DIXON, W. R., and KAPLAN, S. A. 1977a. Pharmacokinetic and biopharmaceutic profile of chlordiazepoxide HCl in healthy subjects: Multiple-dose oral administration. *J. Pharmacokinet. Biopharm.*, 5:25-39.

BOXENBAUM, H. G., GEITNER, K. A., JACK, M. L., DIXON, W. R., SPIEGEL, H. E., SYMINGTON, J., CHRISTIAN, R., MOORE, J. D., WEISSMAN, L., and KAPLAN, S. A. 1977b. Pharmacokinetic and biopharmaceutic profile of chlordiazepoxide HCl in healthy subjects. Single dose studies by the intravenous, intramuscular, and oral routes. *J. Pharmacokinet. Biopharm.*, 5:3-23.

CARRIGAN, P. J., CHAO, G. C., BARKER, W. M., HOFFMAN, D. J., and CHUN, A. H. C. 1977. Steady-state bioavailability of two clorazepate dipotassium dosage forms. *J. Clin. Pharmacol.*, 17:18-28.

DOUGLAS, J. F., LUDWIG, B. J., and SMITH, N. 1963. Studies on the metabolism of meprobamate. *Proc. Soc. Exp. Biol. Med.*, 112:436-438.

DUNDEE, J. W., GAMBLE, J. A. S., and ASSAF, R. A. E. 1974. Plasma-diazepam levels following intramuscular injection by nurses and doctors. *Lancet*, 2:1461.

HOLLISTER, L. E. and LEVY, G. 1964. Kinetics of meprobamate elimination in humans. *Chemotherapia*, 9:20-24.

KAPLAN, S. A., JACK, M. L., ALEXANDER, K., and WEINFELD, R. E. 1973. Pharmacokinetic profile of diazepam in man following single intravenous and oral and chronic oral administrations. *J. Pharm. Sci.*, 62:1789-1796.

KLOTZ, U., AVANT, G. R., HOYUMPA, A., SCHENKER, S., and WILKINSON, G. R. 1975. The effects of age and liver disease on the disposition and elimination of diazepam in adult man. *J. Clin. Invest.*, 55:347-359.

MORSELLI, P. L., PRINCIPI, N., TOGNONI, G., REALI, E., BELVEDERE, G., STANDEN, S. M., and SERENI, F. 1973. Diazepam elimination in premature and full term infants and children. *J. Perinat. Med.* 1:133-141.

RANDALL, L. O. and KAPPELL, B. 1973. Pharmacological activity of some benzodiazepines and their metabolites. In S. Garattini, E. Mussini, and L. O. Randall (eds.), *The Benzodiazepines*, pp. 27-51. New York: Raven Press.

Vest, M. F. and Rossier, R. 1963. Detoxification in the newborn: The ability of the newborn infant to form conjugates with glucuronic acid, glycine, acetate, and glutathione. *Ann. N.Y. Acad. Sci.*, 111:183-198.

12

THE VALUE OF PLASMA CONCENTRATIONS IN ASSESSING THE EFFECTS OF TRICYCLIC ANTIDEPRESSANTS

SAMUEL G. SIRIS, M.D.,
ALEXANDER H. GLASSMAN, M.D., and
FAY STETNER, M.S.

The ability to measure the blood concentrations of tricyclic antidepressants has been one of the major technological advances of the past decade in psychopharmacology. Before this development, all of the landmark antidepressant studies could evaluate the effects of drugs only on the basis of oral dosage. Variability in such factors as patient compliance, gastrointestinal absorption, and hepatic degradation could not be taken into account. Although it is true that measuring plasma levels of antidepressants is not equivalent to direct measurement of activity at the physiologically meaningful site of action, it is a dramatic advance over baseline oral doses in evaluating accurately the usefulness of a drug for various syndromes, the dosage range that may be required for adequate treatment, and the true incidence of side effects at drug concentrations sufficient to be therapeutic.

Investigations using plasma concentrations of tricyclic antidepressants, however, have been hampered because their measurements present certain difficulties. First, the concentrations involved are in nanogram amounts, since the majority of the compounds are sequestered in lipid tissues at the steady state. Not until recently have advances in modern analytic techniques allowed researchers readily to determine such small quantities (Perel et al., 1974). Second, to be meaningful, plasma concentrations must be measured at steady-state conditions. Operationally, this means a patient must be on a dose of a drug for at least five times the half-life of that drug in his system, and have his blood level drawn at a uniform and appropriate interval after his last dose. In the case of imipramine, the average plasma half-life in a patient is about 15 hours and all but the very slowest metabolizers will have reached steady state within a week. Other tricyclic drugs such as nortriptyline (average half-life = 40 hrs) and especially protriptyline (average half-life = 140 hrs) require considerably more time to reach steady state. Studies in which there was insufficient time for steady-state conditions to be achieved must be interpreted with extreme caution, and the utility of plasma level feedback for clinical purposes is correspondingly dubious. Third, most tricyclics have active metabolites that must be taken into consideration. It is no accident, then, that the first tricyclic to have its plasma concentration measured was nortriptyline (Asberg et al., 1971), a compound with no known active metabolites. The unexpected finding with nortriptyline, now confirmed in four out of six studies (Asberg et al., 1971; Kragh-Sorensen, Asberg, and Hansen, 1973; Kragh-Sorensen et al., 1976; Ziegler et al., 1976), was that nortriptyline exhibited a "therapeutic window" of effective plasma concentrations. Below 50 ng/ml the drug was not useful as an antidepressant; above 150 ng/ml, the favorable results obtained between 50 and 150 ng/ml were once again lost. Impressive confirmation of this thesis was obtained in a study in which nonresponding depressed patients with plasma levels in excess of 180 ng/ml were either maintained on their dosage or had their dosage decreased in a double-blind fashion (Kragh-Sorensen et al., 1976). Those patients who had their dosages decreased were the ones who improved. Preliminary data now available suggest that protriptyline may also demonstrate the phenomenon of a therapeutic window (Whyte et al., 1976), although more detailed studies still need to be done to confirm this because of protriptyline's unusually long half-life. Findings of such therapeutic windows certainly must caution us in our explorations and inferences with regard to tricyclic compounds, especially those which have active metabolites whose biological action needs to be taken into account.

Our own work with imipramine began with a study in which patients with endogenous depressions were treated with a standard dose of 3.5 mg/kg (Glassman et al., 1977). Patients' clinical outcomes were rated, and plasma levels of imipramine and its known active metabolite desmethylimipramine were measured at steady state. Under these conditions, the median combined plasma concentrations of these compounds was 180 ng/ml. But the range of combined concentrations extended from 40 to 1200 ng/ml, a striking thirtyfold variation. What we had administered as a uniform oral dose had certainly been translated into a highly variable drug load in the patients' circulation. It is noteworthy that a sizable percentage of patients who had received seemingly substantial oral doses nevertheless were found to have plasma drug levels that were quite low. Furthermore, it was observed that other substances entering the patients' systems could markedly influence imipramine plasma concentrations through enzyme induction, enzyme inhibition, and possibly other mechanisms. For example, the addition of a regular dose of 100 mg of Seconal as a sleeping pill could cause a stable imipramine level of 200 ng/ml to fall to 70 ng/ml. Similarly, smokers are noted generally to stabilize at imipramine levels considerably lower than nonsmokers receiving comparable dosage. On the other hand, the addition of methylphenidate (Ritalin), 10 mg t.i.d. (three times daily), could result in a steady-state concentration of 200 ng/ml jumping to 900 ng/ml, a level that might be toxic in a child (Garrettson, Perel, and Dayton, 1969).

Arbitrarily, in our study of clinical outcome in endogenously depressed

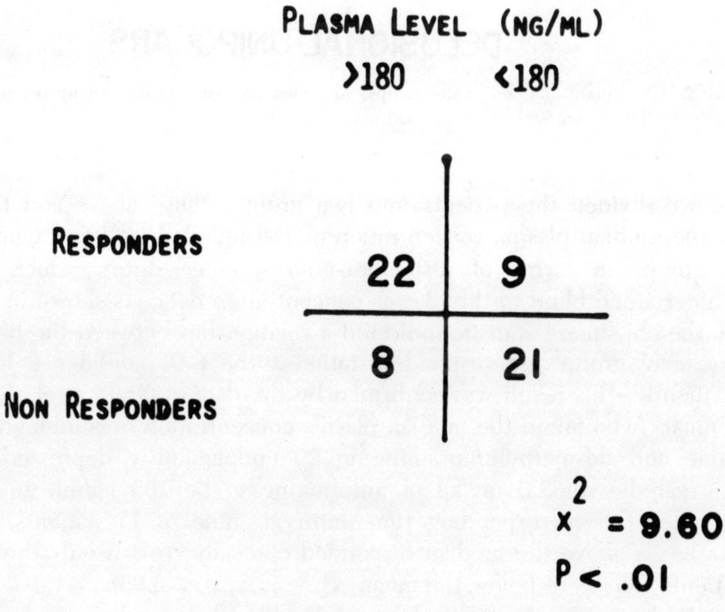

Figure 1. Chi-square analysis of the total sample, comparing responders and nonresponders above and below median plasma levels.

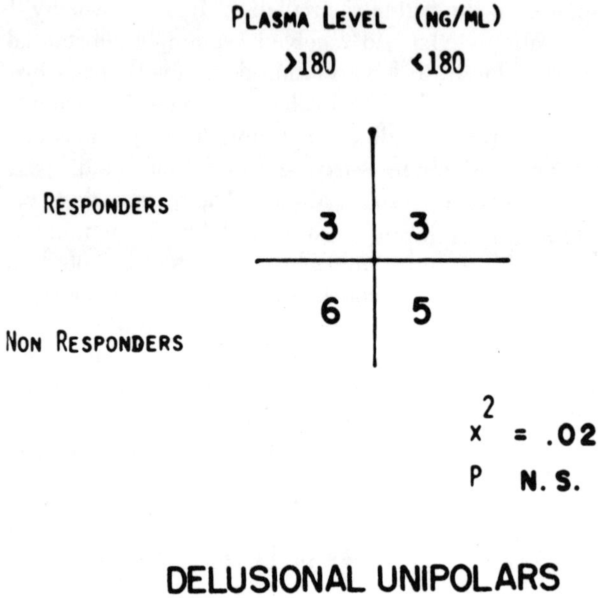

Figure 2. Chi-square analysis of the sample of delusional patients comparing responders and nonresponders above and below median plasma levels.

adults, we divided the patients into two groups: those above and those below the median plasma concentration of 180 ng/ml. We then examined these groups in terms of responder-nonresponder status, which had been ascertained blind to the plasma concentration data. As shown in Figure 1, the chi-square statistic indicated a relationship between the higher plasma level group and responder status at the 0.01 confidence level. Subsequently, this result was confirmed by the data of Gram et al. (1976) in Denmark who found the median plasma concentration of combined imipramine and desmethylimipramine in 23 endogenously depressed patients treated with 3.5 mg/kg of imipramine to be 185 ng/ml. In that study, after the corresponding time interval, nine of 11 patients with plasma levels above the median responded clinically, versus only three of 12 patients who were below the mean ($x^2 = 5.32$, $p < 0.05$).

Our display of the data, based on subdividing the population according to plasma drug concentration, allowed a second observation to emerge. As shown in Figure 2, it became apparent that the response pattern of patients who were delusional was unlike the pattern of patients who were nondelusional. Although six of 17 (35 percent) of the delusional patients were responders, the rate of response was essentially the same among patients who had blood levels above 180 ng/ml as among those whose plasma concentrations were below that level. This rate of response, of course, is similar to the rate of response of depressives to placebo in many double-blind studies. Unfortunately, these earlier studies did not subdivide the patient group into delusional versus nondelusional categories, so that the rate of placebo response in the pure subset of delusional depressives is not known. The nondelusional depressive patients, in our data then, when considered alone, had an even more striking relationship between clinical response and plasma imipramine concentrations ($x^2 = 17.22$, $p < 0.001$). This observation was further supported by seven of 13 nondelusional nonresponders at blood levels of less than 180 ng/ml becoming responders when their plasma concentrations were raised to exceed 180 ng/ml. Such a discrepancy between the patterns of response of delusional and nondelusional depressive patients suggests that the two groups might be suffering from different disease entities from the psychopharmacologic perspective (Kantor and Glassman, 1977). It may be noted, parenthetically, that to date 14 of 17 delusional depressives not responding to imipramine have responded well to electroconvulsive therapy.

Figure 3 depicts response rates when our nondelusional patient population was divided into thirds on the basis of plasma imipramine concentra-

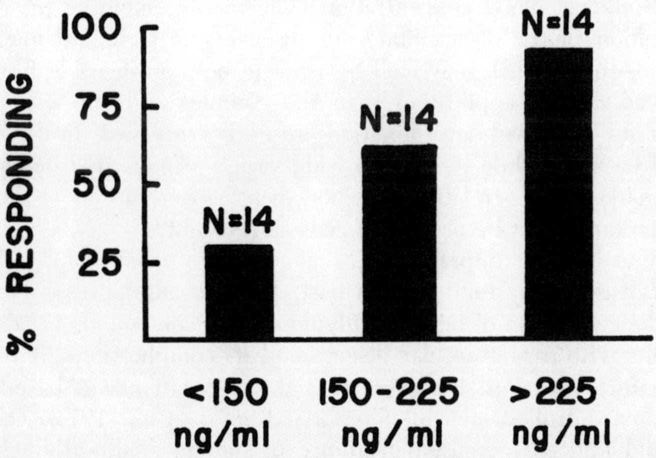

Figure 3. Forty-two nondelusional patients divided into three equal groups by plasma level. Response rates calculated independently for lowest, middle, and highest plasma level groups.

tions. Patients with plasma levels of less than 150 ng/ml had a response rate of 29 percent, which again approximates the placebo response rate in most antidepressant studies. Patients with plasma concentrations of between 150 and 225 ng/ml had a response rate of 64 percent, and those above 225 ng/ml responded at a 93-percent rate. A linear relationship between plasma concentration of imipramine and response to treatment at this dosage level is strongly suggested ($x^2 = 12.3$, $p < 0.005$).

The observation that a small number of patients on a standard clinical dosage might achieve plasma levels as much as six times the usual therapeutic concentration (1200 ng/ml versus about 200 ng/ml) naturally led us to consider drug toxicity and side effects. Unwanted or adventitious actions of a drug, like their clinically useful counterparts, may also be thought of as having response curves based on the plasma concentrations. There is no special reason why these other actions of drugs would necessarily begin to occur precisely at the plasma thresholds of clinical utility. Rather, each action of the drug has its own threshold. When the concentration threshold for a particular side effect is less than the therapeutic threshold, that side effect would be an unavoidable concomitant of therapeutic action of the drug in that patient. However, if the side effect threshold is greater than the therapeutic threshold, the drug dose could, at least in theory, be so adjusted as to avoid that side effect. Moreover, if a particular side effect has a threshold relatively near the therapeutic threshold, such a side effect might become a clinically useful marker for adequate clinical blood concentration. The measurement of plasma drug concentrations may thus facilitate our discovery of biological markers for dosage adequacy which may well turn out to be more feasible in terms of widespread clinical application than the complex and still experimental methods of blood level determination presently employed. In this context, it would be worthwhile to study a wide variety of potential biological response markers in correlation to blood drug concentrations to determine which markers might be used with general reliability.

In our work with imipramine, a major interest has been its effects on the cardiovascular system. In the past, tricyclic antidepressants had acquired the reputation of being highly dangerous compounds to administer to patients with cardiovascular disease and its complications. A review of the literature revealed, however, that this reputation was based principally on uncontrolled anecdotal reports (Kantor et al., 1978). One large survey did find an increased incidence of sudden deaths (though not of total deaths) among cardiac patients treated with tricyclics in standard antidepressant usage compared to those not treated with tricyclics (Coull et al., 1970). But this was balanced by another survey which found no such difference (Boston Collaborative Drug Surveillance Program, 1972). Thus, unequivocal evidence of cardiovascular disease as a contraindication to tricyclic use in the usual dosage range does not exist. This is in clear contrast to the overdose situation in which definite propensities for ventricular arrhythmias, sinus tachycardia and bradycardia, first-, second-, and third-degree atrioventricular (A-V) block, bundle-branch block, decreased myocardial contractility, supine hypotension, and asystole have been observed (Thorstrand, 1974; Spiker et al., 1975).

At therapeutic plasma concentrations of imipramine, we found several electrocardiographic changes that occurred frequently. PR intervals, QRS complexes, and QTc intervals were prolonged, ST-T changes were observed, and the heart rates of our patients, taken as a group, increased. In healthy hearts, these changes were not clinically meaningful. In hearts with bundle-branch or partial A-V block, however, imipramine in therapeutic concentrations was capable of producing dangerous degrees of A-V block in some patients. This latter group of patients thus required careful monitoring to determine whether an intracardiac demand pacemaker would be required to enable the continuance of antidepressant therapy. On the other hand, patients who already had indwelling cardiac pacemakers could be treated safely.

Increase in cardiac rate above baseline in our group of patients was statistically significant at therapeutic blood imipramine concentrations, as recorded by 24-hour Holter monitor. This effect was pronounced for patients with relative baseline bradycardia. But in patients with initial rates of 80 or more, the increases were quite modest (about four beats/minute), and several of the patients with baseline rates above 90 actually experienced a decrement in their heart rate on imipramine. Thus, none of the patients who might have been adversely effected by a substantive increment in heart rate experienced that reaction.

The 24-hour Holter monitor recordings in patients with cardiac disease also provided the most striking finding with imipramine, the observation that imipramine has antiarrhythmic properties (Bigger et al., 1977). A series of patients with atrial and ventricular premature depolarizations has now been studied in which the incidence of both has been markedly decreased. So, far from being contraindicated in patients with premature depolarizations, imipramine can actually be helpful in treating these cardiac arrhythmias. Caution must be exercised, however, when imipramine is added to a pre-existing antiarrhythmic drug regimen. In these latter cases, synergistic effects of the imipramine may serve to prolong conduction times unduly, or to lead to an undesirable increase in cardiac irritability. Thus, other antiarrhythmic drugs may need to be discontinued or their dosages decreased when imipramine (and possibly also other tricyclics) are administered.

In our series of patients, we found the most troublesome cardiovascular side effect of imipramine to be orthostatic hypotension (Kantor et al., 1978). We observed a mean systolic drop of 25 mm Hg on imipramine and a mean diastolic drop of 10 mm Hg on imipramine. Twenty-nine of 148 patients (20 percent) had symptoms attributable to these orthostatic changes which were sufficiently severe to warrant alterations of the treatment plan. These symptoms included ataxia, prolonged severe dizziness, and episodes of fainting. We found that the magnitude of orthostatic hypotension in the baseline drug-free state was the best predictor of increase in orthostatic hypotension with imipramine. Increased orthostatic decrements, of course, were most dangerous in older patients and in those suffering from arteriosclerotic cardiovascular disease. Furthermore, we observed that maximal orthostatic changes with imipramine were found at plasma concentrations of 120 ng/ml—a level definitely below the therapeutic range. Subsequent increase to or within the therapeutic range did not then have an additional impact on blood pressure. Additionally, even though initial subjective complaints of dizziness tended to abate over time, the true orthostatic hypotension continued undiminished as long as the patient remained on imipramine. Thus, the emergence of orthostatic hypotension or subjective symptoms of dizziness were not valid indicators of effective plasma concentrations of imipramine.

Summary

It has now been observed that both the therapeutic action and the cardiovascular side effects of tricyclic antidepressants exhibit thresholds of activity based on their plasma concentrations. Since even uniform oral dosage may result in enormously divergent plasma levels of these drugs and their metabolites, the laboratory assessment of these plasma concentrations represents a major methodological advance in allowing us to assess their true psychological and physiological effects. This paper has detailed several of our findings with regard to the actions of imipramine that have been made possible by this development.

REFERENCES

Åsberg, M., Cronholm, B., Sjoqvist, F., and Tuck, D. 1971. Relationship between plasma level and therapeutic effect of nortriptyline. *Br. Med. J.* 3:331-334.

Bigger, J. T., Giardina, E. G. V., Perel, J. M., Kantor, S. J., and Glassman, A. H. 1977. Cardiac antiarrhythmic effect of imipramine hydrochloride. *N. Engl. J. Med.* 296:206-208.

Boston Collaborative Drug Surveillance Program. 1972. *Lancet* 1:529-531.

COULL, D. C., CROOKS, J., DINGIVALL-FORDYCE, I., SCOTT, A. M., and WEIR, R. D. 1970. Amitriptyline and cardiac disease: risk of sudden death identified by monitoring system. *Lancet* 2:590-591.

GARRETTSON, L., PEREL, J., and DAYTON, P. 1969. Methylphenidate interaction with both anticonvulsants and ethyl biscoumacetate. *J.A.M.A.* 207:2053-2056.

GLASSMAN, A., PEREL, J., SHOSTAK, M., KANTOR, S., and FLIESS, J. 1977. Clinical implications of imipramine plasma levels for depressive illness. *Arch. Gen. Psychiatry* 34:197-204.

GRAM, L., REISBY, N., IBSEN, I., NAGY, A., DENCKER, S. J., BECK, P., PETERSEN, G. O., and CHRISTIANSEN, J. 1976. Plasma levels and antidepressive effect of imipramine. *Clin. Pharmacol. Ther.* 19:318-324.

KANTOR, S. J., GLASSMAN, A. H., BIGGER, J. T., PEREL, J. M., and GIARDINA, E. G. 1978. The cardiac effects of therapeutic plasma concentrations of imipramine. *J. Psychiatry*, accepted for publication.

KANTOR, S. J., and GLASSMAN, A. H. 1977. Delusional depressions: Natural history and response to treatment. *Br. J. Psychiatry* 131:351-360.

KRAGH-SORENSEN, P., ÅSBERG, M., and HANSEN, C. 1973. Plasma nortriptyline levels in endogenous depression. *Lancet* 1:113-115.

KRAGH-SORENSEN, P., HANSEN, C., BAASTRUP, P., and HVIDBERG, E. 1976. Self-inhibiting action of nortriptylin's antidepressive effect at high plasma levels. *Psychopharmacologia* 45:305-312.

PEREL, J. M., O'BRIEN, L., BLACK, N. B., BELLWARD, G. D., and DAYTON, P. G. 1974. In *Advances in Biochemical Psychopharmacology*, pp. 201-212. New York: Raven Press.

SPIKER, D. G., WEISS, A. N., CHANG, S. S., RUWITCH, J. E., and BIGGS, J. I. 1975. Tricyclic antidepressant overdose: Clinical presentation and plasma levels. *Clin. Pharmacol. Ther.* 18:539-546.

THORSTRAND, C. 1974. Cardiovascular effects of poisoning with tricyclic antidepressants. *Acta Med. Scand.* 195:505-514.

WHYTE, S., MACDONALD, A., NAYLOR, G., and MOODY, J. 1976. Plasma concentrations of protriptyline and clinical effects in depressed women. *Br. J. Psychiatry* 128:384-390.

ZIEGLER, V., CLAYTON, P., TAYLOR, J., CO, B., and BIGGS, J. 1976. Nortriptyline plasma levels and therapeutic response. *Clin. Pharmacol Ther.* 20:458-463.

IV.
STUDIES WITH SPECIAL POPULATIONS

13

KINETICS OF ANTIEPILEPTIC DRUGS IN CHILDREN

W. EDWIN DODSON, M.D.

Concentrations of antiepileptic drugs (AEDs) vary widely when standardized dosages are given to infants and children (Dodson et al., 1976; Morselli, 1977). In general, children require relatively larger dosages of AEDs than adults to achieve effective, anticonvulsant concentrations in plasma (Svensmark and Buchthall, 1964; Borofsky, Louis, and Kutt, 1973; van der Kleijn et al., 1976). Studies of pharmacokinetics among adults indicate that drug concentrations vary greatly among patients taking standardized dosages (Travers, Reynolds, and Gallagher, 1972). Disease states, interpersonal variation in rate of drug metabolism, drug interaction, and noncompliance usually account for this variability. In children, in whom the pharmacokinetics of AEDs are even more diverse, the greater variability results from the same factors, in addition to differences in drug distribution and drug absorption.

To speak of the kinetics of drugs in children is to oversimplify. In fact, several distinct subpopulations require definition. Among newborns, those with transplacentally acquired anticonvulsants are usually healthy babies who have been exposed *in utero* to the metabolic inducing effects of AEDs. In contrast, newborn infants with neonatal seizures have no prior exposure to AEDs and are likely to have a variety of associated metabolic disturbances that influence drug elimination (Volpe, 1977). During the newborn period, dramatic changes occur in the organ systems responsible for the detoxification of drugs. The overall hepatic systems which effect the transport, biotransformation, and conjugation of AEDs mature rapidly in the newborn period (Klinger, 1977). Over the first two to four weeks of life, there are concurrent increases in the glomerular filtration rate and

The author is the recipient of National Institutes of Health Career Academic Award No. 1-K07-NS11074. This work was supported by a grant from the National Foundation—March of Dimes.

renal tubular secretory capacity (Guignard et al., 1975). By the end of the first month of life, infants' relative ability for hepatic and renal detoxification of drugs usually exceeds that of adults and causes accelerated drug clearance. After the first month, kinetics are more stable, but interpatient variability in drug distribution, drug absorption, and drug elimination plays a large role in producing individual differences in drug requirements.

Although the AEDs have a high therapeutic index when seizure control and lethal effects are compared, the therapeutic index is considerably smaller when the toxicities of cognitive and behavioral side effects associated with drug intoxication are weighed against efficacy (Plaa, 1975; Reynolds, 1975). Particularly, the adverse effects on cognitive function and behavior indicate that drug intoxication should be prevented in children (Stores, 1975). Although AEDs usually are administered for long periods of time, the possibility that chronic exposure even at therapeutic, nontoxic concentrations may have adverse effects on development has not been well studied. In any event, a lengthy duration of treatment increases the danger for overt intoxication and underscores the need for prudent prescribing and reassessment to minimize long-term adverse effects.

Since the mid-1960s, knowledge of pharmacokinetics of AEDs has grown tremendously as a result of improved methods of measuring drug concentrations (Dodson et al., 1976). The first spectrophotometric techniques of drug measurement were vulnerable to interfering chromagens and required relatively large volumes of blood. These problems limited the usefulness of spectrophotometric techniques in studying the kinetics of AEDs among infants and children. With the development of gas-liquid chromatography, radioimmunoassay and, more recently, immunoenzymatic methods (EMIT,® Syva), it has become possible to carry out repeated measurements of AED concentrations in infants and children for kinetic studies. The more recent techniques are sensitive enough to measure AED concentrations in saliva, an assay that indicates the unbound concentration of phenytoin in plasma.

Definition of Terms

Preliminary to a further discussion of the kinetics of AEDs, several terms and relationships need to be defined (Table 1) (Greenblatt and Koch-Weser, 1975a, b; Gibaldi and Levy, 1976a, b). When a patient begins taking a drug, it accumulates in the body until net drug intake equals output and a steady state is reached. Under steady-state conditions the

Table 1
Definitions and Relationships of Terms

$$C_{\bar{p}}^{ss} = \frac{\text{infusion rate}}{\text{clearance rate}} \qquad \text{(I)}$$

$$C_{\bar{p}}^{ss} = \frac{F \bullet D}{\tau} \bullet \frac{1}{Vd \bullet k_{el}} \qquad \text{(II)}$$

$$K = Vd \bullet k_{el} \qquad \text{(III)}$$

$$K = \frac{F \bullet D}{C_{\bar{p}}^{ss} \bullet \tau} \qquad \text{(IV)}$$

$$T_{1/2} = \frac{0.693}{k_{el}} \qquad \text{(V)}$$

$$C_{\bar{p}}^{ss} = \frac{F \bullet D}{\tau} \bullet \frac{T_{1/2}}{Vd(0.693)} \qquad \text{(VI)}$$

$C_{\bar{p}}^{ss}$ is average concentration in plasma at steady state in mg/ℓ. F is bioavailability. D is dose in milligrams. τ is the time interval between doses in hours. Vd is the apparent volume of distribution in liters. k_{el} is the first-order elimination rate constant with dimensions of per hour (hr^{-1}). $T_{1/2}$ is the half-life in hours.

average plasma concentration ($C_{\bar{p}}^{ss}$) is stable. This concentration is related directly to the infusion rate and inversely to the elimination rate (I and II). The bioavailability (F) is the fractional absorption of any dose relative to an intravenous test dose. The apparent volume of distribution (Vd) is a mathematical term that describes an apparent volume in the body in which a drug is dissolved. Vd is formally defined as the amount of drug in the body divided by the concentration in plasma. It is thus a term that summarizes the net effects of drug binding to proteins in plasma and to tissues as well as the effects of the pKa and lipid solubility of a drug relative to the pH and lipid content, respectively, of various body compartments. The product of the volume of distribution times the elimination rate constant is the clearance (K) (III). Clearance provides a relative measure of the influence of both drug distribution and elimination rate on drug concentration at steady state. By rearranging equation I, clearance may be calculated from steady-state concentrations if assumptions are made about bioavailability (IV). Most data regarding drug clearance in populations of children and adults are calculated by this method. For comparative purposes the relative volume of distribution and the relative clearance are used. These are the Vd or K divided by either the patient's weight or surface area.

The concept of the half-life (T½) of a drug is essential to understanding kinetic differences among patients and the times required for a drug to equilibrate to a steady-state concentration. The T½ is the time required for a drug concentration to fall to 50 percent of an original value. If treatment is initiated at standardized doses, five half-lives are required for the drug concentration to nearly reach the concentration that occurs at theoretical steady state. Thus, sufficient time must be allowed for the drug to reach a stable concentration when treatment is initiated or altered. If the T½ of a drug is prolonged because of drug interaction or disease, the average drug concentration will increase. Conversely, if metabolism is accelerated and T½ reduced, the average drug concentration will be reduced. The elimination rate constant (k_{et}) is a mathematical expression of the T½. Both of these terms summarize the rates of all of the processes by which a drug is being eliminated. When the half-life is substituted for k_{el}, it may be seen that under steady-state conditions the plasma concentration is directly proportional to the T½ (VI). These pharmacokinetic terms are reviewed in greater detail elsewhere (Greenblatt and Koch-Weser, 1975a, b; Gibaldi and Levy, 1976a, b).

The type of elimination kinetics demonstrated by the processes that eliminate a drug also influences the T½ (Greenblatt and Koch-Weser, 1975a, b). Most AEDs are eliminated according to first-order kinetics, that is, a constant fraction of the AED is eliminated per unit of time and the half-life is independent of dose or concentration. The elimination of phenytoin, however, almost wholly depends upon biotransformation by enzyme systems. These systems may become saturated at concentrations close to the therapeutic range. Thus, at high concentrations when the enzyme systems are saturated, elimination proceeds according to zero-order kinetics, at a constant amount per unit of time. Thereafter, when the concentration has fallen to a level below that which saturates the enzyme system, first-order elimination is resumed. If dosage is not reduced during the period of zero-order kinetics, drug accumulation will continue and drug intoxication will ensue.

Similarities of AED Kinetics Among Children and Adults

Certain principles of kinetics of AEDs among children may be generalized from data obtained in adults. These generalizations are supported by personal observations and are largely undocumented in the pediatric literature. For example, the effects of renal and hepatic disease on AED concentration among children are comparable to those observed among adults (Karlin and Kutt, 1970; Blaschke et al., 1975). In renal disease there is reduced binding of phenytoin to plasma proteins, and lower steady-state concentrations are obtained per unit dosage because of the accelerated elimination of phenytoin (Odar-Cederlöf, Lunde, and Sjöqvist, 1970; Letteri et al., 1971; Dodson et al., 1976). Although general trends can be anticipated, as among adults with systemic illness, the magnitude of pharmacokinetic deviance of a particular child is unpredictable. Thus, measurements of AED concentrations and protein binding may be required to assure adequacy of therapy.

The kinetics of the acute administration of anticonvulsants in treating status epilepticus may be contrasted to the chronic administration of AEDs to prevent the recurrence of seizures. In the former circumstance, transiently high concentrations of drug are desired and AEDs should be administered intravenously. Because diazepam and phenytoin are absorbed slowly after intramuscular injection, these agents should be given intravenously when prompt attainment of high concentrations is necessary (Dodson et al., 1976).

For the prophylaxis of seizures, stable AED concentrations are desired. Wide fluctuation in drug concentrations may precipitate either toxicity or loss of anticonvulsant effect. Fortunately most AEDs have absorption and/or elimination kinetics that facilitate the achievement of stable drug concentrations with the use of relatively simple once- or twice-daily dosage schedules. The major exceptions to this principle are primidone and valproic acid, both of which are rapidly absorbed and have short half-lives (Glazko, 1975; Rowan et al., 1975; Jeavons, Clark, and Maheshwari, 1977). Even with these compounds, frequent administration may not always be required. In the former case, the parent compound, primidone, is metabolized to phenylethylmalonamide and phenobarbital, both of which are anticonvulsant and have longer half-lives than primidone. It has also been suggested that a longer-lived, anticonvulsant metabolite of valproic acid may accumulate in plasma and limit the need for frequent administration (Kupferberg, 1977). Phenytoin is absorbed slowly and has saturation kinetics in children (Morselli, 1977). Even among those children with rapid elimination, slow absorption counteracts the need for excessively frequent administration. Furthermore, saturation kinetics act to prolong the half-life of phenytoin when concentrations are in the therapeutic range. These kinetic properties rarely make it necessary to administer phenytoin more often than twice daily. Among older children, once daily administration often can be achieved without causing unduly wide swings in plasma phenytoin concentrations.

Drug measurements are particularly useful in monitoring therapy during transitions to more simplified dosage regimens. The advantages of simplified dosage schedules are self-evident; simple regimens increase convenience and thereby reduce a tendency to noncompliance. In addition, when dosages are taken privately at home, the potential stigmata associated with taking medication at school can be circumvented.

The same drugs that cause drug interactions among adults may also produce drug interactions among children (Kutt, 1975; Vree et al., 1975). The addition of carbamazepine to the regimen of a child previously taking phenytoin may be associated with the reduction in phenytoin concentration. The interaction of phenobarbital and phenytoin is unpredictable. Although on the average no net change in phenytoin concentration occurs when phenobarbital is added, certain patients may experience a significant change in phenytoin concentration, and thus the interaction is unpredictable (Müller et al., 1977). Among children, the co-administration of phenytoin with primidone results in phenobarbital-to-primidone ratios higher than those of primidone alone. This indicates that phenobarbital usually should not be administered simultaneously to children who are taking primidone and phenytoin. Isoniazid also inhibits the elimination of primidone in children; a higher steady-state concentration of primidone results, lowering the ratio of phenobarbital to primidone (Sutton and Kupferberg, 1975). The co-administration of isoniazid with phenytoin in children may also inhibit the biotransformation of phenytoin, causing phenytoin accumulation to toxic concentrations. In summary, drug interactions involving AEDs are prevalent among children and often unpredictable. Whenever another medication is added or deleted, the possibility of a drug interaction must be considered.

Many of the signs of drug intoxication are similar among children and adults (Plaa, 1975). Children, like adults, develop tolerance to barbiturate-induced sedation when treatment is initiated (Stores, 1975). This side effect can be minimized by starting with lower dosage, but then the time required to reach effective concentrations is obviously longer. It is useful to forewarn parents of this potential side effect to encourage perseverance and compliance when treatment with barbiturates is begun.

Barbiturate-induced hyperactivity is a more troublesome side effect. In general, the hyperactivity and behavior disturbances that result from barbiturate treatment do not subside with continued therapy, although dosage reduction occasionally may be helpful if toxic concentrations have been reached. After weighing the disadvantages of the behavior disturbance against the advantages of seizure control, an alternative AED is often selected.

Children, like adults, usually demonstrate a progression of dose-related side effects of phenytoin (Wilder, Buchanan, and Serrano, 1973; Kutt and Penry, 1974). These are nystagmus, ataxia, and mental disturbances which appear at concentrations of about 20, 30, and 40 μg/ml respectively. Certain children, however, may develop idiosyncratic manifestations of drug toxicity. Unusual manifestations of phenytoin toxicity include bradykinesia, pseudodementia, and chorea (Dodson et al., 1976). The adverse psychiatric effects of phenytoin reported in adults have not been documented clearly in children. On the other hand, a distinct improvement in behavior among certain children with psychomotor seizures often results from treatment with carbamazepine. This "psychotropic" effect of carbamazepine has been documented among institutionalized adults (Singh, Saxena, and Germain, 1977).

Phenytoin elimination among children, as among adults, is also concentration-dependent and has saturation kinetics. For practical purposes, the effects of saturation kinetics are more important in regulating phenytoin concentrations than are age-related kinetic differences in phenytoin elimination. An analysis of the T½ of phenytoin as a function of body weight, without controlling for concentration, indicates no relationship between the T½ of phenytoin and body size. But there is a significant correlation ($r = 0.764$, $p < 0.001$) between half-life and the initial phenytoin concentration at the time of measuring the half-life among infants and children, which emphasizes the importance of the concentration-dependent kinetics of phenytoin. In adjusting phenytoin dosage, small increments should be made as the phenytoin concentration approaches the therapeutic range (Morselli, 1977; Richens, 1977). If the increments are large or unitary, disproportionate rises in concentration will often result in toxicity. The converse occurs when phenytoin dosage is reduced or tapered. Patients who require relatively high concentrations of phenytoin for seizure control are extremely vulnerable to developing drug intoxication because of the near saturation of phenytoin-eliminating processes (Richens, 1977). An error in drug dosage, intercurrent illness, or drug interaction that inhibits phenytoin metabolism may readily lead to intoxication.

Differences in AED Kinetics Among Children and Adults

The kinetics of AEDs in children differ from those of adults in that children have greater average clearance of AEDs, a wider absolute range of variability in AED clearance, and higher incidence of drug malabsorption. Since these differences are age-related, we shall review selected aspects of AED kinetics for different age groups.

The deviance from adult kinetics is greatest among infants. In the immediate neonatal period, children eliminate transplacentally acquired drugs at rates comparable to those observed among adults. Babies not exposed to AEDs *in utero* experience considerable changes in drug-eliminating capacity, and intrapatient kinetic variability is a clinical problem during the first month of life. After the first month, the kinetics of AEDs are more constant for a given patient, but the variability in drug clearance among different children is exceedingly great.

Infants who acquire phenytoin transplacentally usually eliminate it according to zero-order kinetics during the first one to two days of life (Rane et al., 1974). Thereafter a first-order elimination becomes apparent and drug concentrations fall more rapidly. Overall half-lives of transplacental phenytoin have been reported to be 55 to 69 hours, but Rane and associates observed half-lives ranging from 6.6 to 34 hours during the linear phase of phenytoin elimination (Mirkin, 1971; Rane et al., 1974). Less consistently, a similar biphasic elimination occurs for transplacentally acquired phenobarbital and carbamazepine. In newborns the $T_{\frac{1}{2}}$ of carbamazepine acquired transplacentally has been reported to range from 8.2 to 27.7 hours, elimination rates that correspond to the lower end of the range observed among adults chronically taking carbamazepine (Rane, Bertilsson, and Palmer, 1975). Among infants who acquired phenytoin transplacentally, only small amounts of unchanged phenytoin can be recovered in urine. The majority of phenytoin is parahydroxylated and 91 percent of this metabolite is conjugated (Reynolds and Mirkin, 1973; Rane, 1974). Thus, within the first four days of life infants have a well-developed capacity to oxidize and conjugate AEDs following intrauterine exposure.

Data on infants with neonatal seizures indicate the changes in AED kinetics that occur during the first four weeks of life. It should be recalled that in certain nursery populations the most common cause of neonatal seizures is perinatal asphyxia. Thus, associated metabolic disturbances may contribute to impaired drug-eliminating capacity. Painter and associates (1977) found that total intravenous loading doses of 15 to 20 mg/kg, given in divided doses, produced concentrations of phenobarbital and phenytoin of 19.4 μg/l (± 3.4) and 14.9 μg/l (± 2.8) respectively. Treatment with 5 mg/kg/day of phenobarbital causes drug accumulation over the first ten days of therapy, followed by a decline in concentrations thereafter (Figure 1). The greatest variability in phenobarbital concentrations also occurs in the first ten days of treatment. Painter and associates (1977) were unable to maintain therapeutic concentrations of phenytoin by oral administration. Their data suggest a significant gastrointestinal malabsorption of all available preparations of phenytoin among this age group. This type of data emphasizes the need for repeated drug measurements in monitoring AED therapy for neonatal seizures.

Among newborn infants given loading doses of phenytoin and phenobarbital, apparent volumes of distribution are 50 percent greater than the values reported among adults (Table 2). These findings are consistent with reduced binding to plasma proteins and an expanded extracellular volume. Newborns have lower total protein concentrations, and phenytoin binding in plasma in newborns is lower than that reported among adults. Whereas 90 to 94 percent of phenytoin is protein-bound in adults, estimates of phenytoin protein binding in newborns range from 80 to 90 percent. This indicates that among infants unbound phenytoin concentrations are two to three times higher than among adults with comparable total phenytoin concentration in plasma. Such other metabolic differences as higher concentrations of free fatty acids and bilirubin may also contribute to reduced phenytoin binding in babies. Because phenobarbital is generally bound to a much lesser extent (40 to 50 percent), relative differences in phenobarbital binding between infants and adults have relatively insignificant influences on the concentration of unbound phenobarbital.

Among children aged one to 12 months, most reports indicate an accelerated clearance of phenobarbital and phenytoin (Morselli, 1977). The average T½ of phenobarbital among infants is shorter than in adults. Averages of 47 (± 8) and 68 (± 6) hours in infants may be contrasted to average adult half-lives of 83 hours. Among infants, however, individual values have ranged as low as 21 hours and as high as 133 hours (Dodson et al., 1976). Thus, on the average, the $T_{\frac{1}{2}}$ of phenobarbital in infants is about two-thirds the value reported in adults, but there is quite a wide variance from patient to patient. Whereas the Vd of phenobarbital among adults ranges from 0.5 to 0.6 l/kg, among young infants the average Vd is 0.69 l/kg ± 0.16. In slightly older age groups, an average Vd is 0.6 ± 0.09 l/kg, closely approximating that of adults. Compared to the persistent variability in phenobarbital $T_{\frac{1}{2}}$s, the variation in Vd for phenobarbital is relatively transient. Thus it seems that variable elimination rates account for

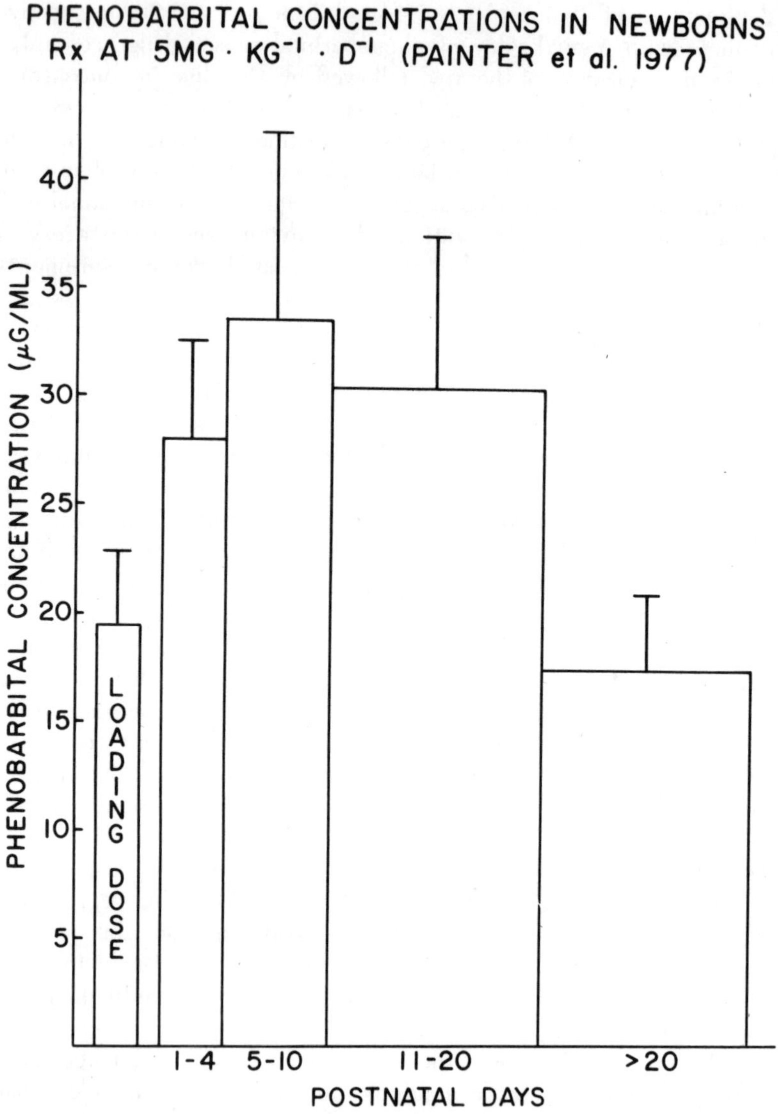

Figure 1. Average concentrations of phenobarbital and standard deviation obtained in newborn infants with seizures. Infants were given initial loading doses totaling 15 to 20 mg/kg and thereafter 5 mg/kg/day of phenobarbital (Painter et al. 1977).

Table 2

Relative Apparent Volumes of Distribution in Newborn Infants and Adults.

	RELATIVE Vd (l/kg)	
	Phenytoin	*Phenobarbital*
Newborns	1.19 ± 0.19 (a)	0.97 ± 0.2 (a)
Adults	0.78 ± 0.11 (b)	0.60 – 0.75 (c)

Sources: (a) Painter *et al.*, 1977; (b) Cranford *et al.*, 1977; and (c) Morselli, 1977.

most of the variance in phenobarbital clearance observed among older infants. Note, however, that both the larger Vd and shorter $T_{\frac{1}{2}}$ of phenobarbital contribute to a two- to fourfold greater clearance of phenobarbital among children aged five years or younger.

The average clearance of phenytoin is at least twice as great in young children as in adults (Figure 2) (Guelen, 1975). More important, however,

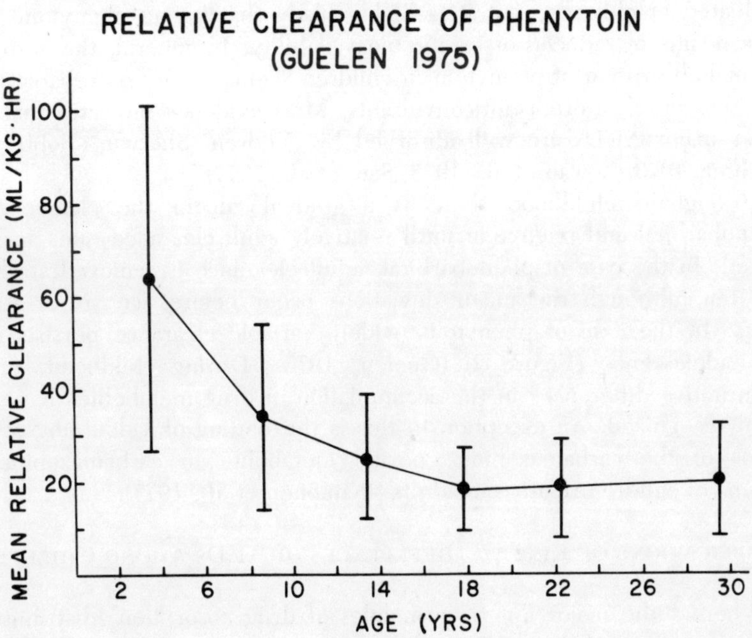

Figure 2. Mean relative clearance of phenytoin as a function of age. Note large standard deviation in younger children (Guelen, 1975).

the standard deviation in phenytoin clearance is 60 percent of the average clearance among young children. Thus initial doses can be expected to err by more than 60 percent from the ideal in one-third of the children who are given phenytoin. This means that considerable titration of dosage of phenytoin is required in this age group.

There is considerable evidence that phenobarbital is well absorbed in children after either oral or intramuscular administration (Morselli, 1977). The absorption of phenytoin is more suspect. The observation that certain infants and children require dosages as high as 20 mg/kg to obtain effective concentration suggests that malabsorption of phenytoin is occurring in a sizeable number of children (Berlet, 1975). In addition, the pediatric suspension of phenytoin is liable to cause dosage errors when inadequately mixed. If the phenytoin settles at the bottom of the bottle, low doses may be administered initially; later, as the bottle is depleted and increasing concentrations of phenytoin are administered per unit volume, drug intoxication may occur. For this reason, we prefer to use the 50-mg phenytoin tablet even for small children or infants. Drug malabsorption may occur when phenytoin is administered concurrently with antacids. The effect of administering phenytoin with food has not been evaluated in children, but it is highly likely that giving phenytoin with milk results in reduced or erratic bioavailability. In general, the gastrointestinal absorption of phenytoin in children seems to be less reliable than the absorption of other anticonvulsants. Most evidence indicates that the other major AEDs are well absorbed by children (Sherwin, Robb, and Lechter, 1973; Rowan et al., 1975; Sato et al., 1977).

Throughout childhood there is a gradual fall in the clearance of phenobarbital and phenytoin until relatively adult clearance rates are obtained. In the case of phenobarbital, adult clearance is achieved at about age ten, although the major deviations occur before age six or seven years. In the case of phenytoin, widely variable clearance persists well into adolescence (Figure 2) (Guelen, 1975). During childhood, major quantitative differences in the accumulation of drug metabolites have not been recognized. An exception to this is the finding of a doubling of the ratios of the carbamazepine epoxide metabolite to carbamazepine in plasma of children relative to adults (Pynnönen et al., 1977).

Implications of Kinetic Differences of AEDs Among Children

Whereas the major kinetic principles of drug absorption, distribution, and metabolism of the AEDs may be generalized from adults to children, the principle of kinetic variability among all patients is demonstrated more dramatically by children than adults. A review of the application of certain rules of thumb for calculating pediatric dosages indicates that interpatient variability among children is so great as to render these rules useless in anything more than a statistical sense. Van der Kleijn and associates found that the Augsberger rule compensated best for the changing relationship between clearance and age when phenobarbital alone was taken (van der Kleijn et al., 1976). However, the standard deviation of the relative clearance is 46 percent of the average relative clearance in a random population of patients taking phenobarbital (Guelen, van der Kleijn, and Woudstra, 1975), thereby negating the value of these types of calculated predictions of dosage requirements. Kinetic data from group studies serve only as a general guide to dosage requirements for initiating therapy with AEDs in children. In at least one-third of young children, the initial estimate of a patient's ideal AED dosage will err 46 and 60 percent for phenobarbital and phenytoin respectively. In cases of medications with predictable linear kinetics, such as phenobarbital, ethosuximide, carbamazepine, or sodium valproate, less "fine tuning" of dosage will be required to achieve effective, nontoxic concentrations than in the case of phenytoin. Because phenytoin kinetics are concentration-dependent and erratic absorption may occur, the measurement of phenytoin concentrations is particularly necessary to the regulation of phenytoin dosage for individual children.

Measurements of drug concentrations and published tables of therapeutic ranges of AEDs are useful adjuncts in treating seizures in children (Kutt and Penry, 1974; Lund, 1974; Rowan et al., 1975; Dodson et al., 1976; Feldman and Pippenger, 1976). Although therapeutic ranges provide general guidelines to effective therapy, they are not absolute indicators of the adequacy of treatment or freedom from toxicity. The lower end of the therapeutic range indicates the concentration above which most responding patients begin to improve. The upper limits of a therapeutic range indicate concentrations above which a majority of patients begin to show toxic side effects. Because of variability in responsiveness of the epileptic process or, conversely, variable sensitivity to the adverse effects of AED, therapeutic ranges constitute only general guidelines for patient management. Among children with neurological impairment and difficult-to-control seizures or systemic disease, repeated drug concentration measurements may reveal that a particular patient's "therapeutic range" deviates significantly from that in the literature. Although therapeutic ranges in general are not statistically derived, the relative rarity of these exceptions is surprising. Nonetheless, AED concentration measurements and published therapeutic ranges serve only as adjuncts to directing therapy. Their value does not supersede the fundamental importance of observation of the patient over time and sound judgment.

REFERENCES

BERLET, H. 1975. Serum levels of phenytoin in children. In H. Schneider, D. Janz, C. Gardner-Thorpe, H. Meinardi, A. L. Sherwin (eds.), *Clinical Pharmacology of Antiepileptic Drugs*, pp. 63-69. New York: Springer-Verlag.

BLASCHKE, T. F., MEFFIN, P. J., MELMON, K. L., and ROWLAND, M. 1975. Influence of acute viral hepatitis on phenytoin kinetics and protein binding. *Clin. Pharmacol. Therap.*, 17:685-691.

BOROFSKY, L. G., LOUIS, S., and KUTT, H. 1973. Diphenylhydantoin in children. *Neurology*, 23:967-972.

CRANFORD, R. E., LEPPIK, I. E., PATRICK, B., ANDERSON, C. B., and KOSTICK, B. 1977. Intravenous phenytoin clinical and pharmacokinetic aspects. *Neurology*, 27:376.

CURLESS, R. G., and WALSON, P. D. 1975. Rapid diphenylhydantoin metabolism in infants. *Ped. Res.* 9:282.

DODSON, W. E., PRENSKY, A. L., DEVIVO, D. C., GOLDRING, S., and DODGE, P. R. 1976. Management of seizure disorders: Selected aspects. Part I. *J. Pediatr.*, 89:527-540.

FELDMAN, R. G., and PIPPENGER, C. E. 1976. The relation of anticonvulsant drug levels to complete seizure control. *J. Clin. Pharmacol.*, 16:51-59.

FERRANDES, B., and EYMARD, P. 1977. Metabolism of valproate sodium in rabbit, rat, dog, and man. *Epilepsia*, 18:169-182.

GIBALDI, M., and LEVY, G., 1976a. Pharmacokinetics in clinical practice. 1. Concepts. *JAMA*, 17:1864-1867.

GIBALDI, M., and LEVY, G. 1976b. Pharmacokinetics in clinical practice. 2. Applications. *JAMA*, 235:1987-1992.

GLAZKO, A. J. 1975. Antiepileptic drugs: Biotransformation, metabolism, and serum half life. *Epilepsia*, 16:367-391.

GREENBLATT, D. J., and KOCH-WESER, J. 1975a. Clinical pharmacokinetics. *N. Engl. J. Med.*, 293:702-705.

GREENBLATT, D. J., and KOCH-WESER, J. 1975b. Clinical pharmacokinetics. *N. Engl. J. Med.*, 293:904-970.

GUELEN, P. J. M. 1975. In H. Schneider, D. Janz, C. Gardner-Thorpe, H. Meinardi, and A. L. Sherwin (eds.), *Clinical Pharmacology of Antiepileptic Drugs*, p. 45. New York: Springer-Verlag.

GUELEN, P. J. M., VAN DER KLEIJN, E., and WOUDSTRA, U. 1975. In H. Schneider, D. Janz, C. Gardner-Thorpe, H. Meinardi, and A. L. Sherwin (eds.), *Clinical Pharmacology of Antiepileptic Drugs*, pp. 2-10. New York: Springer-Verlag.

GUIGNARD, J. P., TORRADO, A., CUNHA, O. D., and GAUTIER, E. 1975. Glomerular filtration rate in the first three weeks of life. *J. Pediatr.*, 87:268-272.

JALLING, B., BOREUS, L., RANE, A. and SJOQVIST, F., 1970. Plasma concentrations of diphenylhydantoin in young infants. *Pharmacologia Clinica*, 2:200-202.

JEAVONS, P. M., CLARK, J. E., and MAHESHWARI, M. C. 1977. Treatment of generalized epilepsies of childhood and adolescence with sodium valproate ("Epilin"). *Dev. Med. Child Neurol.*, 19:9-25.

KARLIN, J. M., and KUTT, H. 1970. Acute diphenylhydantoin intoxication following halothane anesthesia. *J. Pediatr.*, 76:941-944.

KLINGER, W. 1977. In P. L. Morselli (ed.), *Drug Disposition During Development*, pp. 71-87. New York: Spectrum.

KUPFERBERG, H. 1977. Sodium valproate. Presented at Symposium on the Mechanisms of Action of Antiepileptic Drugs, St. Louis, Missouri.

KUTT, H. 1975. Interactions of antiepileptic drugs. *Epilepsia*, 16:393-402.

KUTT, H., and PENRY, J. K. 1974. Usefulness of blood levels of antiepileptic drugs. *Arch. Neurol.*, 31:283-288.

LETTERI, J. M., MELLK, H., LOUIS, S., KUTT, H., DURANTE, P., and GLAZKO, A. 1971. Diphenylhydantoin metabolism in uremia. *N. Engl. J. Med.*, 285:648-652.

LOUGHNAN, P. M., WATTERS, G., and NEIMS, A. 1975. Pharmacokinetics observations of diphenylhydantoin (DPH) in the newborn and young infant. *Pediatr. Res.*, 9:285.

LUND, L. 1974. Anticonvulsant effects of diphenylhydantoin relative to plasma levels. *Arch. Neurol.*, 31:289-294.

MIRKIN, B. L. 1971. Diphenylhydantoin: Placental transport, fetal localization, and possible teratogenic effects. *J. Pediatr.*, 78:329-337.

MORSELLI, P. L. 1977. Antiepileptic drugs. In P. L. Morselli (ed.), *Drug Disposition During Development*, pp. 311-360. New York: Spectrum.

MÜLLER, F. O., HUNDT, H. K. L., AUCAMP, A. K., OLIVIER, L., WESSELS, W., and STEYN, J. M. 1977. Long-term combination therapy with phenytoin and phenobarbital—evaluation of serum levels. In J. K. Penry (ed.), *Epilepsy, The Eighth International Symposium*, pp. 77-80. New York: Raven Press.

ODAR-CEDERLÖF, I., LUNDE, P., and SJÖQVIST, F. 1970. Abnormal pharmacokinetics of phenytoin in a patient with uraemia. *Lancet*, 2:831-832.

PAINTER, J. J., PIPPENGER, C., CARTER, G., and PITLICK, W. 1977. Metabolism of phenobarbital and phenytoin by neonates with seizures. *Neurology*, 27:370.

PLAA, G. C. 1975. Acute toxicity of antiepileptic drugs. *Epilepsia*, 16:183-191.

PORTER, R. J., PENRY, J. K., LACY, J. R., NEWMARK, M. E., and KUPFERBERG, H. J. 1977. The clinical efficacy and pharmacokinetics of phensuximide and methsuximide. *Neurology*, 27:375, 1977.

PYNNÖNEN, S., SILLANPÄÄ, M., IISALO, E., and FREY, H. 1977. Elimination of carbamazepine in children after single and multiple doses. In J. K. Penry (ed.), *Epilepsy, The Eighth International Symposium*, pp. 191-197. New York: Raven Press.

RANE, A., 1974. Urinary excretion of diphenylhydantoin metabolites in newborn infants. *J. Pediatr.*, 85:543-545.

RANE, A., BERTILSSON, L., and PALMER, L. 1975. Disposition of placentally transferred carbamazepine (Tegretol®) in the newborn. *Eur. J. Clin. Pharmacol.*, 8:283-284.

RANE, A., GARLE, M. BORGA, O., and SJÖQVIST, F. 1974. Plasma disappearance of transplacentally transferred diphenylhydantoin in the newborn studied by mass fragmentography. *Clin. Pharmacol. Therap.*, 15:39-45.

REYNOLDS, E. H. 1975. Chronic antiepileptic toxicity: A review. *Epilepsia*, 16:319-352.

REYNOLDS, J. W., and MIRKIN, B. L. 1973. Urinary corticosteroid and diphenylhydantoin metabolite patterns in neonates exposed to anticonvulsant drugs in utero. *Clin. Pharmacol. Ther.*, 14:891-897.

RICHENS, A. 1977. Precise adjustment of phenytoin dosage. In J. K. Penry (ed.), *Epilepsy, The Eighth International Symposium*, pp. 139-148. New York: Raven Press.

ROWAN, A. J., PIPPENGER, C. E., MCGREGOR, P. A., and FRENCH, J. H. 1975. Seizure activity and anticonvulsant drug concentration. *Arch. Neurol.*, 32:281-288.

SATO, S., PENRY, J. K., DREIFUSS, F. E., and DYKEN, P. R. 1977. Clonazepam in the treatment of absence seizures: A double blind clinical study. *Neurology*, 27:371.

SHERWIN, A. L., ROBB, J. P., and LECHTER, M. 1973. Improved control of epilepsy by monitoring plasma ethosuximide. *Arch. Neurol.*, 28:178-181.

SINGH, A. N., SAXENA, B. M., and GERMAIN, M. 1977. Anticonvulsive and psychotropic effects of carbamazepine in hospitalized epileptic patients: A long-term study. In J. K. Penry (ed.), *Epilepsy, The Eighth International Symposium*, pp. 47-55. New York: Raven Press.

STORES, G. 1975. Behavioral effects of anti-epileptic drugs. *Dev. Med. Child. Neurol.*, 17:647-658.

SUTTON, G., and KUPFERBERG, H. J. 1975: Isoniazid as an inhibitor of primidone metabolism. *Neurology*, 25:1179-1181.

SVENSMARK, O., and BUCHTHALL, E. 1963. Dosage of phenytoin and phenobarbital in children. *Dan. Med. Bull.*, 10:234-235.

SVENSMARK, O., and BUCHTHALL, E. 1964. Diphenylhydantoin and phenobarbital, serum levels in children. *Am. J. Dis. Child.*, 108:82-87.

TRAVERS, R. D., REYNOLDS, E. H., and GALLAGHER, B. B. 1972. Variation in response to anticonvulsants in a group of epileptic patients. *Arch. Neurol.*, 27:29-33.

VAN DER KLEIJN, E., GUELEN, P. J. M., VAN WIJK, C., and BAARS, I. 1976. Clinical pharmacokinetics in monitoring chronic medication with antiepileptic drugs. In H. Schneider, D. Janz, C. Gardner-Thorpe, H. Meinardi, and A. L. Sherwin, (eds.), *Clinical Pharmacology of Antiepileptic Drugs*, pp. 11-33. New York: Springer-Verlag.

VOLPE, J. J. 1977. Neonatal seizures. *Clin. Perinatol.*, 4:43-64.

VREE, T. B., HENDERSON, P. T., VAN DER KLEIJN, E., and GUELEN, P. J. M. 1975. Drug interactions at the metabolic level: A reality in drug treatment of epilepsy. In H. Schneider, D. Janz, C. Gardner-Thorpe, H. Meinardi, and A. L. Sherwin (eds.), *Clinical Pharmacology of Anti-Epileptic Drugs*, pp. 34-54. New York: Springer-Verlag.

WILDER, B. J., BUCHANAN, R. A., and SERRANO, E. E. 1973. Correlation of acute diphenylhydantoin intoxication with plasma levels and metabolite excretion. *Neurology*, 23:1329-1332.

14

SOME SPECIAL CONSIDERATIONS FOR PSYCHOPHARMACOLOGY IN THE ELDERLY

WILLIAM E. FANN, M.D.
and
JEANINE C. WHELESS

Until recently, it was generally assumed that psychiatric disorder was an inevitable concomitant of aging and that mental ailments exhibited by elderly patients could not be successfully treated. Precise psychiatric diagnoses were rare, and the wastebasket diagnosis of "senility" implied no hope for improvement; orthodox medical treatment was often denied older patients because it was thought that little could be achieved (Exton-Smith and Windsor, 1971; Carver, 1974). When psychopharmacological intervention occurred, it focused upon impaired brain-tissue function. Even when elderly patients presented with symptoms of a predominantly depressive or paranoid nature, these symptoms were assumed to be merely prodromal to the emergence of an underlying cerebral disease (Carver, 1974; Fann, Wheless, and Richman, 1974, 1976). In fact, before effective screening methods were instituted, almost 90 percent of all geriatric patients committed to state mental hospitals were given diagnoses of "senility" or "hardening of the arteries," regardless of the problem (Whanger, 1974). Even today, a considerable amount of pathological behavior may be dismissed by family and physicians as "just old age."

Although old age is usually defined as over age 65, the choice of chronologic age is arbitrary and does not necessarily correspond to biologic age, the functional integrity of the organism (Lamy and Kitler, 1971). Health surveys indicate that organic disorders do not take a significant toll until individuals reach the age of 75 years or beyond (Busse and Pfeiffer, 1969), and some authorities propose classifying those less than 75 years of age as "young" and considering no one "old" until age 80 (Lamy and Kitler, 1971). Consequently, when one is discussing the psychopharmacology of late life, the functional disorders may occur anytime during the latter part of the life span and, in fact, predominate in persons under the age of 70 (Young, 1972), whereas organic conditions are more likely to emerge after age 75. Some studies have indicated about 30 percent prevalence of diagnosable psychiatric disorders in the elderly with the likelihood that about 15 percent of the aged population will become severely disabled by psychiatric disturbance (Kral, 1973). The rapidly increasing number of older citizens will bring increasing requirements and demands for psychiatric care.

Emotional decompensation often accompanies progressive loss of intellectual function secondary to senility, to the extent that the geriatric years present a special risk for the development of additional psychopathology superimposed upon chronic brain syndrome. Manifestations of psychiatric disorders of the elderly are frequently atypical, however, and co-existent anxiety, depression, or psychosis may go undiagnosed and untreated. Improvement ascribed to alteration of brain function following the use of psychotherapeutic agents is often the result, in fact, of the effects of the medication on neuroses or psychoses existing alone or concurrently with a chronic brain syndrome (Fann, Wheless, and Richman, 1974, 1976).

Aging per se is an important variable when one prescribes therapeutic agents (Shock, 1967; Bellville et al., 1971). With increasing age, physiological and pathological changes profoundly affect the pharmacological activity of drugs. While senescence alters drug effects, drug effects simultaneously alter senescent functions. Despite the interest in various aspects of aging, few comprehensive and well-controlled studies on the relation of aging to drug responses have been reported.

Evidence accumulated over the past decade supports the generally accepted view that the probability of a patient's sustaining an adverse reaction increases with age (Seidl et al., 1966; Smith, Seidl, and Cluff, 1966; Hurwitz, 1969a, b). More than 21 percent of patients 70 to 79 years of age (Hurwitz, 1969a) and almost 25 percent of patients 80 and above (Seidl et al., 1966) have been reported to have adverse reactions to drugs. Gender may also play a role in drug response. Salzman and Shader (1973) report that methylphenidate is a more effective antianxiety agent for females than males whereas the opposite is true for diazepam. Furthermore, the incidence of adverse reactions is higher in elderly women than in elderly men (Hurwitz, 1969a; Davison, 1973).

Geriatric patients lack reserves with which to offset disturbances of body balance and are thereby less capable of reversing untoward effects

(Timiras, 1972). Because of multiple system decompensation, the aged are also the group at greatest risk for developing drug interactions, synergisms, and antagonisms due to multiple drug use associated with their several ills. Frequently, the aged are prescribed a polypharmacy of medical and psychotropic drugs, sometimes receiving different medication from different physicians. Elderly patients often add to these proprietary drugs, concerning which they receive no medical advice beyond television or magazine advertising. As a result, they tend to be chronically medicated and overmedicated (Fann and Wheless, 1976). Discontinuation of all medication to evaluate the patient's drug-free baseline state is a useful strategy, both diagnostically and therapeutically (Davis et al., 1973; Janowsky, El-Yousef, and Davis, 1974; Verwoerdt, 1976a).

Geriatric Pharmacology

Age influences drug response. The action of a drug may be modified by the effect of age on systems that determine the concentration of the drug at its site of action, or by age-related changes that affect, directly or indirectly, systems and tissues involved in its mechanism of action.

Although little is known about variation with age in the absorption of drugs, it is generally believed that reduced or delayed gastrointestinal absorption occurs with increasing age (Bender, 1965a, 1968; Freeman, 1974; Fann and Wheless, 1976), while parenteral routes seem to promote higher than expected blood levels of the drug (Bender, 1974). In fact, it is not uncommon to find unabsorbed tablets in the stools of geriatric patients (Bendkowski, 1970). The factors implicated in these alterations include reduction in gastric pH with corresponding decrease in drug solubility, reduction in size of the absorbing surface, reduced mesenteric blood flow, impairment of enzyme systems responsible for transport across gastrointestinal membranes (Bender, 1968, 1974; Hollister, 1977). It should be emphasized, however, that reduced absorption with age is not a consistent finding. Reports indicate enhanced absorption of cysteine and methionine in old animals, possibly attributable to the greater demands for these sulphur amino acids during senescence (Penzes, Simon, and Winter, 1968a, b; Winter, 1971).

The extent to which a drug is protein-bound in the plasma, distribution patterns of blood flow, the ability of the drug to pass through various membranes, and specific properties of tissue affinity and binding influence the availability and distribution of a drug once it reaches the circulation (Bender, 1974). Percentage of fat relative to body weight is generally increased in the elderly, creating a potential for increased storage and duration of action of fat-soluble drugs (Karasu and Murdofsky, 1976; Hollister, 1977). Drugs are bound in circulation to plasma proteins, particularly albumin; inasmuch as plasma albumin decreases with advancing age, a proportionate reduction in the amount of bound drug may be assumed (Bender, 1974). The increased incidence of adverse effects in geriatric patients may result from an increased amount of unbound drug being available for increased pharmacologic effect (Freeman, 1974; Hollister, 1977).

An asymmetrical redistribution of blood flow occurs with age. Distribution toward coronary and cerebral circulation is favored at the expense of flow to hepatic and renal systems, thus potentially diminishing the metabolic and excretory capacity of these organs (Bender, 1965b; Goldman, 1970; Karasu and Murdofsy, 1976).

Major enzyme systems responsible for drug biotransformation are located in liver microsomes. Consistent with the observation that serum and tissue levels of barbiturates and other centrally acting agents are lower in youthful and middle-aged animals than in either infant or very old animals, it has been hypothesized that microsomal enzyme activity increases during the early stages of development and decreases with advancing age. Kato et al. (1964) report that the metabolic capacity of older rats is only 50 percent of the maximum capacity which is reached at a young age.

Concentration of a drug in the blood depends upon the rate at which it is eliminated. A progressive decline in renal function with age is particularly pronounced after the age of 50. Glomerular filtration rate and renal plasma flow decline significantly and linearly with age (Davis and Shock, 1950; Shock, 1967; Hansen, Kampmann, and Laursen, 1970) and at advanced old age may be reduced to one-third that of a healthy young person; this degree of impairment, however, may not be apparent on ordinary tests of serum creatinine concentrations (Hansen, Kampmann, and Laursen, 1970; Hollister, 1977). Lower dosages of drug may produce the required concentration and half-life may be prolonged (Verwoerdt, 1976a; Exton-Smith and Windsor, 1971). For example, mean plasma half-life values of antipyrine and phenylbutazone were 45 percent and 20 percent greater, respectively, in geriatric patients. Considering elderly females alone, half-life of antipyrine was 78 percent longer (O'Mallery et al., 1971).

Changes in drug activity with age are frequently observed in the absence of changes in blood or tissue drug levels. These differences can be attributed to the physiological and pathological status of the tissue or systems involved directly or indirectly as part of the drugs' mechanism of action. These include changes in the number of receptors and the concentration of substrate, variations in the structural features and integrity of the responsive tissue, and alterations in homeostatic capacity (Bender, 1974).

Age-related changes in pharmacologic action of psychotropic drugs result from functional and anatomical changes in the central nervous system (CNS) such as decreased cerebral metabolism, intracellular or extracellular accumulation of pigment, progressive loss in total number of functioning neurons, and alterations in neurotransmitter mechanisms (Hamilton, 1966; Jonec and Finch, 1975; Emerson and Wingo, 1975; Robinson, 1975b). Kupferberg and Way (1963) report that enhanced lethal effect of morphine in young animals seems to be associated with increased brain levels and brain-to-plasma ratio of the drug. Drawing from similarities in drug response between very young and very old patients, one may hypothesize that an increase in the permeability of the blood-brain barrier occurs with aging.

Age-related changes in the activity of drugs with central nervous system effects have been attributed to a reduction in the number of receptor cells. This assumption is supported by the observation that the action of stimulant compounds is inhibited with advancing age, while the action of depressants is potentiated (Bender, 1964). The stimulant effect of amphetamine, for example, is less marked in older persons, and they seem better able to tolerate its effects. In contrast to the reduced stimulant activity, however, the appetite-depressant action appears to be of greater magnitude in old animals. Furthermore, barbiturates may tend to stimulate rather than sedate geriatric patients. This paradoxical response has been attributed to the fact that centers stimulated by barbiturates are relatively less affected by advancing age than are centers that are depressed by the compounds (Bender, 1965a, 1974).

A well-known feature of the aging organism is that homeostatic mechanisms are impaired so that physiological balance is more precarious. The aged have restricted powers of adjustment to high and low temperature, limited regulatory mechanisms for maintaining blood-sugar levels, decreased ability to restore acid-base equilibrium, and reduced tolerance to orthostatic stress. Thus, functional flexibility to changes in the internal environment imposed by drugs is reduced (Bender, 1965a; Davison, 1965; Exton-Smith and Windsor, 1971). For example, the elderly have impaired capacity to respond effectively to orthostatic stress, and this particular homeostatic loss may be aggravated by phenothiazines and antidepressants (Verwoerdt, 1976a). Undesired drug reactions may have more drastic immediate effects, as well as more serious long-term consequences (Davison, 1965; Exton-Smith and Windsor, 1971).

During the period from age 50 through advanced old age, 25 to 30 percent of body cells and capacities are lost, and this loss proceeds at a progressive, irreversible rate of about 1 percent a year. The decline in cells and their function suggests that drug dosages should be reduced for old persons by about 10 percent from the standard 20- to 60-year level at age 65, 20 percent at age 75, and 30 percent at age 85 (Freeman, 1974).

Clinical Use of Drugs in the Geriatric Patient

Several general principles should serve as a basis for drug prescription to the elderly. Geriatric patients often present with a bewildering array of behavioral symptoms complicated by physical illness, prescribed and non-prescribed drugs, and sensory deficits (Raskind and Eisdorfer, 1976). The physician needs to distinguish between changes that are significant and caused by disease or mental disorder and those that are due to "old age." Furthermore, many diseases and psychiatric ailments have different manifestations and clinical courses in the aged. Since diagnostic techniques for identifying these disorders in the elderly are not clearly defined (Davison, 1965; Gershon, 1973), the physician is often faced with a complex diagnostic challenge. Frequently, a useful diagnostic tool is the withdrawal of all medication in order to evaluate the patient's drug-free baseline. Iatrogenic illness is common in the elderly and many physical and behavioral complaints may abate once medication is discontinued.

Enormous variation exists in responses of the elderly to medications, and response is likely to vary from a hypothetical norm. For many drugs, in fact, each prescription should be regarded as an individual therapeutic experiment (Exton-Smith and Windsor, 1971). The safety margin between therapeutic and toxic dosage of many drugs is narrow and the safest course, therefore, is to start with low doses (generally one-third to one-half the recommended adult dosage) and increase gradually in small increments ("start low and go slow"). With lower dosages, improvement may progress more slowly than would be expected for a younger patient. A common error is the discontinuation of medication because of apparent ineffectiveness when the problem is inadequate dosage or treatment period (Karasu and Murdofsky, 1976).

Because of variations in the homeostatic mechanisms of the elderly, side effects are quite frequent and may be severe; side effects increase not only in incidence but also in severity with increasing age (Exton-Smith and Windsor, 1971; Raskind and Eisdorfer, 1976). Once adverse reactions develop, they tend to be more incapacitating than in younger patients.

Multiple pathology is the rule rather than the exception in the elderly; the concomitant presence of several physical and psychiatric disorders often results in polypharmacy which may cloud clinical signs so that it may be impossible to differentiate among intended drug effects, side effects, and placebo effects (Verwoerdt, 1976a). Furthermore, adverse drug reactions and errors in administration increase in direct proportion to the number of drugs prescribed (Smith, Seidl, and Cluff, 1966; Ayd, 1973; Robinson, 1975a). Every effort should be made to limit drug treatment to a minimum. Individual therapists will have their own drug experiences and preferences, but it is better to know and use a few drugs well than many poorly. Physicians also need to be sensitive to the placebo potential of pharmacological treatment—many older patients respond well to the attention and concern that accompany the prescribing of medication, and placebo may be efficacious treatment (Webb, 1971; Davison, 1973; Karasu and Murdofsky, 1976; Verwoerdt, 1976a).

Patients maintained on psychotropic drugs should be reviewed regularly to ascertain whether they are taking their medication as prescribed, and for dosage adjustment. The physician needs to be aware of the possibility of the development of insidious, progressive side effects or of physical illness which would require additional drug treatment, with the subsequent increased risk of drug-drug interactions (Verwoerdt, 1976a).

Antipsychotic Agents

The most commonly used antipsychotic agents are the phenothiazines. These drugs are indicated for the agitated, delusional, hallucinating geriatric patient and are often effective in reducing the symptomatic intensity of a core psychotic process. About 70 percent of disturbed elderly patients respond favorably to phenothiazines (Hamilton, 1966). The aging process, however, causes a variability in clinical response to these drugs with an increased sensitivity to their desired action and a decreased tolerance to side effects. Common side effects include hypotension, sedation, extrapyramidal symptoms and anticholinergic effects such as dry mouth, blurred vision, and urinary retention. Adverse reactions may occur at essentially therapeutic dosages; the initial dosage should be one-third to one-half of that recommended for adults. It is seldom necessary to exceed 300 mg/day, and 75 to 100 mg/day is the average geriatric dose. If an aged patient is very intolerant to drugs, a dose of 10 mg three times a day is sufficient (Exton-Smith and Windsor, 1971). High dosages of the antipsychotics, especially those with strong atropine-like properties like the piperazine derivatives, often exacerbate psychotic symptoms associated with anticholinergic toxicity. The common practice of increasing dosage when confronted with persisting or worsening psychotic symptomatology would be particularly unfortunate in these cases and would further aggravate the problem (Davis et al., 1973; Fann, Wheless, and Richman, 1974, 1976; Janowsky, El-Yousef, and Davis, 1974).

Deciding on the most appropriate antipsychotic agent for a geropsychiatric patient is difficult. Thioridazine (Mellaril) and chlorpromazine (Thorazine), which are strong sedative and hypotension-inducing phenothiazines, may be life-threatening to patients with compromised cerebrovascular or cardiovascular function. On the other hand, elderly patients seem to be particularly vulnerable to the extrapyramidal effects of such agents as haloperidol (Haldol), butaperazine (Repoise), perphenazine (Trilafon), and trifluoperazine (Stelazine). If parkinsonism does develop as a result of neuroleptic therapy, prescription of additional anticholinergic agents may lead to development of severe anticholinergic toxicity. Generally, conservative use of one of the less sedating, less hypotension-inducing agents, such as haloperidol or perphenazine, is an appropriate initial therapy, with a switch to thioridazine or chlorpromazine if extrapyramidal reactions develop. Prescription is complicated by the fact that there is substantial commonality of side effects among the neuroleptics, so that particular deleterious effects cannot be indisputably assigned to the individual agents (Fann, Wheless, and Richman, 1974, 1976; Janowsky, El-Yousef, and Davis, 1974).

Fifty percent of all patients between 60 and 80 years of age receiving phenothiazines develop extrapyramidal symptoms (Hamilton, 1966), ranging from mild tremors to gross, choreoathetoid, disabling symptoms. Geriatric patients are particularly susceptible to the development of these side effects, which may appear secondary to even moderate doses of neuroleptics. The most common extrapyramidal syndrome in patients over 50 is parkinsonism (Bender, 1964; Hamilton, 1966; Eisdorfer, 1975) whose symptoms include rigidity, slowing of movement (bradykinesia), pill-rolling tremor, salivation, mask-like facies, and a gait characterized by short, fast steps (*marche petit pas*). The drug-induced parkinsonism is symptomatically similar to idiopathic or postencephalitic Parkinson's disease and responds similarly to treatment with antiparkinson agents (Davis et al., 1973). Akathisia, the next most frequent reaction, must not be mistaken for increased agitation with subsequent increase in dosage of the offending agent (Hamilton, 1966; Eisdorfer, 1975).

Neuroleptics, administered chronically in high doses, may also cause disfiguring, often irreversible extrapyramidal symptoms known collectively as tardive dyskinesia. These disorders consist of involuntary, gross, choreoathetoid movements of the extremities, face, and tongue. Withdrawal of antipsychotic medication tends to increase the frequency and intensity of the symptoms. Increasing dosage of the neuroleptic temporarily suppresses the symptoms, but probably increases the underlying neuropathology. Although the hyperkinetic state sometimes remits spontaneously, tardive dyskinesia tends to be irreversible and attempts at controlling the disorder pharmacologically have been disappointing (Fann, Davis, and Lake, 1973; Janowsky, El-Yousef, and Davis, 1974; Eisdorfer, 1975). Tardive dyskinesia may occur in up to 60 percent of the patients in psychogeriatric wards (Fann, Davis, and Janowsky, 1972); furthermore, Barton and Hurst (1966) reported that 80 percent of their sample of elderly demented patients were receiving long-term antipsychotics unnecessarily. Consequently, reduced dosages, "drug holidays," and patterns of drug withdrawal are recommended with the expectation that a reduction in the total quantity of drug administered may reduce the probability of developing tardive dyskinesia (Eisdorfer, 1975).

Certain phenothiazines, especially chlorpromazine, block activity of the adrenergic-membrane transport system which actively takes up, in addition to norepinephrine, a variety of ring-substituted bases, including the antihypertensive agent guanethidine (Ismelin). Guanethidine is actively transported by the "norepinephrine pump" and becomes concentrated in the adrenergic neuron where it exerts a selective blocking action on sympathetic postganglionic neurons. By blocking pump activity, certain phenothiazines prevent accumulation of guanethidine, thereby antagonizing its antihypertensive effects (Janowsky et al., 1973; Fann, 1973a, b; Davis et al., 1973; Ban, 1975).

Recent studies indicate that antacid gels containing hydroxides and silicates of magnesium or aluminum interfere with the absorption from the gastrointestinal tract of a variety of drugs, including chlorpromazine and other neuroleptics. Concomitant administration of one of the antacids and a major tranquilizer may reduce the effectiveness of the antipsychotic by impairing its absorption (Fann et al., 1973; Fann, 1973a, b).

Antiparkinson Agents

Anticholinergic agents, including benztropine mesylate (Cogentin) and trihexyphenidyl (Artane), as well as atropine and scopolamine, have been used to treat Parkinson's disease and the parkinsonian symptoms that emerge as side actions of antipsychotic agents. The side effects of anticholinergic agents are numerous and include dry mouth, blurred vision, nasal congestion, constipation, mydriasis, urinary retention, urinary-tract dilation, ataxia, aggravation of glaucoma, confused state, and extrapyramidal symptoms. The agitated or confusional state seen at toxic levels of these agents may easily be misinterpreted as a functional change or physical illness in the patient and thus lead to an exacerbating increase in the dosage of medication. In addition, ileus, urinary obstruction, or other physical side effects caused by the anticholinergic drugs may lead to more serious physical complications, such as urinary-tract infection and dehydration. When prescribing anticholinergic drugs to geriatric patients, it is usually best to begin with low doses and to administer them infrequently and cautiously. As with many other medications, toxic side effects of the anticholinergics may occur at lower doses in the elderly than they might in younger adults (Davison, 1973; Janowsky, El-Yousef, and Davis, 1974).

Strang (1965) compared the effectiveness of trihexyphenidyl and orphenadrine in the treatment of geriatric parkinsonism. He reported that tolerance to trihexyphenidyl is particularly low in patients older than age 70; the drug caused more side effects than orphenadrine and was likely to result in mental disturbances.

Because drug-induced extrapyramidal symptoms may be particularly severe and disabling in the aged, it has become almost universal practice to prescribe an antiparkinson agent prophylactically whenever neuroleptics are indicated. Recent studies, however, have cast some doubt on the necessity of prescribing these agents for all patients who receive neuroleptics (Fann, Lake, and Richman, 1975). Not all patients who receive neuroleptics develop the parkinsonlike syndrome, and not all patients who develop the syndrome continue to display extrapyramidal symptoms over a long period. Moreover, recent evidence indicates that patients for whom antiparkinson and antipsychotic agents are prescribed concurrently are at greater risk of developing tardive dyskinesia (Fann and Lake, 1974). The elderly are particularly susceptible to anticholinergic toxicity, and on a milligram/kilogram basis, the antiparkinson medications are more potent in producing anticholinergic changes than the phenothiazines (Davis et al., 1973). A possible alternative to anticholinergic antiparkinson agents is amantadine, a putative dopaminergic agent that is effective and seems to manifest fewer side effects at the usually prescribed dosage (200 to 300 mg/day) than the anticholinergics (Fann and Lake, 1975). It is nevertheless better to withhold antiparkinson agents until their need is demonstrated (Fann and Lake, 1974; Eisdorfer, 1975).

Tricyclic Antidepressants

Major depression, the most common psychiatric illness of the elderly, is also the disorder that most often responds favorably to drug therapy. In the elderly, however, depressions often are overlooked or accepted as "just growing old" because of the similarity of depressive symptomatology to the stereotype of the listless, pessimistic, withdrawn aged person. Furthermore, masked depression may present as somatic complaints or hypochondriasis (Raskind and Eisdorfer, 1976). Symptoms of anxiety are often manifestations of underlying depressive illness and frequently the two conditions co-exist (Hollister, 1973; Gershon, 1973; Fann and Wheless, 1977). Brodie et al. (1975) prescribed either fluphenazine or nortriptyline and promazine to elderly patients suffering from irritability, loss of initiative, agitation, and insomnia. The combined drug regimen was superior, and the authors concluded that patients who presented with predominantly anxious symptomatology were concomitantly depressed.

The tricyclic antidepressants include nonsedative (protriptyline, imipramine) and sedative (amitriptyline, doxepin) agents. The nonsedative types are indicated in the treatment of retarded depression characterized by hypoactivity and hypomentation. Sedative antidepressants are effective in cases of depression with agitation. Patients who appear senile, confused, and depressed respond dramatically to tricyclic antidepressants with improvement in both cognitive function and depressive symptoms (Fann and Wheless, 1975). These medications are most useful in mild to moderate depression; because there is a latency period of from ten days to four weeks before onset of therapeutic action, they may be contraindicated when depression is unusually pronounced.

When tricyclic antidepressants are administered to aged patients, the clinician can expect therapeutic efficacy at lower dosages and greater incidence of unpleasant side effects than when these drugs are prescribed to younger individuals. Consequently, an antidepressant should be started in lower than normal doses with a slower increase in dosage and with careful monitoring of baseline physical state and side effects. An initial dose of amitriptyline (Elavil) or imipramine (Tofranil) of 10 mg twice daily (b.i.d.), with slow increases over a period of one to two weeks to 50 mg b.i.d. or less would be prudent. Certain elderly patients, however, may require higher dosages (200 mg or more) to gain therapeutic effect (Fann and Wheless, 1976). Lower dosages may prolong the latency period and produce a less rapid escalation of improvement, but the decreased incidence of side effects makes the additional wait worthwhile (Webb, 1971).

The biology of aging predisposes the geriatric patient to an aggravation of problems related to the anticholinergic side effects of the tricyclics. For example, elderly male patients with benign prostatic hypertrophy may be susceptible to the development of drug-induced urinary-tract dilatation or urinary retention. Similarly, glaucoma, diagnosed and undiagnosed, may be aggravated by the mydriatic effects of these agents. Dry mouth can cause substantial discomfort to the denture wearer. Blurred vision and confusion can be particularly distressing to the geriatric patient, who is always alert to real and imagined perceptual or intellectual decrements.

The cardiovascular effects of the tricyclic antidepressants are the main hazard of use in the aged. Arrhythmias, myocardial infarctions, serious hypotensive episodes leading to cerebrovascular accidents, and related problems occur with increased frequency in individuals with diminished cardiovascular or cerebrovascular function who receive antidepressants. Baseline electrocardiogram is advisable before initiating tricyclic therapy. Provisions should be made for monitoring pulse and blood pressure when these agents are administered to geriatric patients (Prange, 1973; Fann and Wheless, 1976).

Neurologic symptoms associated with administration of tricyclics include paresthesias, numbness, incoordination, ataxia, neuropathies, seizures, and tinnitus. Although the elderly are not necessarily more susceptible to the neurologic side effects of these agents, neuromuscular disorders common to old age may dominate the physician's thinking and lead him or her away from an accurate diagnosis of drug effect. A mistaken diagnosis of idiopathic cerebrovascular accident or other primary neurologic disorder may be made, rather than a diagnosis of drug toxicity. Further complicating the problem, the cardiovascular effects of these agents may themselves precipitate cerebrovascular accidents following hypotensive episodes.

Tricyclic antidepressants may cause increases or decreases in blood-sugar levels, changes in gastrointestinal motility, and libidinal changes as well as weakness, drowsiness, and soporific responses. Since these symptoms often occur spontaneously with advancing age, their correct identification as drug side effects requires special care (Janowsky, El-Yousef, and Davis, 1974).

The tricyclics are frequently administered to patients who have hypertension secondary to old age. Although the general effect of these agents is to lower blood pressure, they block the effects of the antihypertensive agent guanethidine (Ismelin). This probably occurs through blockade of the "norepinephrine pump" of the presynaptic adrenergic neuron which transports guanethidine to its site of action. When a hypertensive, depressed patient whose blood pressure is controlled by guanethidine is given a tricyclic, blood pressure may return to hypotensive levels. Consequently, blood pressure should be monitored weekly and dosage of guanethidine adjusted accordingly, or another hypotensive agent should be prescribed when a tricyclic and hypertensive agent are used concurrently (Fann, 1973a, b; Fann and Lake, 1974; Janowsky, El-Yousef, and Davis, 1974).

Monoamine Oxidase Inhibitors

Mainly because of their numerous side effects, the monoamine oxidase (MAO) inhibitors have been relegated to a relatively minor role in the treatment of depression since the introduction of the tricyclic antidepressants. Deleterious effects of the MAO inhibitors include anxiety, agitation, manic symptoms, exacerbation of psychotic episodes, weakness, drowsiness, nausea, diarrhea, abdominal pain, constipation, edema, tachycardia, blurred vision, impotence, chills, and headache. Cerebrovascular defect, cardiovascular disease, hypertension, or history of severe headache are contraindications for the use of these drugs. The MAO inhibitors are also contraindicated in patients receiving CNS depressants, narcotics, alcohol, diuretics, antiparkinsonian agents, anesthetics, amphetamines, tricyclic antidepressants, and sympathetic amines. These drugs are frequently prescribed individually or in combination to the elderly, who may also inadvertently ingest them while taking proprietary agents (Janowsky, El-Yousef, and Davis, 1974; Fann and Wheless, 1975). Generally, the MAO inhibitors are unsuitable for use in the elderly (Prange, 1973; Davison, 1973). The correlation between diminished MAO levels and antidepressant effects, however, and the recent finding that there may be an age-related increase in brain MAO activity (Nies et al., 1973; Robinson, 1975b) suggest that MAO inhibitors may be especially effective in alleviating depression in certain elderly patients.

Tranylcypramine (Parnate) is a clinically effective antidepressant that is highly effective in inhibiting MAO within the adrenergic neuron. It diminishes intraneuronal breakdown of norepinephrine, thereby making more of this transmitter substance available for release by indirect-acting pressor amines, such as tyramine and amphetamine and its congeners. Through inhibition of MAO, such compounds as tranylcypramine and pargyline, an antihypertensive agent, potentiate the pharmacologic action of pressor amines. Because of this interaction, patients given tranylcypramine or pargyline may experience a hypertensive crisis after eating foods containing large amounts of tyramine (i.e., certain cheeses, chicken liver, beer, pickled herring, and certain wines) or after ingesting such sympathomimetic amines as amphetamines (Fann, 1973a, b; Prange, 1973; Janowsky, El-Yousef, and Davis, 1974; Fann and Wheless, 1975). Since many of these sympathomimetic compounds are readily available in decongestants and other proprietary cold remedies, this interaction is likely and warrants the clinician's studied attention. As preventive measures, the physician should avoid prescription of such combinations and advise the geriatric patient and his or her family of the potential hazards of self-prescription.

Lithium Carbonate

Although the onset of manic episodes or manic-depressive episodes usually occurs in middle age, it is not uncommon to find patients of 65 years and older who present with either initial or recurrent manic episodes. Lithium is remarkably efficacious in the treatment of acute manic episodes and in preventing recurrent mania and depression. Geriatric patients are more susceptible to the side effects of lithium and often respond therapeutically to lower than normal doses. Whereas the half-life of lithium in a middle-aged adult is about 24 hours, half-life of lithium is as long as 36 to 48 hours in the aged patient (Davis, 1974) and even longer if glomerular filtration rate is seriously impaired. Consequently, a patient may achieve an adequate blood level on a smaller oral dose. Although the usual serum level of lithium required for effective treatment of mania is 1.2 to 1.5 mEq/l of serum, the level required in the elderly is often only 1.0 to 1.4 mEq/l or less. Furthermore, toxicity may occur in elderly patients at serum levels as low as 1.5 to 1.7 mEq/l, whereas toxicity rarely occurs in younger patients when the serum level is below 2.0 mEq/l (Fann and Wheless, 1976; Raskind and Eisdorfer, 1976). Minor side effects of lithium carbonate include nausea, vomiting, diarrhea, mild tremor, anorexia, and occasional edema. More serious effects include ataxia, dysarthria, dystonias, polyurea and polydypsia, confusion, hyperreflexia, obtundation, muscle spasms, coma, and even death (Davis and Fann, 1971). Sodium-depleting diuretics and low salt intake may cause serum sodium levels to fall below normal physiological levels, creating a selective increase in the reabsorption of lithium and thus increasing lithium blood levels to possibly toxic proportions. An elderly patient who becomes ill, weakened, and anorectic may not eat, may become hyponatremic, and subsequently develop lithium toxicity. Furthermore, since lithium is excreted by the kidneys, geriatric patients with compromised renal function may be at risk to retain lithium and develop toxicity (Janowsky, El-Yousef, and Davis, 1974). For example, an oral dose of 1500 mg/day might be prescribed to a young patient to achieve an antimanic blood level of 1.2 to 1.5 mEq/l, whereas a geriatric patient might require only 600 to 900 mg to achieve the same blood level. Nevertheless, principal attention in evaluating lithium dosage should be directed to symptoms of toxicity rather than to blood levels per se (Davis et al., 1973). A conservative regimen would involve initial dosage of one 300 mg lithium carbonate tablet daily with triweekly or daily serum lithium carbonate determinations (Janowsky, El-Yousef, and Davis, 1974). Increases in dosage should be made only after the initial blood level has stabilized; dosage should then be raised slowly with careful monitoring of side effects.

The confused, withdrawn state associated with lithium toxicity may be mistaken for other medical problems or senility in the elderly. Since lithium is administered chronically as well as acutely, lithium toxicity may occur months or years after therapy has been initiated. Symptoms of toxicity include a worsening of the usual fine tremor, which develops into a coarse tremor, drowsiness, slurred speech, chorea and choreoathetoid movements. There is a pitressin-resistant, diabetes insipidus-like syndrome characterized by a spontaneous increase in water intake and urine output, fasciculation, nystagmus, and an increase in gastrointestinal symptoms (Davis et al., 1973; Janowsky, El-Yousef, and Davis, 1974). Frequently, the patient's family attributes the symptoms to "old age" and may not seek medical attention until the patient actually becomes comatose.

Antianxiety Agents and Soporifics

Antianxiety agents include a broad range of chemically heterogeneous compounds which have similar clinical effects. Ethanol, barbiturates, meprobamate, and benzodiazepines, and even paraldehyde and hydroxyzine are classed as anxiolytics. These clinically effective compounds are indicated for relieving anxiety and reducing its unpleasant somatic components; they are not efficacious in treating psychotic symptoms and tend to increase confusion, disorientation, and incontinence. Such drugs as chlordiazepoxide (Librium), diazepam (Valium), and flurazepam (Dalmane) are virtually suicide-proof. Physical dependence may occur, but does so generally only with extremes of dosage and duration of treatment (Hollister, 1973). At very high dosages, benzodiazepines may produce severe unsteadiness of gait, drowsiness, orthostatic hypotension, and coma. Ataxia, nystagmus, and incoordination are clinical signs that suggest chronic overdosage (Verwoerdt, 1976b). Withdrawal symptoms may be mistaken for the onset of psychosis in elderly patients (Fann, Wheless, and Richman, 1974, 1976).

Antianxiety agents have a narrow therapeutic range between a dosage that effectively relieves symptoms and one that produces severe decrements in performance. These drugs may exacerbate agitation by loosening cognitive function (the so-called "disinhibition effect") and they must, therefore, be administered with caution to geriatric patients. Some elderly individuals are extremely intolerant of chlordiazepoxide and initial dosage should be very low (i.e., 5 mg three times/day)—a dosage of 60 to 75 mg of chlordiazepoxide may produce cerebellar ataxia in the elderly, whereas 600 mg is often required to produce this reaction in younger patients (Exton-Smith and Windsor, 1971). Meprobamate is useful in controlling anxiety and mild agitation in geriatric patients because it does not cause the muscular instability that may occur with benzodiazepines. Tybamate, a shorter-acting agent, may be used during the day (Verwoerdt, 1976b).

Salzman et al. (1975) treated men aged 60 and older with diazepam or placebo for two weeks. Diazepam had sedative and moderate antidepressant effects and caused a decrease in memory in all patients, but the effects were less marked in the relatively younger patients. Placebo had an antianxiety effect in the relatively older patients and was associated with decreased fatigue, improved memory, and improved motor function. Older subjects experienced greater reduction in anxiety with placebo; younger subjects required active medication. These findings suggest that physicians should consider using placebo in treating relatively older anxious patients (Salzman et al., 1975). Salzman and Shader (1973) also report that diazepam is a more effective antianxiety agent in men than in women.

Barbiturates and related sedative-hypnotic compounds frequently are prescribed to the elderly for treatment of anxiety, insomnia, convulsions, and mild hypertension. These agents often produce confusion, disorientation, disinhibition of psychopathology, and paradoxical excitement in geriatric patients, and the CNS-depressant effects of these medications may lead to ataxia and falling, with subsequent trauma. With prolonged use a clinical picture that mimics arteriosclerotic dementia may occur, with intellectual impairment, slurred speech, and unsteady gait. Depressed and anxious individuals are at risk of developing habituation to the sedative hypnotics. Methaqualone (Quaalude), for example, has been reported to cause physiologic addiction when used in essentially therapeutic dosages (Bridge and Ellinwood, 1973). Withdrawal symptoms may mimic other physical illness or the onset of psychosis. Accidental death may easily occur when sedatives are prescribed injudiciously or are taken repeatedly by an increasingly bewildered geriatric patient (Freeman, 1974; Janowsky, El-Yousef, and Davis, 1974). Because of their low ratio of therapeutic effectiveness to lethality and their high abuse potential, these agents are not generally recommended for the treatment of geriatric patients (Fann, Wheless, and Richman, 1974, 1976; Janowsky, El-Yousef, and Davis, 1974; Fann and Wheless, 1976).

Elderly persons normally require less sleep than younger adults and may regularly awaken during the night. This pattern does not necessarily constitute insomnia nor require chemotherapeutic intervention (Karasu and Murdofsky, 1976; Exton-Smith and Windsor, 1971). Consequently, hypnotics should not be prescribed routinely or indefinitely. With all hypnotics, some degree of hangover is common, and muddleheadedness and ataxia may result (Davison, 1973). Flurazepam (Dalmane) and diazepam (Valium), given at bedtime, are effective soporifics and safer than sedative-hypnotics. Paraldehyde is rapid in action, rapidly excreted by the lungs, and has no deleterious effects on cardiovascular or respiratory systems, but it is distasteful (Bender, 1964; Verwoerdt, 1976b). Chloralhydrate is safe—it does not significantly suppress rapid eye-movement sleep, leaves little hangover or ataxia, and carries a reduced risk of habituation (Verwoerdt, 1976b).

In a blind controlled trial of four sedative drugs in the treatment of geriatric patients for insomnia, meprobamate and dichloralphenazone were significantly better than amylobarbitone sodium or promazine. Additionally, patients preferred these agents because they caused less morning drowsiness (Exton-Smith, Hodkinson, and Cromie, 1963).

Phenobarbital, a sedative variously prescribed for anxiety, as an anticonvulsant, and as a hypotensive agent in mild essential hypertension, accelerates liver microsomal metabolism of certain drugs including chlorpromazine, heparin, coumarin, warfarin, corticoids, and diphenylhydantoin, thereby lowering blood levels of these agents. Concomitant prescription of phenobarbital to augment the soporific action of chlorpromazine may actually antagonize the clinical effect of chlorpromazine, including sedation (Curry et al., 1970; Fann, 1973a, b; Janowsky, El-Yousef, and Davis, 1974). Other compounds in the group of sedative-antianxiety agents show these same interactions with other therapeutic agents and the clinician should be aware of such possibilities.

Stimulant Compounds

The psychostimulants, including amphetamine and methylphenidate, are frequently prescribed to increase alertness and overcome drug-induced sedation. The use of these agents is controversial, however, because they can produce numerous side effects such as excessive stimulation, rage reactions, activation of psychotic symptoms, insomnia, increased blood pressure, tachycardia, anorexia, agitation, anxiety, and tremulousness. The elderly have diminished capacity to cope with drug-induced tachycardia and hypertension and have an increased liability for cerebrovascular accidents and myocardial infarctions. In high doses, psychostimulants cause a paranoid psychosis virtually indistinguishable from paranoid schizophrenia (Griffith et al., 1972). Furthermore, withdrawal from these agents frequently leads to depression of equal or greater severity than the original depression, lethargy, and dysphoria which is best relieved by reinstituting psychostimulant ingestion (Janowsky, El-Yousef, and Davis, 1974). Clinicians are urged to avoid this self-defeating cycle.

Methylphenidate (Ritalin) has been found to retard liver microsomal metabolism of certain compounds, including the anticonvulsant diphenylhydantoin, tricyclic antidepressants, phenothiazines, and anticoagulants such as coumarin and warfarin. Methylphenidate prescribed to counteract drug-induced sedation blocks liver metabolism of the sedative drug, thereby increasing blood level of the sedative and resulting in increased sedation. Neuronal uptake of guanethidine, an antihypertensive agent, is also blocked by methylphenidate. A patient whose blood pressure is controlled with guanethidine therapy may become hypertensive while ingesting psychostimulants (Fann, 1973a, b; Janowsky, El-Yousef, and Davis, 1974).

The psychostimulants generally are not recommended for use in the treatment of geriatric patients because the beneficial mood-related effects offset rapidly, potent pressor side effects are routine, and there is high risk for development of tolerance or dependency.

Rejuvenators

Gerovital H_3, a specially formulated preparation of procaine hydrochloride, has been widely publicized as a "rejuvenating" drug and is currently receiving much attention and clinical trial in the United States. Anna Aslan of Rumania, the originator of the drug, claims that it has "anabolic" and "eutropic" effects, revitalizes tissue, and can restore intellectual and physical ability to geriatric patients (MacFarlane, 1973). Studies have shown the drug to be an effective monoamine oxidase inhibitor that seems to have selective affinity for certain of multiple forms of MAO (MacFarlane, 1973; Zung et al., 1974). Since depression in older patients and the aging process itself have been correlated with high MAO activity (Nies et al., 1973; Robinson, 1975b), the beneficial results ascribed to the preparation—especially in alleviating depression—may be due to its inhibition of MAO. Other reported actions of Gerovital H_3 include beneficial effects on skin tone and turgor, stabilization of blood pressure, alleviation of depression and psychotic symptoms, and improvement in symptoms of senility (MacFarlane, 1973). Furthermore,

Gerovital H_3 is a weak, reversible, competitive inhibitor and does not cause the adverse effects associated with the use of irreversible MAO inhibitors (MacFarlane, 1975). Although it is clinically prescribed in some European countries, this compound is still in the experimental stages in the United States.

Nöotropics

The nöotropic drug, piracetam, is one of a recently reported new category of therapeutic compounds, which supposedly increase neuronal cellular repair and intraneuronal protein synthesis. They thereby activate, protect, and restore the working of the impaired nerve cell while improving the function of healthy neurons. Their activity is supposedly preferentially situated at the cortical levels. Although there have been positive reports of efficacy of these compounds from clinical trials in Europe and in this country (Abuzzahab, Merwin, and Sherman, 1973), a definite statement of their value cannot be made at this time.

Summary

Psychotropic drugs are clearly useful in the treatment of geriatric patients. Advancing age influences the action of medication, however, and the physical and metabolic state of the elderly impairs the predictability of drug effects. Pharmacological principles depend upon an evaluation of known drug effects projected against the tissue, organ, and system changes that occur with senescence. Deleterious drug effects are more common in elderly than in young patients as a result of the multiplicity of psychotropic and medical agents required, chronic drug use, and interaction of drugs with drugs or of drugs with physiological systems altered by age. Geriatric patients are frequently prescribed a vast polypharmacy by several physicians who do not communicate with each other, and the patients often add proprietary drugs to their medication regimen. Consequently, it is often prudent to obtain a drug-free baseline when evaluating the mental status of geriatric patients and recommending treatment. Many symptoms may disappear when medication is discontinued.

It is especially important that the physician use thorough diagnostic techniques in treating the elderly with psychotropic drugs and be knowledgeable of drug side effects and interactions. He or she should be aware that patients presenting symptoms of "senility" or "hardening of the arteries" may actually exhibit these symptoms as a result of drug side effects or drug toxicity. The possibility that a drug is having deleterious effect on the patient should always be considered, and the geriatric patient should be carefully monitored for such reactions.

In past years an unwarranted therapeutic nihilism concerning prognosis for geriatric psychiatric patients often resulted in these patients' receiving minimal or no treatment. Although these patients present special age-related problems, they often respond dramatically to treatment with psychotherapeutic agents. With expeditious instatement of therapy, the prognosis for geropsychiatric patients can be good.

REFERENCES

ABUZZAHAB, F. S., MERWIN, G. E., and SHERMAN, M. C. 1973. A controlled investigation of piracetam versus placebo on the memory of geriatric patients. *Pharmacologist*, 15: 237.

AYD, F. J. 1973. Rational pharmacotherapy: Once-a-day dosage. *Dis. Nerv. Syst.*, 34:371-378.

BAN, T. A. 1975. Drug interactions with psychoactive drugs. *Dis. Nerv. Syst.*, 36:164-166.

BARTON, R. and HURST, L. 1966. Unnecessary use of tranquilizers in elderly patients. *Br. J. Psychiatry*, 112:989-990.

BELLVILLE, J. W., FORREST, W. H., MILLER, E., and BROWN, B. W. 1971. Influence of age on pain relief from analgesics. *JAMA*, 217:1835-1841.

BENDER, A. D. 1964. Pharmacologic aspects of aging: A survey of the effect of increasing age on drug activity in adults. *J. Am. Geriatr. Soc.*, 12:114-134.

BENDER, A. D. 1965a. A pharmacodynamic basis for changes in drug activity associated with aging in the adult. *Exp. Gerontol.*, 1:237-247.

BENDER, A. D. 1965b. The effect of increasing age on the distribution of peripheral blood flow in man. *J. Am. Geriatr. Soc.*, 13:192-198.

BENDER, A. D. 1968. Effect of age on intestinal absorption: Implications for drug absorption in the elderly. *J. Am. Geriatr. Soc.*, 16:1331-1339.

BENDER, A. D. 1974. Pharmacodynamic principles of drug therapy in the aged. *J. Am. Geriatric Soc.*, 22:296-303.

BENDKOWSKI, B. 1970. Choice of antibiotics for elderly patients. *Practitioner*, 205:85-89.

BRIDGE, T. P., and ELLINWOOD, E. H. 1973. Quaalude Alley: A one-way street. *Am. J. Psychiatry*, 130:217-219.

BRODIE, N. H., MCGHIE, R. L., O'HARA, J., VALLE-JONES, J. C., and SCHIFF, A. A. 1975. Anxiety/depression in elderly patients: A double-blind comparative study of fluphenazine/nortriptyline and promazine. *Practitioner*, 215:660-664.

BUSSE, E. W., and PFEIFFER, E. 1969. Introduction. In E. W. Busse and E. Pfeiffer (eds.), *Behavior and Adaptation in Late Life*. Boston: Little, Brown.

CARVER, E. J. 1974. Geropsychiatric treatment: Where, why, how. In W. E. Fann and G. L. Maddox (eds.), *Drug Issues in Geropsychiatry*. Baltimore: Williams & Wilkins.

CURRY, S. H., DAVIS, J. M., JANOWSKY, D. S., and MARSHALL, J. H. L. 1970. Factors affecting chlorpromazine plasma levels in psychiatric patients. *Arch. Gen. Psychiatry*, 22:209-215.

DAVIS, J. M. 1974. Use of psychotropic drugs in geriatric patients. *J. Geriatr. Psychiatry*, 7:145-164.

DAVIS, D. R., and SHOCK, N. W. 1950. Age changes in glomerular filtration rate, effective renal plasma flow and tubular excretory capacity in adult males. *J. Clin. Invest.*, 29:496-507.

DAVIS, J. M., and FANN, W. E. 1971. Lithium. *Ann. Rev. Pharmacol.*, 11:285-302.

DAVIS, J. M., FANN, W. E., EL-YOUSEF, M. K., and JANOWSKY, D. 1973. Clinical problems in treating the aged with psychotropic drugs. In C. Eisdorfer and W. E. Fann (eds.), *Psychopharmacology and Aging*. New York: Plenum Press.

DAVISON, W. 1965. Drug hazards in the elderly. *Gerontologia Clinica* (Basel), 7:257-264.

DAVISON, W. 1973. The hazards of drug treatment in old age. In J. C. Brocklehurst (ed.), *Textbook of Geriatric Medicine and Gerontology*. New York: Churchill Livingstone.

EISDORFER, C. 1975. Observations on the psychopharmacology of the aged. *J. Am. Geriatr. Soc.*, 23:53-57.

EMERSON, G. M., and WINGO, W. J. 1975. Mitochondrial function: Age, sex, liver/brain compared. *Fed. Proc.* 34:277.

EXTON-SMITH, A. N., HODKINSON, H. M., CROMIE, B. W. 1963. Controlled comparison of four sedative drugs in elderly patients. *Br. Med. J.*, 2:1037-1040.

EXTON-SMITH, A. N., and WINDSOR, A. C. M. 1971. Principles of drug treatment in the aged. In I. Rossman (ed.), *Clinical Geriatrics*. Philadelphia: J. B. Lippincott.

FANN, W. E. 1973a. Interactions of psychotropic drugs in the elderly. *Postgrad. Med.*, 53:182-186.

FANN, W. E. 1973b. Some clinically important interactions of psychotropic drugs. *South. Med. J.*, 66:661-665.

FANN, W. E., DAVIS, J. M., and JANOWSKY, D. S. 1972. The prevalence of tardive dyskinesia in mental hospital patients. *Dis. Nerv. Syst.*, 33:182-186.

FANN, W. E., DAVIS, J. M., JANOWSKY, D. S., SEKERKE, H. J., and SCHMIDT, D. M. 1973. Chlorpromazine: Effects of antacids on its gastrointestinal absorption. *J. Clin. Pharmacol.*, 13:388-390.

FANN, W. E., DAVIS, J. M., and LAKE, C. R. 1973. Attempts at pharmacological management of tardive dyskinesia. In C. Eisdorfer and W. E. Fann (eds.), *Psychopharmacology and Aging*. New York: Plenum Press.

FANN, W. E., and LAKE, C. R. 1974. Treatment of drug-induced disorders in the elderly: An appraisal of treatment. In W. E. Fann and G. L. Maddox (eds.), *Drug Issues in Geropsychiatry*. Baltimore: Williams & Wilkins.

FANN, W. E., and LAKE, C. R. 1975. Amantadine vs. trihexyphenidyl in drug-induced parkinsonism. *Clin. Pharmacol. Ther.*, 17:233.

FANN, W. E., LAKE, C. R., and RICHMAN, B. W. 1975. Drug-induced parkinsonism: A reevaluation. *Dis. Nerv. Syst.*, 36:91-93.

FANN, W. E., WHELESS, J. C., and RICHMAN, B. W. 1974. Psychopharmacological treatment of disorders of senescence. *N.C. Med. J.*, 35:672-677.

FANN, W. E., WHELESS, J. C., and RICHMAN, B. W. 1976. Treating the aged with psychotropic drugs. *Gerontologist*, 16:322-328.

FANN, W. E., and WHELESS, J. C. 1975. Depression in elderly patients. *South. Med. J.*, 68:468-473.

FANN, W. E., and WHELESS, J. C. 1976. Effects of psychotherapeutic drugs on geriatric patients. In E. Usdin and I. Forrest (eds.), *Psychotherapeutic Drugs*, vol. 1. New York: Marcel Dekker.

FANN, W. E., and WHELESS, J. C. 1977. Pharmacological treatment of the moderately anxious and depressed patient. In W. E. Fann, I. C. Karacan, A. D. Pokorny, and R. L. Williams (eds.), *Phenomenology and Treatment of Depression*. New York: Spectrum Publications.

FREEMAN, J. T. 1974. Some principles of medication in geriatrics. *J. Am. Geriatr. Soc.*, 22:289-295.

GERSHON, S. 1973. Antianxiety agents. In C. Eisdorfer and W. E. Fann (eds.), *Psychopharmacology and Aging*. New York: Plenum Press.

GOLDMAN, R. 1970. Speculations on vascular changes with age. *J. Am. Geriatr. Soc.*, 18:765-779.

GRIFFITH, J. D., CAVANAUGH, J., HELD, J., and OATES, J. 1972. Amphetamine psychosis. *Arch. Gen. Psychiatry*, 26:97-100.

HAMILTON, L. D. 1966. Aged brain and the phenothiazines. *Geriatrics*, 21:131.

HANSEN, J. M., KAMPMANN, J., and LAURSEN, H. 1970. Renal excretion of drugs in the elderly. *Lancet*, 1:1170.

HOLLISTER, L. E. 1973. Uses of psychotherapeutic drugs. *Ann. Intern. Med.*, 79:88-98.

HOLLISTER, L. E. 1977. Prescribing drugs for the elderly. *Geriatrics*, 32:71-73.

HURWITZ, N. 1969a. Predisposing factors in adverse reactions to drugs. *Br. Med. J.*, 1:536-539.

HURWITZ, N. 1969b. Admissions to hospital due to drugs. *Br. Med. J.*, 1:539-540.

JANOWSKY, D. S., EL-YOUSEF, M. K., DAVIS, J. M., and FANN, W. E. 1973. Antagonism of guanethidine by chlorpromazine. *Am. J. Psychiatry*, 130:808-810.

JANOWSKY, D. S., EL-YOUSEF, M. K., and DAVIS, J. M. 1974. Side effects associated with psychotropic drugs. In W. E. Fann and G. L. Maddox (eds.), *Drug Issues in Geropsychiatry*. Baltimore: Williams & Wilkins.

JONEC, V., and FINCH, G. E. 1975. Aging and uptake of catecholamines by striatal and hypothalamic synaptosomes in mice. Abstract 333, *Fed. Proc.*, 34:277.

KARASU, T. B., and MURDOFSKY, C. A. 1976. Psychopharmacology of the elderly. In Bellak and Karasu (eds.), *Geriatric Psychiatry*. New York: Grune and Stratton.

KATO, R., VASSANELLI, P., FRONTINO, G., and CHIESARA, E. 1964. Variation in the activity of liver microsomal drug-metabolizing enzymes in rats in relation to the age. *Biochem. Pharmacol.*, 13:1037-1051.

KRAL, V. A. 1973. Psychiatric problems in the aged: A reconsideration. *Can. Med. Assoc. J.*, 108:584-589.

KUPFERBERG, H. J., and WAY, E. L. 1963. Pharmacologic basis for the increased sensitivity of the new born rat to morphine. *J. Pharmacol. Exp. Ther.*, 141:105-112.

LAMY, P. P., and KITLER, M. E. 1971. Drugs and the geriatric patient. *J. Am. Geriatr. Soc.*, 19:23-33.

MACFARLANE, M. D. 1973. Possible rationale for procaine (Gerovital H_3) therapy in geriatrics: Inhibition of MAO. *J. Am. Ger. Soc.*, 21:414-418.

MACFARLANE, M. D. 1975. Procaine HCl (Gerovital H_3): A weak, reversible fully competitive inhibitor of monoamine oxidase. *Fed. Proc.*, 34(1):108-110.

NIES, A., ROBINSON, D. S., DAVIS, J. M., and RAVARIS, L. 1973. Changes in monoamine oxidase with aging. In C. Eisdorfer and W. E. Fann (eds.), *Psychopharmacology and Aging*. New York: Plenum Press.

O'MALLERY, K., CROOKS, J., DUKE, E., and STEVENSON, I. H. 1971. Effect of age and sex on human drug metabolism. *Br. Med. J.*, 3:607-609.

PENZES, L., SIMON, G., and WINTER, M. 1968a. Intestinal absorption and utilization of radiomethionine in old age. *Exp. Geront.*, 3:257-263.

PENZES, L., SIMON, G., and WINTER, M. 1968b. Autoradiography of intestinal absorption of sulphur-labelled methionine in senescence. *Exp. Geront.*, 3:321-325.

PRANGE, A. J. 1973. The use of antidepressant drugs in the elderly patient. In C. Eisdorfer and W. E. Fann (eds.), *Psychopharmacology and Aging*. New York: Plenum Press.

RASKIND, M., and EISDORFER, C. 1976. Psychopharmacology of the aged. In L. L. Simpson (ed.), *Drug Treatment of Mental Disorders*. New York: Raven Press.

ROBINSON, D. S. 1975a. Pharmacokinetic mechanisms of drug interactions. *Postgrad. Med.*, 57:55-62.

ROBINSON, D. S. 1975b. Changes in MAO with human development and aging. *Fed. Proc.*, 34(1):103-107.

SALZMAN, C., and SHADER, R. I. 1973. Use of psychotropic agents in the normal elderly. In C. Eisdorfer and W. E. Fann (eds.), *Psychopharmacology and Aging*. New York: Plenum Press.

SALZMAN, C., SHADER, R. I., HARMOTZ, J., and ROBERTSON, L. 1975. Psychopharmacologic investigation in elderly volunteers: Effect of diazepam in males. *J. Am. Geriatr. Soc.*, 23:451-457.

SHOCK, N. W. 1967. Current trends in research on the physiological aspects of aging. *J. Am. Geriatr. Soc.*, 15:995-1000.

SEIDL, L. G., THORNTON, G. F., SMITH, J. W., and CLUFF, L. E. 1966. Studies on the epidemiology of adverse drug reactions. III. Reactions in patients on a general medical service. *Bulletin of Johns Hopkins Hospital*, 119:299-315.

SMITH, J. W., SEIDL, L. G., and CLUFF, L. E. 1966. Studies on the epidemiology of adverse drug reactions. V. Clinical factors influencing susceptibility. *Ann. Intern. Med.*, 65:29-40.

STRANG, R. R. 1965. Comparative study of trihexiphenidyl (Artane) and orphenadrine (Disipal) in treatment of geriatric parkinsonism. *J. Am. Geriatr. Soc.*, 13:756.

TIMIRAS, P. S. 1972. *Developmental Physiology and Aging*, pp. 542-563. New York: Macmillan.

VERWOERDT, A. 1976a. *Clinical Geropsychiatry*, pp. 119-131. Baltimore: Williams & Wilkins.

VERWOERDT, A. 1976b. *Clinical Geropsychiatry*, pp. 147-158. Baltimore: Williams & Wilkins.

WEBB, W. L. 1971. The use of psychopharmacological drugs in the aged. *Geriatrics*, 26:95-103.

WHANGER, A. D. 1974. Drug management of the elderly in state hospitals. In W. E. Fann, and G. L. Maddox (eds.), *Drug Issues in Geropsychiatry*. Baltimore: Williams & Wilkins.

WINTER, D., DOBRE, V., and OERIU, S. 1971. Cystein-S^{35} absorption in old rats. *Experimental Gerontology*, 6:367-371.

YOUNG, J. P. R. 1972. Acute psychiatric disturbances in the elderly and their treatment. *Br. J. Clin. Pract.*, 26:513-516.

ZUNG, W. W. K., GIANTURCO, D., PFEIFFER, E., WANG, H.-S., WHANGER, A., BRIDGE, T. P., and POTKIN, S. G. 1974. Pharmacology of depression in the aged: Evaluation of Gerovital H_3 as an antidepressant drug. *Psychosomatics*, 15:127-131.

15

ALCOHOL AND SEDATIVE DRUGS—DRUG INTERACTIONS

K. D. CHARALAMPOUS, M.D., and D. S. McCAUL

Ethanol

Absorption

The absorption of ethanol occurs throughout the gastrointestinal tract; about 20 percent of an oral dose may be absorbed through the stomach, the rest through the intestines and colon (Pawan, 1972). Absorption occurs so rapidly that about one-half of a dose may be absorbed within 15 minutes (Ritchie, 1975). Whereas gastric absorption depends on the type of beverage, concentration, gastric emptying, and the presence of food, intestinal absorption seems to be independent of ethanol concentration and digestive products. Although ethanol absorption is rapid and apparently complete, significant amounts of ethanol are found in the proximal jejunum and ileum following ingestion (Halstead, Robles, and Mezey, 1973). This may be due to recirculation from the vascular space into the gut lumen. In general, however, complete absorption is believed to require from two to six hours or more (Ritchie, 1975).

Distribution

After oral ingestion of ethanol, peak plasma concentrations are seen within one to three hours, and total clearance from the body occurs after eight to 12 hours (Haggard, Greenberg, and Carroll, 1941). Ethanol is distributed throughout the body water, and brain concentration quickly approaches that of the blood. Comparable concentrations of ethanol are found in the blood, urine, saliva, and alveolar air (Ritchie, 1975).

Metabolism

Ethanol is primarily oxidized to acetaldehyde in the liver by three enzyme systems of which alcohol dehydrogenase (ADH) seems to be the principal one (Mezey, 1976). The K_m (Michaelis constant) value *in vitro* is lower than that for any of the other ethanol-oxidizing systems and is comparable to the apparent *in vivo* K_m obtained at low blood ethanol concentrations. In addition, pyrazole markedly inhibits ethanol metabolism *in vivo* and has been shown to be a specific inhibitor of hepatic ADH. The oxidation of ethanol by ADH is dependent upon NAD^+ as a cofactor and thus will generate NADH. A second system is that of catalase whereby ethanol is oxidized in the presence of an H_2O_2-generating system. Although this system appears to be of little significance in ethanol metabolism, it is important in the elimination of methanol. The third most controversial system is the microsomal ethanol-oxidizing system (MEOS) which is similar to the mixed-function oxidase system responsible for drug hydroxylations. This system has requirements for NADPH and oxygen such that $NADP^+$ and H_2O are the products of the oxidation. Cytochrome P-450 is also associated with the system and it has been shown that ethanol will bind to and alter the absorption spectrum of this macromolecule. In addition, H_2O_2 may be generated from NADPH and oxygen by an NADPH oxidase of the MEOS. This would suggest a further role for the catalase reaction. The problem remains unresolved, but it is estimated that, in general, 70 to 80 percent of the absorbed ethanol is metabolized by ADH with the remaining drug being metabolized by the MEOS (Lemberger and Rubin, 1976). The acetaldehyde produced is further metabolized to acetate by an NAD^+-dependent mitochondrial acetaldehyde dehydrogenase present in human liver. Acetate is then used as acetyl CoA in pathways of intermediary metabolism or is completely oxidized to CO_2 and H_2O via the Krebs cycle.

Excretion

The rate of elimination of ethanol from the blood varies (Mezey, 1976). The variation tends to occur among individuals more so than within the same individual at different times. Variation in elimination of 70 to 150 mg/kg body weight/hour is about average in human studies. Normally only 2 percent of the administered dose of ethanol is exhaled unchanged, yet this may approach 10 percent with excessive intake (Lemberger and Rubin, 1976). As much as 5 to 10 percent of a dose may also be excreted unchanged in the urine, and in some species the glucuronide or sulfate conjugate may be excreted. The extent to which ethanol is eliminated through exhalation of CO_2 depends on the dose, and up to 95 percent of a low dose has been eliminated in this way.

Chloral Hydrate

Chloral hydrate [$CCl_3CH(OH)_2$] is a hydroxylated trichloro derivative of acetaldehyde (Harvey, 1975b). The halogenation increases lipid solubility and enhances its activity in the central nervous system (CNS). Its margin of safety is too narrow for use as a general anesthetic, but the sedative and hypnotic effects of chloral hydrate are therapeutically useful.

Absorption

Both chloral hydrate and its metabolite trichloroethanol (TCE) are absorbed rapidly and completely through the gastrointestinal tract (Marshall and Owens, 1954). Following an oral dose in humans, plasma chloral hydrate is not demonstrable, but TCE is present within five minutes, reaching peak plasma levels within 1.5 hours.

Distribution

After oral administration, chloral hydrate has been reported to be present in cerebrospinal fluid, milk, and amniotic fluid but not in the plasma (Harvey, 1975b). However, TCE is found throughout the body tissues (Cabana and Gessner, 1970). A comparison of lipid solubilities showed a partition coefficient in benzene/water of 3.5 for TCE while chloral hydrate showed a value of 0.03. In mice, the ratio of brain-to-body TCE concentrations was found to be 3.5 times the value found for chloral hydrate five minutes after administration.

Metabolism

Chloral hydrate is reduced primarily by hepatic alcohol dehydrogenase to trichloroethanol in the presence of NADH (Sellers et al., 1972a). Elimination of the TCE then takes place via glucuronide conjugation, and no conversion of TCE to chloral hydrate via the ADH has been demonstrated. Chloral hydrate is also converted to trichloroacetate (TCA) via an aldehyde dehydrogenase, but purified human acetaldehyde dehydrogenase has not been shown to metabolize chloral hydrate. Chloral hydrate has also been shown to be reduced by human erythrocytes. There has been no characterization of the enzyme responsible, but the apparent K_m for the reaction is one order of magnitude less than that found with horse liver ADH. In addition, consideration of the maximal velocity based on erythrocyte mass suggests that this process contributes more to the overall reduction of chloral hydrate than does the hepatic ADH.

Following intraparenteral (i.p.) administration of chloral hydrate in mice, at least 56 percent of the dose was found to be reduced to TCE with a half-life equal to 22 minutes (Cabana and Gessner, 1970). The blood half-life of chloral hydrate was found to be 12 minutes. No TCA was formed from TCE, but 12 percent of the chloral hydrate was converted to TCA. About 9 percent of the administered dose appeared to be protected from metabolic degradation, and half of this was excreted unchanged in the urine. Approximately 23 percent of the administered chloral hydrate seems to undergo some unknown process of metabolism.

Excretion

The disappearance of TCE from the blood of mice shows a half-life ($T_{\frac{1}{2}}$) of 211 minutes (Cabana and Gessner, 1970). The rate of TCE formation is ten times this, and the accumulation of this metabolite is responsible for the continued hypnotic effect of chloral hydrate. Urinary metabolites account for less than 8 percent of the administered dose of chloral hydrate in humans six hours after oral dosing (Sellers et al., 1972a). Of these, about 80 percent was conjugated TCE, 10 percent free TCE, and 10 percent TCA. The slow rate of renal clearance of TCE may be due to its high lipophilicity since this is associated with significant renal tubular reabsorption. In addition, plasma TCE is 40 percent protein-bound and this may partially explain low clearance values. To a lesser extent, metabolites of chloral hydrate have also been found in the feces and bile (Cabana and Gessner, 1970).

Interaction with Ethanol

Experiments with mice have been performed using several ethanol-chloral hydrate combinations so as to characterize the interaction with regard to degree of potentiation (Gessner and Cabana, 1970). The time taken to induce loss of the righting reflex was used to calculate ED_{50} (mean effective dose) values, while LD_{50} values reflect the incidence of fatality. All doses were administered by the i.p. route. The ED_{50} for ethanol was found to be 2666 mg/kg, that of chloral hydrate 244 mg/kg. Thus chloral hydrate alone is more than ten times as potent as ethanol in inducing loss of righting reflex. Analysis of the effects of administered combinations showed significant potentiation of hypnotic effects for mixtures containing a wt/wt ratio of chloral hydrate:ethanol greater than 1:7. Onset of effect was found to be quickest for a ratio of 1:1.5, while duration was minimal with a ratio of 1.76:1. The latter ratio was a combination associated with maximum potentiation. Potentiation was further maximized when ethanol was administered two minutes before chloral hydrate injection. When lethality was measured, chloral hydrate alone (LD_{50} = 741 mg/kg) was 5.5 times more toxic than ethanol alone (LD_{50} = 4115 mg/kg). Partial antagonism was found for ratios from 1:5 to 1:15, 1:10 being maximal. No deviation from simple additive effects was found when the drugs were given in 1:1.14 and 1:1 wt/wt combinations. Significant potentiation of lethality was found when they were given in equimolar (3.6:1) amounts. The therapeutic ratio and standard safety margin, however, were found to be greater than those for equivalent hypnotic doses of chloral hydrate or ethanol alone. Thus, chloral hydrate and ethanol were shown to interact with a potentiation of both hypnotic and lethal effects when administered in the proper relative concentrations.

The interaction between TCE and ethanol was then studied in a similar manner. Following i.p. administration, the ED_{50} of TCE was 199 mg/kg which is significantly lower than that for chloral hydrate (Gessner and Cabana, 1970). In addition, with intravenous (i.v.) administration, TCE was found to have a hypnotic potency 1.31 times that of chloral hydrate (Cabana and Gessner, 1970). Since the plasma half-life of chloral hydrate was about one-twentieth of TCE's, one would expect increasing levels of this metabolite, which would suggest that it may be responsible for the observed potentiation. Nevertheless, no deviation from additivity was seen when several combinations of TCE and ethanol were administered (Gessner and Cabana, 1970). In addition, chloral hydrate and TCE were also shown to interact only with simple additivity over a range of combined dosages. Thus, the potentiation seemed to result primarily from the relative concentrations of ethanol and chloral hydrate rather than from TCE directly.

Equimolar amounts of chloral hydrate and ethanol when given i.p. to mice led to a 29.9-percent increase in the rate of chloral hydrate disappearance (Cabana and Gessner, 1970). The rate of TCA formation remained constant, so that less was formed overall. The only process seen responsible for the increased rate of chloral hydrate disappearance was an 84-percent increase in the rate of TCE formation. In addition, the unaltered rate of TCE conjugation and elimination resulted in greater accumulation of TCE. Under these conditions, it was found that 70 percent of the administered chloral hydrate was reduced to TCE, in contrast to the 50 percent found in the absence of ethanol.

The effects of TCE and chloral hydrate on the disappearance of ethanol have also been studied in mice (Gessner, 1973). Ethanol administered i.p. at 139 mg/kg showed first-order elimination from the blood with a half-life of 3.6 minutes. When equimolar doses of chloral hydrate or TCE were administered simultaneously with this dose of ethanol, the blood half-life of ethanol increased to 26.9 and 18.9 minutes respectively. In addition, the rate of chloral hydrate reduction to TCE was increased by 83 percent when administered with ethanol. This may be compared to the 86-percent decrease in ethanol elimination when administered with chloral hydrate. The rate constants for these two processes do not differ significantly, which may be taken as evidence for a 1:1 coupling of the oxidation of ethanol with the reduction of chloral hydrate by ADH.

TCE has been shown to inhibit ethanol oxidation by rat-liver homogenates, human ADH, and horse-liver ADH (Gessner, 1973). Thus, the decrease in elimination of ethanol when administered with TCE or chloral hydrate is probably caused by direct inhibition of ADH. Chloral hydrate, however, has a greater effect on ethanol metabolism *in vivo* than does TCE. TCE is more lipophilic and exhibits a larger distribution throughout the body. Moreover, the TCE released from the reduction of chloral hydrate will be localized at the enzyme which it is inhibiting. Thus, chloral hydrate may not directly inhibit ethanol metabolism, but its administration could lead to more efficient inhibition by TCE. The direct role of increased levels of ethanol in the potentiation of hypnotic effects is questionable. Ethanol is only one-tenth as potent as chloral hydrate while TCE is about 1.2 times as potent as chloral hydrate. Calculations show that the contribution of ethanol would be raised from 2.1 to 11.1 percent of the total hypnotic action of the two drugs. Thus, raised ethanol levels contributed to a degree but not as much as enhanced TCE levels. TCE also led to a 37-percent decrease in the rate of methanol elimination when these drugs were administered in equimolar amounts (Gessner, 1973). Although this effect is markedly less than the effect on ethanol elimination, it indicates that TCE does not specifically inhibit ADH since methanol oxidation in mice is through a hepatic peroxidative enzyme system that involves catalase.

Studies of the metabolism of ethanol and chloral hydrate in the human have produced similar results (Sellers et al., 1972a). Chloral hydrate was administered per os (p.o.) at 15 mg/kg followed by 0.5 g/kg of ethanol p.o. thirty minutes later. In addition, 15 mg/kg of chloral hydrate were administered p.o. for seven days, followed by 0.5 mg/kg of ethanol p.o. 12 hours after the last dose. These procedures differ from those used with mice, however, and they are not expected to show potentiation since the ratio of chloral hydrate to ethanol is 1:33 wt/wt. Since the half-life of chloral hydrate was 12 minutes in mice, only 18 percent of the administered dose would be expected to be present after 30 minutes, while 43 percent of the dose would be present as TCE (assuming that one may compare men and mice) (Gessner, 1973). This, in addition to the simple additivity exhibited by TCE and ethanol, suggests that differences would be found in the metabolic interactions.

Nevertheless, the results were qualitatively similar, as raised and prolonged plasma TCE levels were found in human subjects treated with ethanol (Sellers et al., 1972a). The rate of TCE elimination was unaffected by ethanol, yet was slower than that found in rats ($T_{\frac{1}{2}}$ = 8.2 hours). Lower levels of TCE glucuronide in the plasma were also found, and this resulted in less conjugated TCE in the urine. Total urinary TCE was also decreased, but the concentration of unchanged TCE in the urine was greater than that found with chloral hydrate alone. Significantly lower levels of TCA in the plasma were also demonstrated. The decrease in TCE conjugation is difficult to explain. This impairment by ethanol was not found in the experiments with mice, and any suggestion as to a mechanism is speculative. Ethanol may interfere with glucuronide transferase directly, or reduced concentrations of NAD^+ may decrease the NAD^+-dependent production of UDP-glucuronide. A similar cofactor dependence may also explain the reduced production of TCA from chloral hydrate. This conversion is known to require such high levels of NAD^+ that the enzyme should be very sensitive to changes in available NAD^+.

In the experiment with human subjects, peak blood ethanol concentrations were reached earlier and showed higher levels when administered after chloral hydrate (Sellers et al., 1972a). The rates of elimination of both ethanol and acetaldehyde were not altered, yet blood acetaldehyde levels were found to be decreased significantly for 4.5 hours. The blood ethanol concentration following administration was also seen to depend on TCE levels at the time of ingestion. After the seven-day administration of chloral hydrate, ethanol treatment resulted in a similar decrease in acetaldehyde levels, yet the peak level of ethanol was not much different. Although these results are in accord with the *in vivo* inhibition of ADH by TCE, other studies with mice have pointed toward an additional inhibition of acetaldehyde dehydrogenase (Creaven and Roach, 1969). Ethanol was administered one hour after chloral hydrate, and blood acetaldehyde was measured from five to 50 minutes after the injection of ethanol. The blood acetaldehyde levels rose up to 300 percent after five minutes and then declined rapidly. The peak acetaldehyde levels were quite transitory and dependent on the ratio of chloral hydrate to ethanol administered.

Clinical studies of the interaction of chloral hydrate and ethanol have shown that ethanol leads to greater impairment on pursuit rotor tests when chloral hydrate is given beforehand (Sellers et al., 1972b). Under these conditions, maximal impairment occurs during the time when ethanol levels are dropping, whereas, with ethanol alone, maximal impairment develops with rising ethanol concentrations in the blood. Chloral hydrate followed by ethanol leads to greater increases in heart rate and skin temperatures than when ethanol is administered alone. Also, systolic pressure increases with this drug combination at one hour and then decreases after three hours. Neither drug alone showed any effect on diastolic blood pressure. One subject, given ethanol after seven days of chloral hydrate, showed profound vasodilation within 15 minutes and continued with an "acetaldehyde syndrome" for 1.5 hours. This included increased heart rate and pulse pressure, palpitations, anxiety, and facial flushing. Nevertheless, his blood acetaldehyde levels were only one-half of those reached with ethanol alone. Since this occurred with chronic chloral hydrate administration only, metabolites of chloral hydrate may have been responsible. TCE accumulation is not significantly greater under these circumstances, but TCE accumulation increases since it is highly bound to plasma albumin and shows a blood half-life of 67 hours. It should also be noted that although acetaldehyde is bound up to 30 percent to plasma proteins, it is not displaced by TCA.

The metabolic interaction of chloral hydrate and ethanol helps to explain the mechanism of potentiation between these drugs. The oxidation of ethanol occurs according to an ordered mechanism. The ADH-NAD^+ complex must be formed before ethanol can bind to the enzyme. However, it is dissociation of the ADH-NADH complex which is rate-limiting for the production of acetaldehyde. Likewise, the reduction of chloral hydrate depends on the formation of an ADH-NADH complex before the reaction can take place. Thus, chloral hydrate should be metabolized more quickly in the presence of ADH-NADH, which explains the increased TCE concentration found with ethanol administration. It would also make sense that ethanol administered before chloral hydrate would have a stronger effect than ethanol administered later, since more time would be available for the production of NADH and the ADH-NADH complex.

The Barbiturates

The Family

The barbiturates studied most often for their interaction with ethanol include barbital, phenobarbital, pentobarbital, amobarbital, hexobarbital, and thiopental. These compounds, listed in order of increasing lipophilicity, are derivatives of the inactive barbituric acid (Saunders, 1974). As substitutions are made at C-5 on the barbiturate ring, lipid solubility increases as does rapidity of onset, shortness of duration, and extent of metabolization. Thiopental is produced by replacing the C-2 oxygen atom with sulfur, and this results in a very fast-acting drug. All of these compounds are comparatively weak acids (pKa 7.5 to 8.5) and are sparingly soluble in water. The barbiturates are used for their hypnotic, anticonvulsant, and anesthetic actions, although small doses given for severe pain are capable of producing hyperalgesia.

Absorption

The barbiturates are absorbed throughout the gastrointestinal tract, and their rate of absorption has been directly related to differences in lipid solubility (Kakema et al., 1967a). Highly lipophilic compounds are absorbed rapidly through the stomach while the less lipid soluble compounds (e.g., phenobarbital) may show rising plasma concentrations several hours after an oral dose. This dependence on lipophilicity is especially true in the stomach where a low pH results in the majority of species being in the unionized state. At alkaline pH, however, absorption constants were comparable for the various drugs studied. That is, when the barbiturates are predominantly in the ionized state their rates of absorption are similar. With rat intestines, pH profiles of absorption showed maximal rates at the pKa of each drug, that is, at a point at which the acids are half ionized (Kakema et al., 1967b). The order of binding to intestinal mucosa was similar to that of absorption rates. In addition, pH mucosal-binding profiles resembled those for albumin binding. Thus, intestinal absorption seems to depend more on protein-moiety affinity than on lipophilicity. Other studies indicate that dissolution time is rate-limiting for the oral absorption of the intermediate and short-acting barbiturates (Sjögren, Solvell, and Karlsson, 1965). Absorption may be slowed by stomach contents, but the extent of absorption is not altered (Smith et al., 1973). Absorption is apparently complete for each class though rates will differ. Secobarbital (comparable to amobarbital and pentobarbital) showed 90-percent absorption within 1.5 hours after oral administration to nonfasting human subjects, and was detected in the blood for 108 hours (Clifford, Cookson, and Wickham, 1974).

Distribution

The distribution of barbiturates is affected primarily by lipid solubility, protein-binding, and the degree of ionization. In general, the degree of

protein-binding is reflected in the degree of lipophilicity, with about 50 percent of the phenobarbital in plasma being protein-bound. The differences in the anesthetic actions of thiopental and pentobarbital may be explained in terms of their distributions (Goldstein and Aranow, 1960). Upon intravenous administration, thiopental in brain fluid equilibrated immediately with plasma thiopental, and the levels of both fell as the drug diffused into other tissues and body water. Pentobarbital brain:plasma concentrations equilibrated more slowly and brain levels leveled off as the plasma level decreased. Thiopental has been shown to distribute throughout body tissues and its serum concentration is 75 percent bound to protein. This accounts for only 20 percent of the administered thiopental after brain levels have fallen; most of the drug is deposited in body fat. Pentobarbital, in contrast, is evenly distributed throughout body tissues including fat when plasma levels are falling (Brodie et al., 1953). As a result of more even distribution, pentobarbital levels in the brain remain higher than those of thiopental, resulting in a more prolonged anesthesia. Overall, barbiturate distribution is uniform so that the volume of distribution of barbital is essentially that of the total body water when measured 24 hours after administration. Plasma pH affects the distribution of barbiturate in that, with alkalinization, more of the ionized form is present, and plasma concentrations increase with corresponding decreases in tissue concentrations (Waddell and Butler, 1957). This results in an increase of barbiturate available for renal excretion.

Metabolism

The metabolism of barbiturates is to some extent related to their lipid solubilities. The excretion of unchanged drug in the urine of humans is found to be 65 to 90 percent of the administered barbital, 10 to 30 percent of phenobarbital, 0 to 3 percent of pentobarbital, and 0 to 1 percent of amobarbital (Harvey, 1975a)—the more lipophilic compounds seem to be more extensively metabolized. The short duration of action of the very lipophilic derivatives is, however, primarily due to their rapid redistribution. The four basic metabolic routes of biotransformation occur primarily through microsomal enzymes. Oxidation or removal of the substituents at C-5 is the most important pathway; it leads to the formation of polar compounds that may appear in the urine as both free and conjugated metabolites. N-dealkylation contributes little to the elimination of short-acting compounds as the oxidation at C-5 occurs more rapidly. This reaction is important for barbiturates which yield active compounds upon demethylation (e.g., mephobarbital to phenobarbital). Desulfuration of the thiobarbiturates occurs but is also of less significance than the oxidation reaction. Hydrolytic cleavage of the barbiturate ring is known to occur but it is of little significance (Harvey, 1975a).

Excretion

The barbiturates are eliminated primarily through the renal system, yet they may also be secreted into the bile (Lemberger and Rubin, 1976). After intravenous administration in rats, 28 percent of a dose of pentobarbital and 18 percent of phenobarbital were found in the bile as polar metabolites which would then be eliminated in the feces. Renal clearance was shown to be independent of plasma barbiturate concentrations, but dependent on urinary flow rate (Lous, 1954). The rate of urinary excretion is influenced by several factors. Plasma half-lives of the barbiturates increase with decreasing lipid solubility, primarily because of concomitant decrease in the rate of redistribution. Higher lipid solubilities will also lead to slower excretion, however, as a result of increased reabsorption from renal tubules. Binding to plasma proteins reduces the drugs' availability to glomerular filtration, but this does not explain the mechanism of long-acting barbiturates since they are less protein-bound. Changes in physiologic pH may alter the rate of barbiturate excretion as described above. Finally, the rate of urinary excretion will also depend on the rate of production of more polar metabolites in addition to the excretion of unchanged barbiturate.

Interaction with Ethanol

A relatively early study on ethanol-barbiturate interactions in rats used a representative group of barbiturates in an attempt to measure altered barbiturate toxicity and distribution (Coldwell, Wiberg, and Trenholm, 1970). Induction time was shortened and sleeping time lengthened by the simultaneous i.p. administration of 3 g/kg of ethanol with the long-acting barbital and phenobarbital, the intermediate-acting amobarbital and pentobarbital, and the short-acting thiopental. The effects were most pronounced with the long-acting, least-metabolized barbiturates, which suggests that altered drug metabolism may not be as relevant to the interaction as lipid solubility. The barbiturates' lipid solubility is slightly increased by ethanol at physiological concentrations, and their solubilities are several times greater in 15-percent ethanol than in water (Coldwell et al., 1971). Thus, ethanol could increase the rate of absorption of barbiturates into the blood and alter their distribution and excretion.

Coldwell and his co-workers (Thomas et al., 1972) have used ^{14}C-

labeled pentobarbital (30 mg/kg) to study the effects of ethanol (3 g/kg), with both drugs injected simultaneously i.p. in rats. Measurements of distribution into blood, liver, diaphragm, heart, lung, kidney, skeletal muscle, duodenum, and brain showed no differences one hour after administration. After three hours, however, higher concentrations of pentobarbital were found in all tissues except kidney and duodenum. This enhancement was observed during the overall decrease in tissue levels, and it was reflected in a significant difference between the blood-concentration versus time curves from two to four hours after administration. In addition, the area under the curve for the pentobarbital-ethanol mixture was found to be greater than that for pentobarbital alone. The Thomas group concluded that ethanol did not cause any apparent redistribution since the changes in pentobarbital levels occurred in all tissues to about the same extent. No metabolites of pentobarbital were detected in the brain; since the relative increase in brain pentobarbital concentration paralleled the rise in blood levels, ethanol does not seem to specifically affect the blood-brain barrier with respect to pentobarbital. The induced increase in brain pentobarbital levels indicates the possibility of more than simple additive drug effects. Additionally, pentobarbital had no significant effect on ethanol blood levels (Coldwell, Wiberg, and Trenholm, 1970). Ethanol decreased the renal excretion of radioactivity from three to six hours after dosage, and by 12 hours the net excreted radioactivity was the same for both groups (Thomas et al., 1972). The elimination of an acidic metabolite with an intact barbiturate ring was shown to be reduced in the ethanol-plus-pentobarbital group. Since significant levels of this metabolite were not seen in the plasma, it was concluded that the increased blood and tissue levels concomitant with decreased elimination were caused by an inhibition of pentobarbital metabolism by ethanol.

In another study, Rubin et al. (1970) administered 5 g/kg of ethanol to rats by gastric intubation and followed this with 40 mg/kg of ^{14}C-pentobarbital i.p. two hours later. The plasma half-life of pentobarbital was doubled and the total-body elimination half-life tripled in the ethanol-treated group. Again, the investigators concluded that ethanol inhibits the metabolism of pentobarbital. Similar results were obtained in humans when a dose of 6 mg/kg of ^{14}C-pentobarbital was given p.o., followed by 1 g/kg of ethanol p.o. six hours later, and 24 g of ethanol every two hours thereafter (Rubin et al., 1970). The plasma-level curves showed an immediate doubling in plasma pentobarbital half-life upon administration of ethanol. Thus, ethanol may interact with pentobarbital during its elimination so as to stabilize blood pentobarbital levels, and subsequently alter the barbiturate's pharmacological effect.

The somewhat more extensive studies with phenobarbital have resulted in discrepancies with regard to the effects of ethanol on barbiturate metabolism and distribution. Coldwell, Paul, and Thomas (1973) gave 50 mg/kg oral doses of ^{14}C-phenobarbital alone and with ethanol (3 g/kg) to rats. There was no apparent increase in the absorption of phenobarbital, but during the distribution and elimination phases significantly higher blood levels were found in the ethanol group from four to 15 hours after administration. As in other studies, the investigators found an increase in the area under the blood-level versus time curve. This would indicate either greater absorption or decreased rate of elimination. The half-lives of phenobarbital elimination from the blood were not different between groups ($T_{\frac{1}{2}}$ = 8 h), but this was not surprising since all of the ethanol is expected to be eliminated during the first 12 hours. Liver, heart, muscle, kidney, spleen, fat, and brain concentrations of phenobarbital were increased and reflected increased blood concentrations; tissue levels approached those of control animals as ethanol was eliminated from the blood. An ethanol-induced decrease in renal excretion of radioactivity was believed to explain the increased tissue and blood levels of phenobarbital. In addition, excretion of the metabolite p-hydroxyphenobarbital was decreased in the ethanol-treated rats. The researchers concluded that ethanol inhibits the formation of this metabolite since no significant levels of p-hydroxyphenobarbital were found in the blood or tissues and its concentration in the urine returend to control levels once ethanol was eliminated. In another study using ^{14}C-labeled barbiturates (Coldwell et al., 1971), the ethanol-induced increase in phenobarbital concentrations was greater than that with pentobarbital in cerebral cortex, half-brain, cerebellum, and blood. These levels were measured during the first 20 minutes following i.p. administration of 30 mg/kg of pentobarbital or 50 mg/kg of phenobarbital with saline or 3 g/kg of ethanol.

Further studies of phenobarbital-ethanol interactions used several dosage combinations administered to mice (Curry and Scales, 1974). Dose-response curves were plotted for incidence of death (LD_{50}), induction time for loss of righting reflex, and sleeping time. Analysis of the blood-level curves showed an increased peak level of phenobarbital in less time after administration when given with ethanol (320 g/ml at 15 min versus 450 g/ml at 5 min). The areas under the curve were similar, and ethanol seemed to accelerate the rate of phenobarbital absorption without changing the overall degree of absorption. In contrast, a blood-level curve for ethanol showed that phenobarbital seemed to delay ethanol absorption; the peak concentration appeared later than with ethanol alone. Induction times were decreased and potentiation was greatest at higher relative phenobarbital doses. Sleeping time was decreased as phenobarbital doses increased relative to ethanol. Thus, by increasing initial phenobarbital levels, ethanol decreases induction times. Sleep times are also shortened since the later levels of phenobarbital are lower than those seen in control animals. The LD_{50} measurements showed an antagonism related primarily to the dosage of phenobarbital. The mice seemed to be more resistant to transitory high levels of phenobarbital than to sustained lower levels. Although the study did not determine a mechanism of interaction, it showed that blood levels of ethanol and phenobarbital are relevant parameters of their interaction and pharmacological effect.

The role of ethanol inhibition of barbiturate metabolism in the interactions described above is a subject of controversy. There is good evidence for some sort of interference with the metabolism of these drugs but the mechanism is still speculative. Aniline hydroxylase was shown to be most sensitive to *in vitro* inhibition by ethanol (K_i = 3.0 mM) while pentobarbital hydroxylase was inhibited to a lesser degree (K_i = 90 mM) (Rubin et al., 1970). In addition, cytochrome P-450 reductase activity was inhibited by 35 percent with ethanol *in vitro*. This inhibition is reflected by the capacity of ethanol to bind the cytochrome P-450 with a type-2 spectrum. The same sort of binding is found with aniline; ethanol may interfere with drugs that bind to these sites. In contrast, ethanol does not interfere with the type-1 binding of hexobarbital to cytochrome P-450 (Mezey, 1976). The suggestion is, therefore, that acute doses of ethanol may inhibit the microsomal metabolism of drugs characterized by type-2 rather than type-1 binding.

Corticosterone has been implicated as a mediator in the ethanol-induced enhancement of the effects of barbiturates. Rats were used in a study of microsomal hexobarbital metabolism as affected by acute ethanol (3 g/kg p.o.) (Chung and Brown, 1976). This dose inhibited hepatic hexobarbital hydroxylase activity by 50 percent one hour after administration. Although hepatic microsomal protein content was unchanged, the hepatic cytochrome P-450 level was reduced by 42 percent. Ethanol also was shown to cause a threefold increase in the plasma corticosterone level but had no effect on adrenalectomized rats. In addition, hexobarbital metabolism was not affected by ethanol in adrenalectomized rats. When corticosterone was given i.p. (12.5 mg/kg), hexobarbital hydroxylase activity decreased by 43 percent. Hydroxylase activity decreased by 57 percent when the 12.5-mg/kg dose of corticosterone was given with 3 g/kg p.o. of ethanol. Finally, *in vitro* studies showed that corticosterone inhibits hexobarbital hydroxylase competitively. It is apparent, then, that the interaction of acute ethanol with barbiturates is a complicated matter. The mechanisms of interaction depend on the individual barbiturate given, and they may include alterations in absorption, distribution, metabolism, elimination, and the effects of secondary compounds subject to release by acute ethanol administration.

The effects of chronic ethanol administration on changes in drug metabolism are more easily studied. In human studies, Misra et al. (1971) administered ethanol chronically to nonalcoholic subjects and to abstained alcoholics whose hepatic structure and function had returned to normal. Ethanol intake was balanced with an isocaloric intake of carbohydrate in controlled diets over one month. Disappearance of ethanol from the blood was enhanced in ethanol-treated groups but more so in the alcoholics. A decrease in the plasma half-life of pentobarbital from 35.1 hours to 26.3 hours was found in the nonalcoholic subjects. Chronic ethanol administration has been shown to induce hepatic microsomal pentobarbital hydroxylase which may account for the reduced plasma pentobarbital half-life. This suggests that the tolerance to barbiturates seen in alcoholics may have a metabolic basis in addition to CNS cross-tolerance.

In animals, chronic ethanol administration leads to increases in liver smooth endoplasmic reticulum, cytochrome P-450, cytochrome reductase, and the activities of several microsomal enzymes (Khanna et al., 1976; Lieber and DeCarli, 1972). However, the effects of chronic ethanol administration are diverse and dependent on well-controlled diets. The mechanisms involved are certainly complex, and recent studies are beginning to show that the enzyme-inductive effects of ethanol may not be as important as once believed. In rats, for instance, the difference in ^{14}C-pentobarbital after i.v. administration has been compared between ethanol-treated and pair-fed controls on a high-fat diet (Khanna et al., 1976). Ethanol treatment resulted in a pronounced increase in microsomal protein and several enzyme activities. Nevertheless, no difference was found between the ethanol-treated group and controls with respect to the volume of distribution of pentobarbital or its elimination from the blood. Thus, careful consideration of actual enzyme activities during the interaction of ethanol and barbiturates is necessary before one may conclude that the effects of ethanol result from inhibition of drug metabolism.

The Benzodiazepines

The Family

The benzodiazepines most often used therapeutically include diazepam, oxazepam, chlordiazepoxide, and flurazepam. They are noted for their anticonvulsant, muscle-relaxant, and tranquilizing properties. These CNS depressants produce tolerance in addition to both psychological and physical dependence after prolonged use. The abstinence phenomena vary from minor to major symptoms including agitation, confusion, hallucinations, delirium, and convulsions.

Absorption

After an oral dose, diazepam and chlordiazepoxide appear in the blood within 30 minutes and reach peak plasma levels between two and four hours. The benzodiazepines are poorly soluble in water, with diazepam showing a solubility of 50 μg/ml (pKa = 3.4). Diazepam seems to be completely absorbed after oral administration, as indicated by comparisons of area under the blood-level curves following p.o. and i.v. administration (Kaplan et al., 1973). The absorption of chlordiazepoxide by the oral route was 81 percent in one case (Schwartz, Postma, and Gaut, 1971), and oxazepam is considered to have almost complete absorption (Shull et al., 1976). This, plus good absorbability across everted rat intestinal sac (Kaplan et al., 1973), suggests that dissolution time is rate-limiting for transmucosal absorption of the benzodiazepines. The peak plasma levels of diazepam and the rapidity with which they are reached depend on the means of administration such that i.v. > p.o. > i.m. In addition, this same order is followed with respect to measured clinical effects since they correlate well with diazepam blood concentrations (Hillestad et al., 1974).

Distribution

Whole-body autoradiography has been used in mice to examine the distribution of diazepam and chlordiazepoxide (van der Kleijn, 1969). Brain, kidney, liver, myocardium, and the digestive system showed rapid uptake (3 to 30 minutes) and slow release (30 minutes to 4 hours) following intravenous administration. Adipose tissue differed in that, after rapid uptake, the subsequent decrease in radioactivity also occurred rapidly. Overall, chlordiazepoxide was found to be removed from these tissues more rapidly than diazepam. After both oral and intravenous administration, the ratio of brain:blood radioactivity was higher for diazepam than for chlordiazepoxide. Brain tissue showed a higher affinity for diazepam than for chlordiazepoxide, with rapid uptake into grey matter followed by selective retention in the white matter.

Metabolism

The primary pathways in the metabolism of the benzodiazepines have been elucidated for several species. In the human, the major metabolite of diazepam found in the bloodstream is desmethyldiazepam (Kaplan et al., 1973). This compound is then hydroxylated to form oxazepam, and its glucuronide conjugate is excreted in the urine as the major detectable metabolite. Hydroxylation followed by demethylation is also believed to be a means of elimination. In dogs, the demethylation reaction occurs so rapidly that diazepam is barely detectable and desmethyldiazepam remains as the major blood compound measurable in the blood; moreover, 4-hydroxy derivatives are produced in contrast to the C-3 hydroxylation in man. The biotransformation of chlordiazepoxide occurs through a desmethyl metabolite which is detectable in the plasma (Schwartz, Postma, and Gaut, 1971). Demoxapam is then formed through oxidation of the remaining amine group and this compound is eliminated in the urine. Oxazepam has been reported to be metabolized normally in patients with cirrhosis and acute viral hepatitis (Shull et al., 1976). Since this is not true for diazepam, it implies that extrahepatic means of glucuronidation may be important in the metabolism of oxazepam.

Excretion

The plasma half-life of diazepam after intravenous administration in human subjects varies with age (Klotz et al., 1975). An average half-life of 20 hours in 20-year-olds may be compared to 80 hours in 80-year-olds. Clearance values, however, only ranged from 20 to 32 ml/min and the changes were attributed to increased volumes of distribution. Disappearance of diazepam from the blood is initially rapid as desmethyldiazepam is formed. A second, slower rate of desmethyldiazepam formation occurs 12 hours after intravenous administration and is essentially equal to the overall rate of elimination. This indicates that elimination occurs primarily through demethylation which is dependent upon the rate of return of diazepam from storage sites into the blood. Urinary and biliary excretion of unchanged diazepam is minimal. In addition, 70 percent of the administered dose has been reported to be excreted in the urine while 10 percent is excreted in the feces (Kaplan et al., 1973). Chronic oral administration of diazepam has led to steady-state blood levels after about seven days. Desmethyldiazepam levels plateau later and are significantly higher than those of diazepam. This metabolite shows an apparent biological half-life of 92 hours (Hillestad, Hansen, and Melsom, 1974).

The plasma half-life of chlordiazepoxide has been found to vary from 6.6 to 28 hours in humans (Schwartz, Postma, and Gaut, 1971). Oral administration of demoxepam, the terminal metabolite of chlordiazepoxide, led to half-lives ranging from 14 to 95 hours. Negligible amounts of unchanged chlordiazepoxide were found in the urine. Oxazepam has generally been shown to have a plasma half-life between 2.8 and 5.7 hours (Shull et al., 1976). However, values of 11.4 to 21.2 hours have been reported. Only one percent of the dose is excreted unchanged in the urine; the major metabolite found in the urine is the glucuronide conjugate. From 45 percent to 85 percent of the administered oxazepam has been reported to be excreted in this form after 48 hours.

Interactions with Ethanol

Ethanol-diazepam interactions have been studied extensively with regard to behavioral effects, but differences in methods complicate interpretation and comparison. The work of Linnoila, concerned with psychomotor skills related to driving, has shown that an additive deleterious effect may be produced with dosages of 5 to 10 mg of oral diazepam and 0.5 to 0.8 g/kg of oral ethanol (Linnoila and Mattila, 1973). Neither of these dosages alone significantly affects psychomotor skills. Tests of reaction times and coordination exhibited the most marked additive effects, and self-assessment of skills was also impaired. Peak levels of blood alcohol were reached in about 45 minutes while impairment was seen 30 minutes after ingestion. Since this impairment is rapid, the investigators believed that the combined effect results from interaction at common receptor sites rather than from a metabolic inhibition of drug degradation (Linnoila, 1973a). When diazepam (15 mg/day) and ethanol (0.5 g/kg) were administered for two weeks, greater psychomotor impairment occurred on day 1 than on day 14 (Linnoila, Sarrio, and Maki, 1974). Peak effects again occurred 30 minutes after ingestion. Another study using driving tests showed enhanced impairment when ethanol (0.5 g/kg) was administered ten hours after a 10 mg p.o. dose of diazepam (Linnoila and Hakkinen, 1974). Ethanol was also shown to result in the same degree of impairment whether given simultaneously with diazepam or two hours later (Molander and Duvhok, 1976); in this case, critical flicker-fusion frequency and coordination tests were being measured. In general, however, one sees maximal interaction when the two drugs are given together. Ethanol may lead to a more rapid absorption of diazepam and the distribution of diazepam may also be influenced. Furthermore, the rapidity of increase in plasma levels of diazepam may be more important than the absolute level with regard to behavioral effects (Bliding, 1974).

MacLeod et al. (1977) have produced data on diazepam-ethanol interactions as they affect performance on pursuit rotor tests. Plasma diazepam levels were carefully compared with the decrement in pursuit rotor performance. Ethanol, diazepam, and their combination were shown to impair this performance in increasing degrees. Furthermore, they all produce acute tolerance in that over time the induced impairment begins to wane before drug concentrations have fallen. After an oral 10-mg dose of diazepam, impairment was maximal at 60 minutes and normal skills returned at 120 minutes. With ethanol pretreatment (0.5 g/kg p.o.), the onset of impairment was the same while the degree of impairment increased by 80 percent. In addition, the time for return to normal skills was extended up to 240 minutes. This effect could be caused by raised diazepam levels since pretreatment with ethanol resulted in increased plasma levels throughout elimination, but both drugs probably act together to produce the impairment.

Similar results were obtained from the same study for 10 mg i.v. of diazepam. Performance impairment was maximal at 30 minutes and, by 90 minutes, the effects had disappeared. With ethanol pretreatment, performance remained impaired for 102 minutes, and while the time of maximal impairment was the same the degree of impairment increased by 150 percent. Intravenous administration of diazepam did not produce any major changes in its pharmacokinetic profile; however, plasma diazepam concentrations measured during the distribution phase were lower after ethanol pretreatment. Thus, ethanol appeared to decrease the volume of distribution of orally administered diazepam, whereas the volume of distribution appeared to increase with i.v. administration. In the former case, increased plasma concentrations of diazepam may enhance impairment while, in the latter, the increased volume of distribution may be interpreted to include the brain.

These studies show that the mechanism of ethanol-diazepam interactions may be attributed to altered absorption, altered distribution, simple additivity at common receptors in the CNS, or a combination of these. Since dissolution time is rate-limiting for absorption of diazepam, and diazepam is more soluble in ethanol than in water, it is reasonable that their combination would yield an increased rate of diazepam absorption. This has been demonstrated using 5 mg of diazepam alone and in an ethanol solution providing a 0.07-mg/kg ethanol dose (Hayes et al., 1977). Each subject was used twice, in most instances with an appropriate interval between doses. The result was an increase of plasma diazepam levels at the end of 60 minutes such that concentrations were 85 percent higher than those with diazepam alone.

In another experiment in which 10 mg of diazepam in two gelatin capsules were ingested alone or in combination with 0.8 g/kg of ethanol (Linnoila, Otterstrom, and Anttila, 1974), the serum diazepam levels up to two hours after ingestion were not significantly different between the two groups. This opposite result was most likely due to an increase in dissolution time caused by the gelatin capsules. In addition, it suggests that the enhanced solubility of diazepam in ethanol is responsible for the increased plasma diazepam levels even during part of the distribution phase. This may also be in accord with the differences between p.o. and i.v. administration seen by MacLeod et al. (1977).

The effects of ethanol on diazepam distribution have been studied in a series of experiments with rats (Whitehouse et al., 1975), which showed that ethanol pretreatment facilitates redistribution into adipose and brain tissues. When ethanol (3 g/kg p.o.) was given 30 minutes before diazepam (5 mg/kg p.o.), brain and omental fat diazepam levels increased three- to fivefold, while blood, liver, kidney, and plasma showed levels 1.5 times those in control animals. It would seem then that ethanol increases both the rate of absorption and the redistribution of diazepam, resulting in an increase in the concentration of diazepam available to target tissues.

Other benzodiazepines and their interaction with ethanol have also been studied in human subjects. Saario and Linnoila (1976) administered 30 mg of flurazepam p.o. daily for two weeks. On days 7 and 14, 0.5 g/kg of ethanol was administered orally and increased impairment of coordinative skills was observed. Dosages of 5 to 10 mg of oral nitrazepam have also been shown to interact with 0.5 g/kg of ethanol when the ethanol was given ten hours later (Linnoila, 1973a; Saario, Linnoila, and Maki, 1975). The interaction led to increased impairment of psychomotor ability and coordination. The results of studies with chlordiazepoxide have been contradictory, variously showing no interaction, enhancement, and even antagonism of its effects when administered with ethanol (Kissen, 1974). There are many problems in comparing the methods used in these experiments. Nevertheless, a driving-skills test showed an increase in impairment with 5 to 10 mg p.o. of chlordiazepoxide and 0.5 to 0.8 g/kg p.o. of ethanol (Linnoila, 1973b). In addition, it has been shown that 25 mg of oral chlordiazepoxide as a free base reaches higher serum levels in combination with 0.8 g/kg p.o. of ethanol than chlordiazepoxide administered alone (Linnoila, Otterstrom, and Anttila, 1974). However, this serum concentration difference did not become apparent until two hours post administration. It is believed that chlordiazepoxide is weaker than diazepam in its interaction with ethanol. Studies with the metabolites of chlordiazepoxide and diazepam showed that they do not interact with ethanol to impair psychomotor skills related to driving (Palva, Linnoila, and Mattila, 1976). Apparently only the parent compounds are responsible for enhanced hypnotic effects when administered with ethanol.

Other Sedatives

Meprobamate

Meprobamate is a propanediol carbamate with tranquilizing, sedative, and muscle-relaxant properties. Its sedative actions resemble those of the barbiturates, and large doses may cause physical dependence (Byck, 1975).

Absorption. Meprobamate is well absorbed from the intestinal tract and reaches a peak plasma concentration and systemic effect within one to three hours (Byck, 1975). Gastric absorption is slow, however, and doses have been found in rat stomachs 24 hours after administration (Walkenstein et al., 1958).

Distribution. With the exception of adipose tissue, meprobamate is uniformly distributed throughout body tissues. In mice, the brain and adipose tissues concentrated less activity during the first hour, yet by three hours brain concentration was comparable to body levels. There was also no accumulation of meprobamate in adipose tissue over 24 hours (Walkenstein et al., 1958).

Elimination. The blood half-life of meprobamate is from ten to 12 hours (Byck, 1975). About 90 percent of the administered dose is metabolized to hydroxymeprobamate via microsomal enzymes. Ten percent of the dose is excreted unchanged in the urine, while the rest is found as urinary glucuronide conjugates. In rats, the feces contain about 7 percent of the administered dose (Walkenstein et al., 1958).

Glutethimide

Glutethimide is a cyclic imide closely related to the barbiturates in its chemical structure. It is used as a hypnotic drug and is capable of inducing physical dependence.

Absorption. Glutethimide is variably absorbed from the gastrointestinal tract. A study with human subjects showed peak plasma concentrations from 2.85 to 7.05 μg/ml at times between one and six hours after a 500-mg oral dose (Curry et al., 1971).

Distribution. Upon intravenous administration in rats, general bodily distribution occurred after one minute (Keberle, Hoffman, and Bernhard, 1962), followed by redistribution into fat deposits throughout the first two hours. Only one percent of the dose was found in the CNS while 45 percent could be traced to the gastrointestinal tract. In humans, 54 percent of the plasma concentration was found to be protein-bound (Curry et al., 1971).

Elimination. The metabolism of glutethimide is primarily through hydroxylation and glucuronide conjugation by hepatic microsomal enzymes (Harvey, 1975b). These metabolites then enter the enterohepatic circulation and are slowly excreted into the urine. Twenty-four hours after administration in mice, 50 percent of the dose was found in the urine and 6 percent in the feces (Keberle, Hoffman, and Bernhard, 1962). In human subjects the mean plasma half-life was 11.6 hours (ranging from 5 to 22 hours), with less than two percent of the dose excreted unchanged in the urine (Curry et al., 1971).

Methaqualone

Methaqualone is a quinazoline derivative with a wide spectrum of activities including sedative-hypnotic, anticonvulsant, antispasmodic, local-anesthetic, and weak antihistaminic properties.

Absorption. In the human, oral doses of methaqualone have shown 90- to 99-percent absorption within two hours (Morris et al., 1972; Clifford, Cookson, and Wickham, 1974).

Distribution. At peak blood levels, 58 percent of methaqualone was found to be bound to plasma proteins, and 25 percent of the dose was taken up by erythrocytes (Mitchard and Williams, 1972).

Elimination. Biotransformation of methaqualone involves oxidation of the benzene ring and methyl groups by the hepatic microsomal enzyme system (Stillwell, Gregory, and Horning, 1975). Most of the mono- and dihydroxylated compounds are excreted in the urine as conjugates. Several studies have determined plasma half-lives that range from one to four hours during the distribution phase, and from 16 to 41 hours for the terminal elimination phase (Alvan et al., 1973; Clifford, Cookson, and Wickham, 1974).

Interactions with ethanol. The *in vitro* effect of ethanol on the metabolism of meprobamate has been studied by incubating rat liver slices with radioactive meprobamate at different ethanol concentrations (Rubin et al., 1970). Ethanol at 50 mM caused a 40-percent reduction in meprobamate metabolism, while a 60-percent reduction was reached with 100 mM ethanol. In human studies, ethanol (1 g/kg) was administered 14 hours after a 12- to 15-mg p.o. dose of meprobamate. This was followed by 24 g of ethanol every two hours. The plasma half-life of meprobamate increased two- to fivefold upon ethanol administration. It was concluded that acute doses of ethanol could inhibit the biotransformation of meprobamate.

The effect of chronic ethanol dosing in humans and rats has also been studied (Misra et al., 1971). Both nonalcoholic and stabilized alcoholic subjects were placed on a controlled ethanol diet for one month. Meprobamate was given p.o. in a 10-mg/kg dose before and after the ethanol diet. The percentage of dose excreted in the urine was the same during the control period and after ethanol treatment. The plasma half-life of meprobamate was so reduced, however, that the alcoholic groups averaged a change from 16.7 hours before treatment to 8.1 hours afterward. Likewise, the half-life of meprobamate in nonalcoholics decreased from 13.7 hours to 8.2 hours. A similar experimental design was used with rats so as to measure changes in the liver enzymes. Meprobamate was given i.p. in a 125-mg/kg dose to rats after the animals had been on an ethanol or isocaloric diet for one month. The blood meprobamate half-life in controls averaged 254 minutes while ethanol-fed animals showed a half-life of 138 minutes. In addition, meprobamate metabolism increased to almost double that of controls when it was expressed as activity per weight of liver. At three months, the difference in values was not as great but similar. Mean microsomal meprobamate metabolism was assessed at two months and showed an increase from 1.8 μg of meprobamate/g liver/min in controls to 3.8 μg/g liver/min, while the cytosol fraction showed no activity.

The work of Khanna et al. (1976) is in agreement with these results. Rats were placed on a diet incorporating ethanol (10 to 12 g/kg) or a control diet for four weeks. The mean half-life of meprobamate disappearance from the blood decreased from 62 minutes in control animals to 45 minutes in the ethanol-treated group. The decrease was reflected in a 37-percent increase in meprobamate hydroxylase activity when based on body weight, a 29-percent increase in activity/gram of liver, but no difference in activity/mg of protein. In addition, there were no differences between groups in the volumes of distribution. Ethanol, given chronically, seems to have an inductive effect on liver enzymes that metabolize meprobamate and, given acutely, it may be capable of inhibiting meprobamate metabolism. The latter would then lead to prolonged blood levels and an enhanced pharmacological effect.

The interaction of glutethimide and ethanol has been studied in human subjects with psychomotor tests used in conjunction with measurement of these drugs in bodily fluids (Mould, Curry, and Binns, 1972). One hundred milliliters of vodka were administered with or without 250 mg of glutethimide p.o. No difference in blood ethanol concentrations was noticed up to 75 minutes after administration. From 100 to 165 minutes, ethanol blood levels increased by 30 percent, and the overall mean concentration of ethanol rose by 11 percent. Urinary glutethimide concentrations were significantly lowered by ethanol treatment. These results were reflected by decreased plasma glutethimide levels from one to 2.5 hours after administration. Measurements of reaction time were insensitive to ethanol or glutethimide alone yet were affected by their combination after 1.5 hours; increased ethanol levels were probably the cause. Pursuit rotor and finger-tapping performances were significantly impaired by glutethimide alone and reversed by the concomitant ingestion of ethanol. Thus, these tests were thought to be more sensitive to the effects of glutethimide.

Methaqualone is known to show additive sedative properties when used with ethanol, but there are few pharmacokinetic data on their interaction. Altered plasma levels were expected, however, from data which showed that 0.01% of ethanol would mobilize methaqualone from erythrocytes (Stillwell, Gregory, and Horning, 1975). It was demonstrated that in the presence of ethanol, free methaqualone could potentially be increased from 17 to 22 percent of the total blood methaqualone. Roden, Harvey, and Mitchard (1977) studied the residual blood levels of methaqualone in human subjects, using 0.5 g/kg of ethanol p.o. at 24, 48, and 72 hours after administration of 400 mg of methaqualone p.o. The only significant increase in plasma methaqualone was found at 72 hours. This correlated with a reduction in cognitive skills as measured by the Stroop tests and greater mental and physical sedation using the Visual Analogue Scale (Roden, Harvey, and Mitchard, 1977).

CONCLUSIONS

The data reviewed in this paper present pharmacokinetic changes caused by drug interactions, that is, alterations in certain fundamental parameters (absorption, distribution, metabolism, and excretion). While ethanol directly affects these parameters in individual sedatives, the sedatives themselves cause few changes in the activity of ethanol. This is the result in part of the solvent properties of ethanol. For example, the nearly ubiquitous distribution of ethanol is a result of its combined lipophilic and hydrophilic character which remains unaltered by the sedatives.

Ethanol increases the rate of absorption of lipophilic sedatives by enhancing their solubility. A lipophilic compound permeates membranes readily but gains access to the membrane only while in solution. Thus, solvation becomes rate-limiting for the absorption of these compounds.

This was demonstrated by an ethanol-induced increase in the rate but not in the extent of absorption of diazepam through the gut. The solvation effects of ethanol also partly explain the altered distribution of several sedatives. In the presence of ethanol, phenobarbital reaches a greater concentration in rat brain but for a shorter duration. This indicates an enhanced lipophilicity and is characteristic of shorter-acting barbiturates.

The interaction of ethanol with the fraction of a sedative dose bound to tissues and plasma proteins also contributes to altered plasma and tissue concentrations. With sedatives that accumulate and possess long terminal half-lives, tolerance develops to significant and prolonged blood levels. The ethanol-induced mobilization of erythrocyte-bound methaqualone causes a rise in free methaqualone above levels to which the subject was previously tolerant. This illustrates the capacity of ethanol to alter tissue affinities and may be of importance concerning the effects of ethanol on diazepam distribution. Altered binding properties may even simulate an inhibited sedative metabolism. That is, if the rate of delivery from tissues to the vascular space is decreased, increased tissue concentrations would keep a greater part of the dose from being metabolized and excreted.

Ethanol is a relatively selective and reversible inhibitor of the mixed-function oxidase system; it interferes primarily with drug hydroxylations. The inhibition depends on ethanol's binding to cytochrome P-450 in addition to the complex interaction of ethanol with membranes of the endoplasmic reticulum. The metabolism of meprobamate and some barbiturates seems to be inhibited through this mechanism. This aspect of ethanol-sedative interactions is important since an enhanced pharmacological effect of several sedatives has been shown to coincide with increased blood concentrations. Thus, both the degree and duration of sedative activity may be enhanced following inhibition of the hydroxylating enzymes.

Finally, the elimination of a sedative may be altered by its interaction with ethanol. Renal excretion will vary with changes in blood concentration, protein binding, tubular secretion and reabsorption, and the production of polar metabolites. Thus, the elimination rate will reflect changes in renal excretion but will also reflect the alterations in absorption, distribution, and metabolism considered above.

The interactions of ethanol with sedative drugs involve several different mechanisms at various levels of physiological organization. Different effects may be interdependent and may be explained by changes in one or more of the parameters of absorption, distribution, metabolism, and excretion. The relative contribution of each mechanism may vary with different drugs. Precise definition of the mechanisms of interaction will require detailed pharmacokinetic analysis to differentiate the changes in each system and to assess their relative importance.

REFERENCES

ALVAN, G., LINDGREN, J. E., BOGENTOFT, C., and ERICSSON, O. 1973. Plasma kinetics of methaqualone in man after single oral doses. *Eur. J. Clin. Pharmacol.*, 6:187-190.

BLIDING, A. 1974. Effects of different rates of absorption of two benzodiazepines on subjective and objective parameters. *Eur. J. Clin. Pharmacol.*, 7:201-211.

BRODIE, B. B., BURNS, J. J., MARK, L. C., LIEF, P. A., BERNSTEIN, E., and PAPPER, E. M. 1953. The fate of pentobarbital in man and dog and a method for its estimation in biological material. *J. Pharmacol. Exp. Ther.*, 109:26-34.

BYCK, R. 1975. Drugs and the treatment of psychiatric disorders. In L. S. Goodman and A. Gilman (eds.), *The Pharmacological Basis of Therapeutics*, pp. 188-189. New York: Macmillan.

CABANA, B. E., and GESSNER, P. K. 1970. The kinetics of chloral hydrate metabolism in mice and the effect thereon of ethanol. *J. Pharmacol. Exp. Ther.*, 174:260-275.

CHUNG, H., and BROWN, D. R. 1976. Mechanism of the effect of acute ethanol on hexobarbital metabolism. *Biochem. Pharmacol.*, 25:1613-1616.

CLIFFORD, J. M., COOKSON, J. H., and WICKHAM, P. 1974. Absorption and clearance of secobarbital heptabarbital, methaqualone and ethinamate. *Clin. Pharmacol. Ther.*, 16:376-389.

COLDWELL, B. B., PAUL, C. J., and THOMAS, B. H. 1973. Phenobarbital metabolism in ethanol intoxicated rats. *Can. J. Physiol. Pharmacol.*, 51:458-463.

COLDWELL, B. B., TRENHOLM, H. L., THOMAS, B. H., and CHARBONNEAU, S. 1971. The effect of ethanol on phenobarbitone and pentobarbitone absorption into rat blood and brain. *J. Pharm. Pharmacol.*, 23:947-949.

COLDWELL, B. B., WIBERG, G. S., and TRENHOLM, H. L. 1970. Some effects of ethanol on the toxicity and distribution of barbiturates in rats. *Can. J. Physiol. Pharmacol.*, 48:254-264.

CREAVEN, P. J., and ROACH, M. K. 1969. The effect of chloral hydrate on the metabolism of ethanol in mice. *J. Pharm. Pharmacol.*, 21:332-333.

CURRY, S. H., RIDDALL, D., GORDON, J. S., SIMPSON, P., BINNS, T. B., RONDEL, R. K., and MCMARTIN, C. 1971. Disposition of glutethimide in man. *Clin. Pharmacol. Ther.*, 12:849-853.

CURRY, S. H., and SCALES, A. H. 1974. Interaction of phenobarbitone and ethanol in mice studied from dose response curves and drug concentrations in blood. *J. Pharm. Pharmacol.*, 26:771-777.

GESSNER, P. K. 1973. Effect of trichloroethanol and of chloral hydrate on the *in vivo* rate of disappearance of ethanol in mice. *Arch. Int. Pharmacodyn. Ther.*, 202:392-401.

GESSNER, P. K., and CABANA, B. E. 1970. A study of the interaction of the hypnotic effects and of the toxic effects of chloral hydrate and ethanol. *J. Pharmacol. Exp. Ther.*, 174:247-259.

GOLDSTEIN, A., and ARANOW, L. 1960. The durations of action of thiopental and pentobarbital. *J. Pharmacol. Exp. Ther.*, 128:1-6.

HAGGARD, H. W., GREENBERG, L. A., and CARROLL, R. P. 1941. Studies in the absorption, distribution and elimination of alcohol, 8. *J. Pharmacol. Exp. Ther.*, 71:348-357.

HALSTEAD, C. H., ROBLES, E. A., and MEZEY, E. 1973. Distribution of ethanol in the human gastrointestinal tract. *Am. J. Clin. Nutr.*, 26:831-834.

HARVEY, S. C. 1975a. Hypnotics and sedatives. The barbiturates. In L. S. Goodman and A. Gilman (eds.), *The Pharmacological Basis of Therapeutics*, pp. 97-123. New York: Macmillan.

HARVEY, S. C. 1975b. Hypnotics and sedatives. Miscellaneous agents. In L. S. Goodman and A. Gilman (eds.), *The Pharmacological Basis of Therapeutics*, pp. 124-136. New York: Macmillan.

HAYES, S. L., PABLO, G., RADOMSKI, T., and PALMER, R. F. 1977. Ethanol and oral diazepam absorption. *N. Engl. J. Med.*, 296:186-189.

HILLESTAD, L., HANSEN, T., MELSOM, H., and DRIVENES, A. 1974. Diazepam metabolism in normal man. 1. Serum concentrations and clinical effects after intravenous, intramuscular and oral administration. *Clin. Pharmacol. Ther.*, 16:479-484.

HILLESTAD, L., HANSEN, T., and MELSOM, H. 1974. Diazepam metabolism in normal man. 2. Serum concentration and clinical effect after oral administration and cumulation. *Clin. Pharmacol. Ther.*, 16:485-489.

KAKEMA, K., ARITA, T., HORI, R., and KONISHI, R. 1967a. Absorption and excretion of drugs. 30. Absorption of barbituric acid from rat stomach. *Chem. Pharm. Bull.*, 15:1534-1539.

KAKEMA, K., ARITA, T., HORI, R., and KONISHI, R. 1967b. Absorption and excretion of drugs. 32. Absorption of barbituric acid derivatives from rat small intestine. *Chem. Pharm. Bull.*, 15:1883-1895.

KAPLAN, S. A., JACK, M. L., ALEXANDER, K., and WEINFELD, R. E. 1973. Pharmacokinetic profile of diazepam in man following single intravenous and oral and chronic oral administration. *J. Pharm. Sci.*, 62:1789-1796.

KEBERLE, H., HOFFMAN, K., and BERNHARD, K. 1962. The metabolism of glutethimide (Doriden). *Experientia*, 18:105-111.

KHANNA, J. M., KALANT, H., YEE, Y., CHUNG, S., and SIEMENS, A. J. 1976. Effect of chronic ethanol treatment on metabolism of drugs *in vitro* and *in vivo*. *Biochem. Pharmacol.*, 25:329-335.

KISSEN, B. 1974. Interactions of ethyl alcohol and other drugs. In B. Kissen and H. Begleiter (eds.), *The Biology of Alcoholism*, vol. 3, p. 123. New York: Plenum Press.

KLOTZ, U., AVANT, G. R., HOYUMPA, A., SCHENKER, S., and WILKINSON, G. R. 1975. The effects of age and liver disease on the disposition and elimination of diazepam in adult man. *J. Clin. Invest.*, 55:347-359.

LEMBERGER, L., and RUBIN, A. 1976. *Physiological Disposition of Drugs of Abuse*. New York: Spectrum.

LIEBER, C. S., and DECARLI, L. M. 1972. The role of the hepatic microsomal ethanol oxidizing system (MEOS) for ethanol metabolism *in vivo*. *J. Pharmacol. Exp. Ther.*, 181:279-287.

LINNOILA, M. 1973a. Drug interaction on psychomotor skills related to driving: Hypnotics and alcohol. *Annales Medicinae Experimentalis et Biologiae Fennieae*, 51:118-124.

LINNOILA, M. 1973b. Effects of diazepam, chlordiazepoxide, thioridazine, haloperidol, flupenthixole, and alcohol on psychomotor skills related to driving. *Annales Medicinae Experimentalis et Biologiae Fenniae*, 51:125-132.

LINNOILA, M., and MATTILA, J. J. 1973. Drug interaction on psychomotor skills related to driving: Diazepam and alcohol. *Eur. J. Clin. Pharmacol.*, 5:186-194.

LINNOILA, M., OTTERSTROM, S., and ANTTILA, M. 1974. Serum chlordiazepoxide, diazepam and thioridazine concentrations after the simultaneous ingestion of alcohol or placebo drink. *Ann. Clin. Res.*, 6:4-6.

LINNOILA, M., and HAKKINEN, S. 1974. Effect of diazepam and codeine alone and in combination with alcohol on simulated driving. *Clin. Pharmacol. Ther.*, 15:368-373.

LINNOILA, M., SARRIO, I., and MAKI, M. 1974. Effect of treatment with diazepam or lithium and alcohol on psychomotor skills related to driving. *Eur. J. Clin. Pharmacol.*, 7:337-342.

LOUS, P. 1954. Plasma levels and urinary excretion of three barbituric acids after oral administration to man. *Acta Pharmacol. Toxicol. (Kbh)*, 10:147-165.

MACLEOD, S. M., GILES, H. G., PATZALEK, G., THIESSEN, J., SELLERS, E. M. 1977. Pharmacokinetics and pharmacodynamics of diazepam following ethanol in normal volunteers. In F. A. Seixas (ed.), *Currents in Alcoholism: Biological, Biochemical, and Clinical Studies*, pp. 295-309. New York: Grune & Stratton.

MARSHALL, E. K. and OWENS, A. H. 1954. Absorption, excretion and metabolic fate of chloral hydrate and trichloroethanol. *Bulletin of Johns Hopkins Hospital*, 95:1-8.

MEZEY, E. 1976. Ethanol metabolism and ethanol-drug interactions. *Biochem. Pharmacol.*, 25:869-875.

MISRA, P. S., LEFEVRE, A., ISHII, H., RUBIN, E., and LIEBER, C. S. 1971. Increase of ethanol, meprobamate, and pentobarbital metabolism after chronic ethanol administration in man and rats. *Am. J. Med.*, 51:346-351.

MITCHARD, M., and WILLIAMS, M. E. 1972. Ethanol induced changes in the pharmacokinetics of methaqualone. In S. B. de C. Baker and G. A. Neuhaus (eds.), *Proceedings of the European Society for the Study of Drug Toxicity*, vol. 13. *Toxicological Problems of Drug Combinations*, pp. 110-116. London: Excerpta Medica.

MOLANDER, L., and DUVHOK, C. 1976. Acute effects of oxazepam, diazepam, and methylperone, alone and in combination with alcohol on sedation, coordination and mood. *Acta Pharmacol. Toxicol (Kbh)*, 38:145-160.

MORRIS, R. N., GUNDERSON, M. S., BABCOCK, S. W., and ZAROSLINSKI, J. F. 1972. Plasma levels and absorption of methaqualone after oral administration to man. *Clin. Pharmacol. Ther.*, 13:719-723.

MOULD, G. P., CURRY, S. H., and BINNS, T. B. 1972. Interaction of glutethimide and phenobarbital with ethanol in man. *J. Pharm. Pharmacol.*, 24:894-899.

PALVA, E. S., LINNOILA, M., and MATTILA, M. J. 1976. Effect of active metabolites of chlordiazepoxide and diazepam, alone or in combination with alcohol on psychomotor skills related to driving. *Mod. Probl. Pharmacopsychiatry*, 11:79-84.

PAWAN, G. L. 1972. Metabolism of alcohol (ethanol) in man. *Proc. Nutr. Soc.*, 31:38-89.

RITCHIE, J. M. 1975. The aliphatic alcohols. In L. S. Goodman and A. Gilman (eds.) *The Pharmacological Basis of Therapeutics*, p. 142. New York: Macmillan.

RODEN, S., HARVEY, P., and MITCHARD, M. 1977. The effect of ethanol on residual plasma methaqualone concentrations and behavior in volunteers who have taken Mandrax. *Br. J. Clin. Pharmacol.*, 4:245-247.

RUBIN, E., GANG, H., MISRA, P. S., and LIEBER, C. S. 1970. Inhibition of drug metabolism by acute ethanol intoxication. A hepatic microsomal mechanism. *Am. J. Med.*, 49:801-806.

SARRIO, I., LINNOILA, M., and MAKI, M. 1975. Interaction of drugs with alcohol on human psychomotor skills related to driving: Effect of sleep deprivation or two weeks treatment with hypnotics. *J. Clin. Pharmacol.*, 15:52-59.

SAARIO, I., and LINNOILA, M. 1976. Effect of subacute treatment with hypnotics, alone or in combination with alcohol on psychomotor skills related to driving. *Acta Pharmacol. Toxicol. (Kbh)*, 38:382-392.

SAUNDERS, L. 1974. *The Absorption and Distribution of Drugs*. Baltimore: Williams & Wilkins.

SCHWARTZ, M. A., POSTMA, E., and GAUT, Z. 1971. Biological half life of chlordiazepoxide and its metabolite, demoxepam, in man. *J. Pharm. Sci.*, 60:1500-1503.

SELLERS, E. M., LANG, M., KOCH-WESER, J., LEBLANC, E., and KALANT, H. 1972a. Interaction of chloral hydrate and ethanol in man. 1. Metabolism. *Clin. Pharmacol. Ther.*, 13:37-49.

SELLERS, E. M., CARR, G., BERNSTEIN, J. G., SELLERS, S., and KOCH-WESER, J. 1972b. Interaction of chloral hydrate and ethanol in man. 2. Hemodynamics and performance. *Clin. Pharmacol. Ther.*, 13:50-58.

SHULL, H. J., WILKINSON, G. R., JOHNSON, R., and SCHENKER, S. 1976. Normal disposition of oxazepam in acute viral hepatitis and cirrhosis. *Ann. Intern. Med.*, 84:420-425.

SJÖGREN, J., SOLVELL, L., and KARLSSON, I. 1965. Studies on the absorption rate of barbiturates in man. *Acta Med. Scand.*, 178:553-559.

SMITH, R. B., DITTERT, L. W., GRIFFEN, W. O., and DOLUSIO, J. T. 1973. Pharmacokinetics of pentobarbitone after intravenous and oral administration. *J. Pharmacokinet. Biopharm.*, 1:5-16.

STILLWELL, W. G., GREGORY, P., and HORNING, M. G. 1975. Metabolism of methaqualone by the epoxide-diol pathway in man and the rat. *Drug Metab. Dispos.*, 3:287-296.

THOMAS, B. H., COLDWELL, B. B., SOLOMON RAJ, G., ZEITZ, W., and TRENHOLM, H. L. 1972. Effect of ethanol on the fate of pentobarbital in the rat. *Biochem. Pharmacol.*, 21:2605-2614.

VAN DER KLEIJN, E. 1969. Kinetics of distribution and metabolism of diazepam and chlor-

diazepoxide in mice. *Arch. Int. Pharmacodyn. Ther.*, 178:193-215.
WADDELL, W. J., and BUTLER, T. C. 1957. The distribution and excretion of phenobarbital. *J. Clin. Invest.*, 36:1217-1226.
WALKENSTEIN, S. S., KNEBEL, C. M., MACMULLEN, J. A., and SEIFTER, J. 1958. The excretion and distribution of meprobamate and its metabolites. *J. Pharmacol. Exp. Ther.*, 123:254-258.
WHITEHOUSE, L. W., PAUL, C. J., COLDWELL, B. B., and THOMAS, B. H. 1975. Effect of ethanol on diazepam distribution in rat. *Res. Commun. Chem. Pathol. Pharmacol.*, 12:221-242.

V.

CONCLUSIONS

16

IMPLICATIONS FOR FUTURE CLINICAL RESEARCH

JAMES L. CLAGHORN, M.D.,
ROY J. MATHEW, M.D.,
and
LINDA D. ROBERTS, M.A.

The critical role of discovery in the history of science is emphasized by the laconic, understated comment of Sir Alexander Fleming (1945):

> I am to talk to you about the discovery of penicillin and its development as a therapeutic agent. I have been accused of inventing it but it would be very difficult for a man to invent penicillin, since a mold has been making this substance for thousands of years. . . . All I did was to bring it to the notice of the medical profession . . . and, incidentially, to christen it.

Subsequent steps in Sir Alexander's work included comparative studies of effectiveness and toxicity for penicillin and other antiseptic agents; extraction, purification and other manufacturing concerns; human trials, and ultimately, treatment recommendations.

Early in Fleming's research, absorption, metabolism and excretion data were collected to establish dosing schedules that would keep adequate drug in contact with target microbes. At first, penicillin application was topical because supplies were limited by existing mold-culture technologies; then, as better methods increased supply, injection became possible. Illinois corn-steep liquor was added to 15,000 gallon vats of mold-culture medium, and penicillin became available in quantities sufficient to administer the very large doses necessary for oral use. Subsequently the sulfamides, and then a succession of antimicrobials that attack a broad range of organisms, were identified in nature or synthesized in chemical laboratories. The introduction of penicillin provided the basis for an entire armamentarium against infectious disease; present effort is focused on the development of antiviral agents.

The brief review of penicillin's development and pivotal role in the treatment of disease is not merely a nostalgic glimpse at an enviable bit of research that constituted a medical milestone. It is, rather, a fundamental illustration of a pattern that continually recurs in the ever-expanding, ever-seeking arena of science. Science, for all its incredible advance, futuristic technologies, and modern complexities, cannot be divorced from Bacon's basic principles of "scientific method": discovery, and ultimately progress, cannot be accomplished without keen observation, logical experimentation, and above all, unrelenting curiosity. When discovery is accomplished, as was the case with penicillin, it can become the underpinning for a whole new series of related "discoveries" and consequential theories. These theories in turn can stimulate the research cycle, and an entire new approach to treatment or branch of scientific inquiry may be born.

The development of modern psychopharmacology may be likened to our example of the antibiotic evolution. The Indian snake root *Rauwolfia serpentina*, an ingenious pharmaceutical manufacturer in its own right, gave us reserpine, the first neuroleptic (Carlsson, 1974). Rauwolfia alkaloids in crude, unrefined form were utilized for treatment of insanity in India for thousands of years before the introduction of chlorpromazine. As Fleming "christened" penicillin, chlorpromazine removed the myth and mystery surrounding the use of psychotropic drugs and gave them a "christening."

The synthesis of chlorpromazine, Rp4560, in the Rhone Poulenc laboratories in no way suggested the start of a "new era" or "revolution" at the time. When the new drug's treatment potential was recognized, however, a large number of related agents was developed. The kinetic and dynamic properties of these agents were scrutinized and identified, and the resultant data lent themselves to the construction of theories about the causes and characteristics of psychiatric illness. To briefly reiterate, then, the progression of events in the evolution of psychopharmacology:

1. Discovery of an "interesting agent."
2. Development of similar agents.
3. Kinetic and dynamic study in animals and humans.
4. Theory construction, based on agents' properties, and subsequent research into the processes of mental illness.

From the synthesis of a single agent, chlorpromazine, in 1952, we have developed agents of five chemical classes with varied pharmacological properties: antidepressants of two classes (MAO inhibitors, tricyclics), lithium carbonate, and two classes of minor tranquilizers. Our modern era of psychopharmacology, which has been termed, somewhat controversially by Ronald Fieve (1977), the "third revolution in psychiatry," has given rise to many theories and much research on the underlying processes of psychiatric disorders. If we are to speculate on the future in psychiatric research and attempt to assess forthcoming trends, we must examine the current status of the field; if scientific advancement is based, as we have suggested, on a "building-block" principle, then our present is clearly our window to the future.

One of the most profound and important theories to evolve from psychopharmacological research concerns the relationship of neurotransmitters and schizophrenia. At the observation that neuroleptics block dopamine receptors (a phenomenon that supposedly invokes their antipsychotic properties), it was hypothesized that schizophrenia might be caused by hyperdopaminergia (Crow and Gillbe, 1974). Much emphasis has been given to this notion, and it has even been felt that extrapyramidal effects are intrinsic to antipsychotic potency in neuroleptic agents. The recent finding, however, that clozapine, a benzodiazepine with potent antipsychotic action, has only slight dopamine-blocking potency and does not produce but in fact alleviates extrapyramidal symptoms, indicates that a theory based on a single catecholamine transmitter is unreasonable, and that pharmacological explanation of drug effects is far more complex.

Clozapine blocks dopa and norepinephrine receptors, increases GABA turnover, and seems to get its antipsychotic properties from a neuroleptic action that is unrelated to dopamine uptake. Psychiatrists have long felt that the "schizophrenia syndrome" is a compilation of several conditions; it is quite possible that future research along these lines can break the schizophrenic syndrome into smaller units with variant biochemical etiologies.

Progress in biochemical research is evident in the area of affective disorders. It has been shown that drugs which block both norepinephrine and serotonin uptake are effective in treating depressions. This finding has suggested the existence of at least two types of depression, one associated with low brain serotonin, and the other with low epinephrine; these depressions are indistinguishable from one another upon clinical examination.

The no less than remarkable agent lithium has revolutionized the treatment of manic conditions, and its dynamics hold the key to the biochemistry of bipolar affective disorders. While these dynamics continue to elude active researchers, there are still strong indications that biochemistry will alter the classification of the affective disorders. For example, evidence from several sources indicates the existence of different types of mania. Mendels and Frazer (1974) have shown that the biochemical abnormalities seen in mania are identical to but more pronounced than those seen in depression. Similarly, biochemical researchers have suggested clues for differentiating manic patients according to their lithium response; others claim a basis for underlying serotonin and cholinergic mechanisms. We have also heard that altered osmolarity will change CNS amine concentrations in some amphibians. Whether this finding is relevant to mania remains to be demonstrated (Baxter, this volume).

In our consideration of current research areas, pharmacokinetics must be included. Several researchers (Asberg, Cronholm, and Sjoqvist, 1971; Braithwaite, Goulding, and Theano, 1972; Glassman, Shostak, and Kantor, 1975; Ziegler et al., 1977) have measured the relationship of blood level and clinical response for tricyclic antidepressants. Their results seem to support the notion of a dose-response curve with a narrow accelerated band (a therapeutic "window"); both above and below patients respond poorly. Many reported subjects did badly at dosages in the "window" region, and their oral dose levels varied as much as 30:1 to produce comparable therapeutic blood levels. All the current studies have been of short duration, however, and have raised serious questions about probable results for longer observation times. Winoker and Avery (1976) have shown that doses below 150 mg/day (a dosage at the upper window range in the Ziegler paper) result in an exaggerated mortality from all causes over several years in many age groups; obviously matters of absorption, tolerance, enzyme induction, and protein binding influence these complex blood level relationships. As rapid and slow acetylators affect patients' response to MAO inhibitors, some as yet undetermined factor of subject variability may influence the actions of psychotropic drugs.

To date, the upper limit of effectiveness for the neuroleptics is not clear, but clinicians know that patient behavior will not indicate continued improvement above the established dosages ranges. Further confounding the situation is the observation that penfluridol, a neuroleptic with a half-life of 66 hours in man and negligible blood levels at any time (usual doses are 20 mg/week administered at once), produces persistent antipsychotic effects for 168 hours and side effects for 24 hours. An even more striking lack of blood level relationship is seen with the indole derivative molindone, which is metabolized to 36 separate chemicals in less than three hours while therapeutic effect persists 24 to 36 hours later. These examples may simply be oddities, but they do indeed raise questions about the significance of drug levels in the blood.

Another area of inquiry—neuroendocrinology—has reemerged as a viable field for psychiatric research. Prolactin and growth hormone alterations due to dopamine-blocking effects of neuroleptics have focused concern on the electrochemical transducer cells of the hypothalamus. Unfortunately, the relationship between antipsychotic effect and neuroendocrine effect is uneven: when neuroleptics are stopped, prolactin and growth hormone levels drop quickly to normal, though the symptoms of illness do not so rapidly reappear. Agents with no neuroleptic potency will also alter levels of prolactin and growth hormone, for example, alphamethylparatyrosine; at this time it seems that most endocrine phenomena are best viewed as covarying measures related but not central to the illness.

Currently the most popular and controversial area in clinical research involves the role of amino acids and peptides as central nervous system transmitters. Since the research of Holger Hyden on memory, and Heath's proposed but never confirmed hypothesis that a substance in the circulating blood evokes the thinking disorder schizophrenia, no new events had occurred in the field until the work pioneered by Snyder and Enna (1975). These researchers announced the discovery of opiate receptors in the human brain which are activated by peptides called "endorphins" or "enkephalins"; Wagemaker and Cade (1977) reported the improvement of schizophrenic symptoms in resistant patients who were treated by renal dialysis. This particular finding was critically buffeted by many skeptics, but Palmour et al. (1977), who observed one hundredfold increases from dialysate #1 to #16 in a polypeptide identified as leucine endorphin, have reopened the area of interest.

Continued pursuit of information about the amino acid and peptide messenger substances, whatever the course, will surely cause a merging of the varied lines of neurochemical investigation and provide a single, strong direction. The potential of inquiry for these substances is so great, and the investigational field so fertile, that the romance of American research with the monoamines may well be coming to an end; we are certainly aware that GABA, glycine, taurine, and a wide range of peptides are stimulators, inhibitors, and messenger substances in the brain, and we feel that their role in the etiologies of certain illnesses will emerge as a significant one.

In this discussion of neurochemical theories and investigational highlights, it is important to include a word about the impact of research on and interaction with clinical practice. Growth for this area will be in the application of laboratory technology to routine diagnostic and treatment events. Blood assays as a guide to dosage adjustment will be followed by enzyme assays. Initial work with the latter has proved fruitful:

the availability of pseudocholinesterase measurement has greatly increased the safety of succinylcholine use in electroconvulsive therapy patients. In the future, measurement of monoamine oxidase isoenzymes associated with platelets will improve the speed, safety, and quality of psychopharmacological treatment. Dexamethasone suppression of urinary output of free cortisol is now being used to support the diagnosis of depression, and prolactin assay can be used as an inferential assay of neuroleptic levels. Potentially, peptide assay will also be of value, either as a diagnostic "marker" for selected subjects or as the causative "toxin."

The use of laboratory technology and "mechanism-directed" investigations may have a profound effect on the therapeutic approaches to psychiatric illnesses. For example, clinical experience has traditionally separated a subgroup of schizophrenic individuals from the total; whether identified as "process" or "treatment-resistant," they are clearly set apart. With mechanism-directed investigation, the conclusions may very well be that these individuals have a condition different from that of the group comprised of "reactive" and "responsive" subjects, and that fundamentally different agents are required, not a greater quantity of present treatments. The advent of radically different and more effective therapies may precipitate the release of residual, unimproved hospitalized patients, and provide better social functioning for many in the community who are faring poorly.

Results with the pharmacotherapy of depression give us a 75- to 80-percent improvement rate, with no results from attempts to match subjects to agent. Some degree of specificity of agent to type of depression is likely, however, and it is probable that, with routine assay of serotonin, catecholamine and blood levels, these relationships will clarify and the results improve.

Our final consideration concerns the etiology of anxiety. Pitts and McClure (1967) have demonstrated predictable anxiety symptom production with sodium lactate infusion in vulnerable subjects. Snyder (1975) has identified strychnine-sensitive glycine receptors as the blocking point of the benzodiazepine tranquilizers. Anxiety, however, is pandemic throughout the world, and has even been allowed to roost under the umbrella of "normal" behavior; the close association of anxiety to depression has further confounded efforts to investigate physiological and biochemical origins of the disorder. While the topic has been, at best, sparsely investigated, it is nonetheless ripe for the discovery of dose-response relationships similar to those explored for the tricyclic antidepressants.

We have outlined an array of current theories and areas of investigation which have evolved from the development of psychopharmacology. In keeping with our premise that scientific advancement builds naturally upon the foundations of the present, then directions for the future, we feel, will include expansion and refinement of laboratory procedures for both clinical and research endeavors, and the development of new pharmacological agents whose novel chemical structures will deal with the "resistant" patient, and will be, it is hoped, less conducive to treatment-symptom liabilities. New agents, however, will not be produced solely with therapeutic ends in mind; their potential for research, that is, their ability to play a pivotal role in theory construction, will be of major concern. This last projection (the development of new drugs for research as well as clinical purposes) leads perhaps to the most important implication of all for the field of psychiatry: the merging of clinical and research practices.

Clearly, changes will occur for the patients, who are apt to find themselves in a world in which the "medical model" of laboratory tests, physical appraisal, and medication monitoring along with dietary, exercise, and other general health concerns has become the larger part of their "psychotherapy," but what of the psychiatrist? Will subspecialization be necessary to qualify the "medical" psychiatrist, to set him apart from the social or psychological psychiatrist? We believe so; in our increasingly controlled world, this regulation of practice must soon be upon us. Oddly enough, psychiatry is virtually the last of the medical fields to retain the humanistic and holistic values that typified the turn-of-the-century doctor. Because we treat small numbers and must know our patients well, we are generally well regarded and not frequently the targets of malpractice litigation. Will our science destroy our humanity? While our drugs have alleviated many problems, they have been the cause of others. We are an overmedicated society; with the grim realization of this situation, it has been the concern of psychiatry in recent years to dissuade the public and our colleagues from perfunctorily medicating to cure any and all ills.

As our last comment on the future in psychopharmacological research, we would like to caution against the tendency to impose restrictions on viable areas of inquiry. The fund of information we have before us is infinitely complex, indeed we have merely scratched its surface, and we feel we must grasp and understand this complexity. Newtonian physics served us well in the era preceding the development of atomic energy. The understanding of the mass-to-energy ratio and principles of quantum mechanics required a series of concepts that were free of the constraints imposed by an accurate but less than complete theory; currently we remain trapped in a less than adequate theoretical corset. Single dimension theories abound largely because the complexity of viewing multiple events at the same time has been technologically impossible or mind-boggling. The answers will not be found via the interrelation of one or two messenger substances or one or two endocrines; unrelenting curiosity is our key to discovery, and we urge no restraints on its use.

REFERENCES

ÅSBERG, M., CRONHOLM, B., and SJOQVIST, F. 1971. Relationship between plasma level and therapeutic effect of nortriptyline. *Br. Med. J.*, 3:331-334.

BRAITHWAITE, R. A., GOULDING, R., and THEANO, G. 1972. Plasma concentration of amitriptyline and clinical response. *Lancet*, 1:1297-1300.

CARLSSON, A. 1974. Antipsychotic drugs and catecholamine synapses. *J. Psychiatr. Res.*, 11:57-64.

CROW, T. J., and GILLBE, C. 1974. Brain dopamine and behavior: a critical analysis of the relationship between dopamine antagonism and therapeutic efficacy of neuroleptic drugs. *J. Psychiatr. Res.*, 11:163-172.

FIEVE, R. 1977. The revolution defined: it is pharmacologic. *Psychiatric Annals*, 7:10-18.

FLEMING, A. 1945. The story of penicillin. *Medical Annals District of Columbia*, 14:339-399.

GLASSMAN, A. H., SHOSTAK, M., and KANTOR, S. J. 1975. Plasma levels of imipramine and clinical outcome. *Psychopharmacol. Bull.*, 11:27-8.

MENDELS, J., and FRAZER, A. 1974. Brain biogenic amine depletion and mood. *Arch. Gen. Psychiatry*, 30:447-451.

PALMOUR, R. M., ERVIN, F. R., WAGEMAKER, H., and CADE, R. 1977. Characterization of a peptide derived from the serum of psychiatric patients. Presented to Society for Neuroscience, 7th Annual Meeting, Anaheim, California.

PITTS, F. N., and MCCLURE, J. N. 1967. Lactate metabolism in anxiety neurosis. *N. Engl. J. Med.*, 277:1329-1336.

SNYDER, S. H. 1975. The opiate receptor. *Neurosci. Res. Program Bull.*, 13:1-27.

SNYDER, S. H., and ENNA, S. J. 1975. The role of central glycine receptors in the pharmacologic actions of benzodiazepines. *Adv. Biochem. Psychopharmacol.*, 14:81-91.

WAGEMAKER, H. and CADE, R. 1977. The use of hemodialysis in chronic schizophrenia. *Amer. J. Psychiatry*, 134:684-685.

WINOKER, G., and AVERY, D. 1976. Mortality in depressed patients treated with electroconvulsive therapy and antidepressants. *Arch. Gen. Psychiatry*, 33:1029-1037.

ZIEGLER, V. E., KNESEVICH, J. W., WYLIE, L. T., and BIGGS, J. T. 1977. Sampling time, dosage schedule, and nortriptyline plasma levels. *Arch. Gen. Psychiatry*, 34:613-615.

SUBJECT INDEX

NAME INDEX